Live Right 4 Your Type

Also by the author:

Eat Right 4 Your Type
Cook Right 4 Your Type

DR. PETER J. D'ADAMO

WITH CATHERINE WHITNEY

G. P. PUTNAM'S SONS
NEW YORK

Live Right 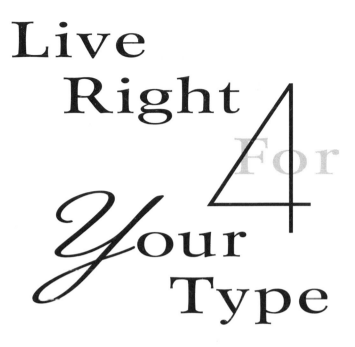 4 *Your* Type

THE INDIVIDUALIZED
PRESCRIPTION FOR
MAXIMIZING HEALTH,
METABOLISM, AND VITALITY
IN EVERY STAGE
OF YOUR LIFE

G. P. Putnam's Sons
Publishers Since 1838
a member of
Penguin Putnam Inc.
375 Hudson Street
New York, NY 10014

Library of Congress Cataloging-in-Publication Data

D'Adamo, Peter.
Live right 4 your type : the individualized
prescription for maximizing health, metabolism, and
vitality in every stage of your life / by Peter J. D'Adamo
with Catherine Whitney.
p.   cm.
Includes bibliographical references.
ISBN 0-399-14673-3
1. Health.   2. Blood groups.   3. Vitality.   4. Self-care,
Health.   I. Title: Live right for your type.   II. Title:
Live right four your type.   III. Whitney, Catherine
(Catherine A.)   IV. Title.
RA776.5 .D325   2000   00-056500
613—dc21

Printed in the United States of America

1   3   5   7   9   10   8   6   4   2

This book is printed on acid-free paper. ∞

For Martha,
to whom all thoughts return

Acknowledgments

IT'S BEEN A BUSY FIVE YEARS SINCE THE PUBLICATION OF *EAT Right 4 Your Type*. In that time, we have seen the blood type theory introduced to millions of readers and translated into more than forty languages. As the diets have gained international acceptance, we have continued to develop ways to make the science accessible and the diets easier to follow, a goal which culminated in *Cook Right 4 Your Type*. We have made full use of the Internet to offer support and education and enable important feedback from tens of thousands of readers around the world, through www.dadamo.com.

This "family secret" that has become such an astounding success story is a testimony to a collaborative process involving many talented and dedicated publishing professionals; the support of doctors, scientists, nutritionists, and other medical specialists; and the valuable input of countless individuals who have shared their ideas and experiences and have helped us constantly refine and update the work. It is impossible to cite each one of you by name, but you have my deepest gratitude.

Live Right 4 Your Type represents years of research and development that have allowed us to take advantage of new genetic breakthroughs and amass the results from hundreds of clinical studies related to blood type and health. A work of this size and scope does not come easy, and I wish to thank a few individuals who have been of inestimable help:

Catherine Whitney, my writer, and her partner Paul Krafin, who have transformed incredibly complex science into lively prose and easy-to-understand guidelines—and who have done so with great enthusiasm and commitment.

My friend and colleague, Dr. Gregory Kelly, who supplied invaluable support, inspiration, and assistance through the gargantuan task of "information prospecting" that a book of this scope required.

My literary agent, Janis Vallely, who has been an invaluable colleague and friend, and is the best advocate one could hope for.

Amy Hertz, my editor at Riverhead/Putnam, who has nurtured my work through three books with patience and skill. And the wonderful staffs at Riverhead and Putnam, whose tireless efforts under the direction of Susan Petersen have produced such great success.

I would also like to acknowledge others who have lent their skill and support to the work: Michael Geoghegan, at Penguin Putnam, for his valued advice; Dr. Klaus Stadler, my editor at Piper-Verlag; Jane Dystel, Catherine's literary agent; Paul Schulick and Thomas Newmark of New Chapter; Dr. Joseph and Lara Pizzorno; Dr. Jules Harran; Ron Rubin of The Republic of T; Dr. Steve Barrie of Great Smokies Diagnostic Laboratories for his support and encouragement; and Dr. Jeffrey Bland, for his thought-provoking afterword.

Many thanks to my staff at 2009 Summer Street for holding down the fort and providing top-quality care to my patients while I wrote this book.

I also wish to single out two special cyber-friends who have done so much to help make www.dadamo.com the friendly place it is: Heidi (^heidi^) Merritt and Steven (s'leve) Shapiro. We also appreciate Heidi's generosity in lending a hand with proofreading.

A special thanks to Eric and Olga Butterworth, for their love and support, and to Robert Messineo, for the sailing adventures.

As always, I am grateful for the wisdom, love, and encouragement of my family: Dr. James and Christl D'Adamo, James and Ann D'Adamo, and Michele D'Adamo.

Special thanks, too, to Marge and Jim Burris, for their constant support and for the generous use of their home on Martha's Vineyard—a welcoming environment for writing this book.

Finally I am thankful to my wife and companion, Martha, and my daughters, Claudia and Emily, who kept me sane as I wrote this book, and make my life the happy adventure that it is.

Contents

Appendices

"Take a sheet of paper and tear it into little pieces. Now you have a divided, fragmented paper. The whole paper is the sum of all the fragments. That is division. But Spirit can be individualized. This means that it may be manifest in many parts, in an infinite number of people, with each containing the essence of the whole. Each is spiritus, and the whole is no less for having been divided."

Eric Butterworth

The Next Step

*E*ACH OF US CARRIES IN OUR BLOOD THE LIVING MEMORY of human history. And someday others will carry our memory into a future we cannot imagine. Humanity is a work in progress, a masterful scaffold that is never quite completed. Quite literally, the way we live today will become a part of the genetic profile of our progeny.

The science of blood type offers us a unique opportunity to examine the past, tinker with it, and pass along an improved version. It provides the knowledge and tools, not only to improve our own lives in the here and now, but to codify those improvements into our genetic hard drive.

When *Eat Right 4 Your Type* was published five years ago, we began with a simple premise: Blood type was the way to explain the many paradoxes in dietary studies and disease survival. Why were some people able to lose weight on a particular diet, while others were not? Why did some people retain vitality late in life, while others deteriorated, mentally and physically? Although as a species humans are mostly alike, we seemed to be most distinguished by our differences. *Eat Right 4 Your Type* was the first diet to explore this biological individuality. Tens of thousands of testimonials, medically certified results, and new genetic research have demonstrated that the Blood Type Diet has become a powerful mainstream tool for living more healthfully.

But *Eat Right 4 Your Type* also opened up new avenues of investigation that took us well beyond the diet itself. If blood type was the key to how we should eat, might it not also be the key to how we should live? This provocative question gained increasing validity with the rapid progress of genetic research, which enabled a study of blood type's cellular influence in every area of human physiology. The result is *Live Right 4 Your Type*, a system-wide blueprint of your individual strengths and weaknesses, based on your blood type. Your blood type has everything to do with how you digest food, your ability to respond to stress, your mental state, the efficiency of your metabolism, and the strength of your immune system. In the pages of this book, we take that knowledge and build a practical construct that will help you:

- choose a lifestyle that agrees with your needs and tendencies
- structure your days to reduce stress and gain more satisfaction
- raise your children in such a way as to maximize their unique potential
- live longer, avoiding the mental and physical deterioration of aging
- fine-tune your dietary strategies to produce new levels of energy and stamina
- overcome the chronic health conditions that may have plagued you and your family for decades
- find emotional balance and the elimination of anxiety and depression
- feel "right" in your body, your mind, and your world

We exist at an exciting moment in our history, when we can both experience and bear witness to a paradigm shift in thought. Our technologies, previously used to explore our similarities, are able to access more advanced means today that allow us to track our variations. The latest, most up-to-date knowledge is free and abundant. In June 2000, the Human Genome Project, a government-sponsored research group whose task is to map the entire human genetic structure; and the biotechnology company Celera announced the completion of a "working draft" of the DNA sequence of the human genome. Their goal is to complete a high-quality version by 2003. Molecular biology gives us the tools to understand our differences in very tangible, physical ways. Knowledge of genetics and biodiversity are expanding at a breathtaking rate. This genetic excavation has enabled us to test the principles of the blood type connection on increasingly deeper levels. Now, as we turn the corner on a new century, we at last know what it means to be true to your type.

Peter J. D'Adamo
September 2000

PART ONE

The Influence of Blood Type

The Unmistakable You

The Blood Type Gene

HAT MAKES ME *ME*, AND YOU *YOU*? THIS IS THE QUESTION that is at the heart of the genetic puzzle. It is also central to our exploration of blood types. What is the animating principle that determines the unique set of characteristics you possess, and the different set that belongs to me?

The key is genetic heritage. Your genetic heritage is the unbroken story line of your life. Even though you are living in the twenty-first century, you share a common bond with your ancestors. The genetic "information" that resulted in their particular characteristics has been passed on to you.

A helpful analogy is the way a computer manages information. Think of the very process of writing this book. As I sit at my computer, only my creative powers and my typing skills limit me. I am free to move words, sentences, or even whole paragraphs around. This information lies in the dynamic portion of my computer, called the RAM (random access memory). Should a sudden power outage occur, or I neglect to save the material to the hard drive, it would all be lost. How-

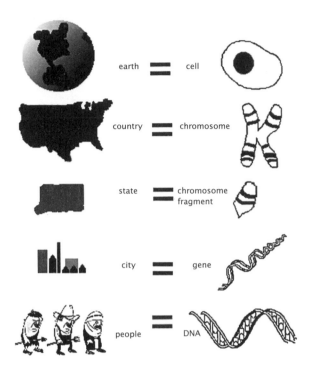

An easy way to envision the relationships within this complex network is to imagine our own relationship to the world. Picture the earth as a human cell. The earth is divided into many nations (chromosomes). Nations are divided into states or provinces (chromosome bands). States have cities (genes), and in those cities live people (DNA).

ever, if I am satisfied with this writing, it will be permanently saved to the hard drive, available for use at a later time.

Your genetic heritage is your biologic hard drive. Embedded within it are the recordings of past "writings" that were saved for later use—along with, in some cases, a few "disk errors." These recordings are stored in your DNA (deoxyribonucleic acid). One of the "saved" pieces of information is your blood type.

What determines your blood type? In genetic lingo, the blood type variations are known as alleles. Every person contains alleles—alternate forms of genes. The alleles determine whether you have blue eyes or brown, are tall or short, have black hair or red, and other distinctions. There are three blood type alleles—A, B, and O. That means there are three variations, or alternatives, for your blood type. However, the influence of your blood type is far greater than that of the gene that gives you eye color. Much of that influence has to do with its location and the way it interacts with other genes.

On the Street Where Blood Type Lives

THE GENE for ABO blood type is located on the q leg of chromosome number 9, around band 34. So the address for your blood type gene is 9q34. It is here that the three basic alleles of the ABO blood system are found, leaving you a Type O, A, B, or AB.[1] The mechanics of blood type's influence have to do with the way genes influence other, seemingly unrelated, genes located immediately adjacent or nearby. This mechanism explains why your blood type can have an impact on such a diverse number of bodily systems—from digestive enzymes to neurochemicals.

We already know of some intimate relationships between the blood type gene and other genes that impact on our health and well-being. For example, in 1984, researchers reporting in the journal *Genetic Epidemiology* presented evidence of a family pedigree in which a major gene for breast cancer susceptibility is located near band q34 on chromosome 9.[2] There is a clear genetic connection between blood type and breast cancer.

Many nutrition experts are baffled when they first hear about the link between blood type and digestion. That's because they are only considering the physical signifi-

Learn more about your personal genetic typography, page 351.

cance of blood type as a surface antigen. Actually, it is not your blood type antigen that is influencing the level of acid in your stomach, but rather the *gene* for your blood type influencing other seemingly unrelated genes located immediately adjacent (or very close) to the ABO blood type gene that can exert an effect on your stomach acid levels. This phenomenon, called gene linkage, isn't well understood yet, but it is well known: Many genes influence the actions of other, seemingly unrelated genes.

Here's another intriguing link that suggests a relationship between blood type and the brain. The gene for the enzyme dopamine beta hydroxylase (DBH), which converts dopamine to noradrenaline, is located right at 9q34. It's literally sitting on top of the gene for blood type.[3] As we will see later, this has vast implications for the association between blood type and stress, mental health, and even personality characteristics.

Your Subtypography

ALTHOUGH THERE are four blood types—O, A, B, and AB—it would be a ridiculous simplification to suggest that there are only four types of people in the world. The reality is far more intricate and complex. Now, let's take it to another level. Subtyping your blood type, especially your secretor status, provides an even greater specificity of identification. Your blood type doesn't just sit inert in your body. It is expressed in countless ways—and the ways in which it is expressed make a difference. A simple analogy would be a water faucet. Depending on the water pressure, the faucet might pour or dribble. You have access to a lot of water or a little water. In the same way, your secretor status relates to how much and where your blood type antigen is expressed in your body.

Secretor: 9q34's First Cousin

Across town from 9q34, on chromosomes 11 and 19, reside the blood type gene's very important first cousins, the blood type secretor genes. Although your secretor gene is independent of your blood type, it influences the way your blood type is expressed. Everyone carries a blood type antigen on their blood cells, but most people (between 80 and 85 percent of the population) have blood type antigens that float around freely in their body secretions. These people are called secretors, because they "secrete" their blood type antigens into their body fluids, such as saliva, mucus, and sperm. If you're a secretor, you can learn your blood type from these other body fluids, as well as from your blood. People who do not secrete their blood type antigens in other fluids besides blood are called, reasonably enough, non-secretors.

Because secretors have more places to put their blood type antigens, they have more blood type expression in their bodies than non-secretors. Your secretor status can have a great influence on the characteristics of your immune system and is associated with a wide variety of diseases and metabolic conditions.

Determining Your Secretor Status

There is a "quick and dirty" method of estimating secretor status. This involves looking at an additional minor blood typing system, called the Lewis Blood Grouping System, which is functionally interlocked with secretor genetics, since the same gene codes for both the secretor type and the Lewis System. In the Lewis System, located on chromosome

19, there are two possible antigens that can be produced, called Lewis^a and Lewis^b. (The a and b antigens of the Lewis System should not be confused with the A and B of the ABO system.) People can type out as one of three varieties: Lewis$^{a+ b-}$, Lewis^{a-b+}, and Lewis^{a-b-}. (A fourth variation, Lewis^{a+b+}, is extremely rare.) The Lewis System can determine secretor status because it has been noted that people who type out Lewis^{a+b-} are also non-secretors, while those who type out as Lewis^{a-b+} are also secretors. The connection between secretor status and the Lewis System occurs because secretors convert all of their Lewis^a antigen into the Lewis^b form (making them Lewis^{b+}), while non-secretors do not (leaving them Lewis^{a+}). The reason I say that this test is quick and dirty is that there are some leftovers that can't be typed this way. People who are Lewis^{a-b-} cannot use this test for determining secretor status. Because they have no ability to produce Lewis substances to start with, they never have +a or +b characteristics on their blood or in their secretions. These individuals can either be secretors or non-secretors of blood type substances, but they will always be non-secretors of Lewis substances. In many instances, Lewis negative individuals have unique interactions with diseases, microbes, or metabolic syndromes. Typically, when I've used the Lewis System to determine secretor status, I've lumped Lewis negative patients and Lewis^{a+} patients into the category of non-secretors. Fortunately, only 6 percent of the Caucasian population and 16 percent of the black population are Lewis^{a-b-}, allowing the greater majority of people to be secretor tested from the same blood sample that we use to test blood type.

The Lewis System

Le (a+b-) = non-secretors
Le (a-b+) = secretors
Le (a-b-) = Lewis negative
(can be either secretors or non-secretors)

Why Secretor Status Matters

We don't yet know precisely why nature made some of us secretors and some of us non-secretors, but we can surmise that secretor status is related to nature's effort to provide some additional layer of protection that didn't exist for the earliest humans. There is some evidence that the non-secretor state is genetically older than the secretor state and may have been more compatible with the digestive needs of hunter-gatherers.

The secretor state was most likely an immunologic adaptation. When you are able to secrete your blood type antigens into saliva, digestive secretions, and other fluids, these secretions appear to create a barrier against environmental elements, such as bacteria, pollutants, and other irritants. Immunologically, non-secretors seem to have more of a "death trap" strategy: They allow pathogenic invaders a way in, and then attack and kill them internally.[4]

These are some of the areas controlled or influenced by your secretor status:

- the degree to which foreign bacteria invade the system
- the adherence of lectins and other blood type–sensitive structures in food to your digestive tissue
- syndrome X or Insulin Resistance Syndrome
- the balance of intestinal bacteria
- predicting the relevance of tumor markers for diagnosing cancer
- blood-clotting capabilities
- the makeup of a mother's breast milk
- susceptibility to Candida-type infections
- immune resistance
- susceptibility to dental cavities
- sensitivity to the bacteria that causes ulcers
- relative risk for the development of inflammatory bowel problems
- an influence in respiratory heath and susceptibility to viruses
- prevalence of autoimmune diseases
- risk factors for cardiovascular disease
- a genetic predictor of alcoholism[5]

Are you a secretor or a non-secretor? We now have an easy way you can test your secretor status. For details, see page 358.

Here's an example of a practical ramification of your secretor status. Let's say you are a Type O about to undergo a surgical procedure. Type O has the lowest concentration of blood-clotting factor, so is more susceptible to bleeding problems. Secretors also have a very low amount of clotting factor. Therefore, if you are a Type O secretor, you have a higher risk of uncontrolled bleeding than if you were a Type O non-secretor.[6]

Here's another example, which has special relevance to Blood Type A. Experience has shown that about 10 percent of the people following the Type A Diet from *Eat Right 4 Your Type* find that they have some problems with the relatively high level of carbohydrates advocated for Type A. Most of these Type A "non-responders" are female. Since *ER4YT* only dealt with A, AB, B, and O types, the diets had to play the odds and assume that the average reader was a secretor, by far the more numerous subtype. No special allowances were made for non-secretors. I've found that, by and large, these non-responders are Type A non-secretors, and their problems are caused by insulin resistance, which often occurs in this subtype. Type A non-secretors may need to increase the percentage of protein in their diets (using such foods as ocean fish and poultry) and downplay the simple carbohydrates. With this in mind, we've adapted the basic Blood Type Diets to reflect secretor-based variations.

The Journey Continues

WE ARE ACCUSTOMED to picturing the course of human evolution as a straight line, with markers along the way that identify significant shifts. In *Eat Right 4 Your Type*, blood type evolution was described in a purposely linear manner, in an effort to communicate the basic idea. However, we know that the evolutionary process is more loop than line, more circular than linear. When we talk of Type O being first, Type A second, followed by Type B, then Type AB, we're not describing a seamless march from hunter to farmer to nomad and beyond. Evolution occurs on an invisible landscape, the actual process spanning eons. The refinements in our species and the many subspecies are the hammer of environmental demands arriving with the force of small taps rather than with thundering blows. These refinements have but one purpose—our survival. Today, as we arrive at a new century, we have the understanding and the tools to maximize our capacity for survival, using the genetic material that nature has supplied.

In Search of Identity

Is There a Blood Type Personality?

HO AM I? THE SIMPLE ANSWER IS ALL THAT I COULD
quickly detail—my age, height, weight, eye and hair color, marital status, number of children, place of residence, occupation. All of the exterior facts of my life. Oh, I am also a Blood Type A.

These are all observable and measurable details about Peter
D'Adamo, but most people would agree that they don't satisfactorily answer the question of who I am. Human beings aren't as easily quantifi-
able as they may seem to be. When someone says, "I'd like to get to
know you," they don't mean they want a listing of my vital statistics or
a copy of my curriculum vitae. They mean they want to know what
I'm *like*, what kind of a personality I have. Am I an extrovert or an intro-
vert? Do I tend to be more emotional or rational? Am I easygoing or
temperamental? Am I generous or selfish? Do I get quickly frustrated,
or am I patient? And so on. The intangible mélange of characteristics
that we call personality is what makes me uniquely me—and you
uniquely you.

Blood type is a marker of individuality, and the study of personality
is in part the study of individuality. Our blood type distinctions also

show us areas of commonality. For example, if you and I are both Type A, we will possess certain neurochemical similarities in the ways we respond to stress.[1]

For hundreds of years, the medical community has separated the mind and body, addressing them as discrete entities, but this split between the mental and the physical is actually an anomaly in the span of history. The understanding we have today that the mind and body are physiologically connected is not a new idea. It has ancient roots. For example, the traditional Indian method of healing, called *ayurveda*, is based on an ancient system of thought encompassing universal forces and life energies. Indian sages proposed five basic elements or transformations of energy: space, air, fire, water, and earth. These elements combine to form three major life forces, or *doshas*: *vata*, *kapha*, and *pitta*. The *doshas* affect life energy—or *prana*—and help to determine a person's body type, constitution, personality, and overall health.

In the second century, the Greek physician Galen distinguished four basic temperaments, called humors: the *sanguine, melancholic, choleric,* and *phlegmatic.* The measure of these humors' longevity is that they are still being used as adjectives in modern language. The humors were thought to derive from various mixtures of the four basic substances found in the body: blood, phlegm, yellow bile, and black bile. Special attention was given to the thickness or thinness of these fluids, particularly blood. Modern science has confirmed a relationship between blood type, blood viscosity, and a variety of chronic anxiety states.

There is no doubt that a connection exists between body and mind—that the ways we think, feel, dream, and imagine are manifested in our complex chemical circuitry. Infused throughout the hardwiring of our systems is our blood type.

I come across this connection all the time in my everyday dealings. People are always eager to share their experiences with the Blood Type Diet when we meet. They tell me how they've lost weight, lowered their cholesterol levels, and found relief from the crippling pain of arthritis. Then, almost as an aside, they'll confide that what's really wonderful is that they don't feel depressed anymore. They begin telling me about the horrible spells of depression that have plagued them for decades. The depression seemed to lift—as if by magic—a little while after they started following the right diet for their blood type.

Does blood type influence behavior? Can blood type play a role in mental health and disease? Is there such a thing as a blood type personality? These are intriguing questions, for which the answer is a qualified yes—if you begin with two basic premises:

Premise #1: The body and mind are integral to the formation of a whole being. The physical functions—immune system, digestive system, circulatory system, endocrine glands, and all other systems—are autonomic, but linked to the mind.

Premise #2: That blood type has an influence on our entire system on a cellular level.

What do we hope to learn from this investigation? We discover the strengths and weaknesses that exist for each of the blood types—the propensities that have an influence on health and well-being.

It is in situations of illness and other forms of physical and emotional stress that this information becomes helpful. Dr. Samuel Hahnemann, the creator of homeopathic medicine, had an interesting concept, which I believe is quite true. Hahnemann noted that almost all individuals have some flaw in their heredity. The most common flaw, which Hahnemann described as *psora*, was derived from the Hebrew word *tsorat*, meaning a crack or fault.

Psora was the line of weakness, the genetic fault line, carried through heredity, by which a person could be expected to become sick. The San Andreas Fault in California is an apt corollary. This crack is a charted weakness in the Earth's geology, a fault line upon which we expect earthquakes to occur.

The blood type and personality correlates assume their proper significance if we consider them in the same way that Hahnemann viewed *psora*. In times of stress, the effects of our blood type genetics on the system's neurochemistry behave as a fault line, the inherent crack beneath the surface. The fault line may remain basically benign when we're healthy, but become inflamed and explode when we're ill or stressed beyond our limits. Our investigation of blood type and the mind is an effort to ease pressure on our fault lines—to keep them in their benign state, and to keep ourselves safe from harm.

Probing the Personality Question

SOMEONE ONCE sent me a matchbook from a singles bar in Japan. It was similar to matchbooks distributed in U.S. singles bars. On the inside cover, there were spaces for a person's name and phone number. Unlike its American counterpart, though, the Japanese matchbook also had a line for blood type. Surveys show that more than 70 percent of

Japanese believe there is a direct relationship between blood type and personality. Talk shows, cartoon characters, and Web sites often carry references to blood type. In 1997, four of the five major private television stations in Japan broadcast blood type–related programs. Job applicants regularly place their blood types on resumés, and it frequently becomes a factor in hiring decisions. Nowhere else on earth is the population so thoroughly imbued with the notion of blood type.[2]

The internationally renowned Japanese cartoon *Sailor Moon*, by Naoko Takeuchi, mentions the blood types of its characters several times throughout the program. When the characters are introduced, Ms. Takeuchi includes their names, birthdays, zodiac signs, blood types, ages, and school names, in that order. Sure enough, the personalities of her characters conform to certain blood type stereotypes. The character Setsuna (Sailor Pluto) is Type A and lists red meat as the thing she hates most in life! We have a copy of *Sailor Moon* at home, and my daughters, both Type A, root for Setsuna as their favorite character.

Ascribing personalities to blood types can be a fun pastime, not unlike astrology. But is there any validity to it? As I was researching and writing *Eat Right 4 Your Type*, I was confounded as to whether or not to believe that blood type had *any* effect on personality. When examining the work of the Japanese author Masahiko Nomi and his detailed characterization of blood type personalities, it seemed that much of the material belonged more to the world of pop culture than in the hallowed halls of science.

The finite truths about personality remain as elusive as humans are diverse. No matter the variety of measuring tools and theories provided by modern psychology, as we draw open the curtains on the twenty-first century, the deepest origins of what we now call personality remain largely a mystery.

One difficulty with any theory of personality is that it tends to be codified into a rigid script. The particular theory determines which labels are ultimately constructed to explain characteristics in line with the model. Even the archetypes we employed in *Eat Right 4 Your Type* to more easily explain the anthropological origins of the ABO blood type groups were intended as loose reference points. Type O became the hunter, to represent the early hunter-gatherers; Type A was the cultivator, in recognition of the agricultural impetus for the emergence of this blood type; Type B was the nomad, because it developed along with the spread of populations to new environments; Type AB became the enigma, for the simple reason that we don't yet know why this more recent blood type came into being. For many people, however, their blood type labels became as personalized as their astrological signs, a further means to identify and explain innate characteristics. In the end, however, the exquisite mystery of human nature is lost in a rather superficial analysis of "types."

For this reason, I have remained rather skeptical and resolutely cautious about exploring the blood type–personality connection. However, the overwhelming evidence of studies clearly marking neurochemical blood type differences has finally given me an opportunity to consider the question of personality in a different way. If the very mechanisms that control behavior, temperament, and mental health are influenced by blood type, it becomes legitimate to extend the analysis to the question of personality.

Blood Type and Personality: The Existing Theories

THE RELATIONSHIP between blood type and temperament has been a subject of study since the 1920s, when a psychology professor named Takeji Furukawa began to explore whether blood type could be a marker of some kind that would translate into psychological qualities. Furukawa published some of his work in the German *Journal of Applied Psychology* in the early 1930s, and influenced several European psychologists to begin examining the relationship of blood type to temperament.[3]

However, the connection between blood type and personality didn't really gain widespread attention until the 1970s, when a journalist named Masahiko Nomi single-handedly popularized the notion that ABO blood type is a key to personality. Nomi's book, *What Blood Types Reveal about Compatibility* (Ketsueki de wakaru aisho) was a huge success in Japan, and remains so—it's now in its 240th printing. His later book, *You Are Your Blood Type*, became a major international success.[4] Nomi went on to write more than sixty-five books, either alone or with his son, Toshitaka.

Many of Nomi's characterizations are based on the simple observation of thousands of individuals, often for days at a time. While this method may not be sufficient to meet strict scientific standards, it is certainly meaningful. Consistent observation is going to reveal some clear trends. My father, James D'Adamo, formed many of his conclusions about blood type from observing and cataloging information about thousands of his patients, accumulated over the long years of his practice. Only later were many of his conclusions confirmed by genetic research and laboratory studies.

In 1997, Peter Constantine published *What's Your Type?* (Plume), a book about blood type and personality.[5] While tipping his hat to Nomi, Constantine's simple yet insightful look at personality seems to take more of its inspiration from the work of European psychologists of the 1930s, '40s and '50s. Drawing heavily on the work of the French psychologist Leone Bourdel and the Swiss specialist Fritz Schaer, Constantine's blood type personality profiles seem mostly to be in harmony with Nomi's profiles. Then there are times that they differ dramatically.

Nomi portrays Type B as a "non-stereotypical thinker," and "not very ambitious." Constantine characterizes Type Bs as "rational, sober, and pragmatic—inveterate organizers with an energetic drive to reach goals." Both Nomi and Constantine characterize Type Bs as "individualists."

Nomi and Constantine are in agreement about Type O and extroversion—especially with regard to Type O's speaking their minds. They also agree that Type A is more likely to be introverted, with a rather heightened sensitivity to public opinion—although Constantine considers Type A more "reserved and calm" than Nomi would suggest.

Constantine describes Type AB as maintaining a balance of introversion and extroversion—a positive mixture of opposites. Nomi views the introversion and extroversion as being less well-balanced, describing Type AB as good at adapting to human relations, but in general "inwardly emotional," with feelings of distance from society. On the whole, Constantine and Nomi's characterizations are actually quite similar. The most consistent trait noted by both is a tendency toward extroversion in Type O and introversion in Type A.

Two leading twentieth-century psychologists, Raymond Cattell and Hans Eysenck, were the first to open up scientific investigations into the link between blood types and personality. Cattell's work focused on examining the individual differences in cognitive abilities, personality, and motivation. He is best known for his 16 Personality Factor (16PF) personality assessment device, one of the most widely used and recognized personality tests in the world.

Cattell studied blood types using his 16PF system in 1964 and 1980. A sample of 323 Caucasian Australians was broken down into seventeen genetic systems and twenty-one psychological variables, including seven blood groups. Cattell found that Blood Type ABs are significantly more self-sufficient and group-independent than Type O, Type A, or Type B. Blood Type A is more prone to serious anxiety than is Blood Type O.[6] These findings correlate exactly with other findings regarding stress and mental disorders.

Eysenck, a German psychologist and professor of psychology at

London University, pioneered the theory that genetic factors play a large part in determining the psychological differences between people. His major contribution is his theory of personality, known as the PEN System (Psychoticism, Extroversion, and Neuroticism). According to Eysenck, these variables are the result of physiological and chemical preferences. For example, introverts have higher levels of activity in the cortico-reticular loop of the brain, and so are chronically more cortically aroused than are extroverts. If so, crowds and noise would very quickly create a sensory overload for such an individual.

Eysenck compared differences in nationality to personality characteristics and was able to make distinctions about blood types in specific populations. He used earlier studies, which showed significant differences in the frequency of particular blood types among European introverts and extroverts, and between highly emotional and more relaxed people. These results showed that emotional behavior was significantly more common in Type B than in Type A, and that introversion was more common in Type AB than in any of the other blood types.[7]

Eysenck looked at two population samples—one British, the other Japanese. Since previous studies had shown that Japanese population samples were more naturally introverted and more neurotic than British

Blood Type–Personality Characterizations

	TYPE O	TYPE A	TYPE B	TYPE AB
Masahiko Nomi	Extroverted Strong Expressive	Introverted Perfectionist Restrained	Free-thinking Independent Lacking ambition	Sensitive Distant Passive
Peter Constantine	Extroverted Outspoken	Introverted Reserved Calm	Pragmatic Organized	Balance of extroversion and introversion
Raymond Cattell	Stable	Prone to anxiety	Self-sufficient	Alienated
Hans Eysenck	Extroverted	Calm	Highly emotional	Introverted
Blood Type–Personality Test at www.dadamo.com	Extroverted Practical Decisive Lives in the present	Introverted Sensitive to the needs of others	Feeling Flexible Spontaneous Subjective	Feeling Intuitive

samples, he predicted that the Japanese would have a higher proportion of Type AB and a lower ratio of Type A to Type B. This was confirmed by looking at the established blood type frequencies for the two countries.[8]

The Blood Type Personality Project

ABOUT A YEAR AGO, a visitor posted an interesting piece on my Web site bulletin board. Using Carl Jung's personality types as a basis, she had conducted a small study correlating blood types to personality test results.

Carl Jung was the first to identify the two fundamentally different attitudes of extroversion and introversion—the opposing characteristics that have sometimes been assigned to Type O and Type A. To embody these attitudes, Jung identified two types of mental processes: *perceiving:* the taking in of information; and *judging:* the organizing and prioritizing of information to arrive at decisions. Each of the processes had variations, which Jung called orienting functions—either *rational* (thinking and feeling) or *irrational* (sensing and intuition).[9] Jung's work was seminal to twentieth-century personality theory and was used as the basis for the development of the Meyers-Briggs Type Indicator, a widely used personality test.[10]

My Web site visitor wrote the following about her study:

"From a sample group of about 45 MBA students, I found that Blood Type O scored significantly higher than the rest in 'sensing,' using the five physical senses to gather information; and in the 'sensing/thinking' combination, indicating that they are more detail- and fact-oriented, logical, precise, orderly, rule- and procedure-conscious, dependable, responsible, and good at objectively observing and organizing than the rest (of the sample). Blood Type O also had a preference for learning through reading and writing. I believe that the tendency to sense and get facts right stems from the inbred hunter-gatherer need to observe and accurately assess the environment in order to insure survival.

"The only really significant finding for Blood Type A was that they had a higher need for autonomy than any of the other types. It may have stemmed from a genetic imperative to establish a separate identity. Coming from generations of people who worked mostly alone, they needed to do so, needed to be certain of themselves. They were self-sufficient farmers in a loosely woven society of agrarian communities.

"Blood Type Bs were the most interesting. They scored significantly higher on 'intuiting,' indicating a preference for sixth sense information; and they scored high on the 'intuiting/feeling' combination, indicating that they tend to be 'insightful, mystical, idealistic, personal, creative, original, globally oriented, people-oriented, and good at imagining.' They also learned best through listening, then reflecting on and interpreting what they had observed. Perhaps the nomadic life of the steppes contributed to long hours given over to talk, as well as ample time for meditation and reflection."

I liked the way this visitor made the association between blood type personality and the anthropological imperatives the blood types faced. We readily accept that our purely physical characteristics evolved over time as adaptations to changing environments. Logic dictates that our personality characteristics had to make adaptations, too. With that in mind, I decided to perform a study.

Since the Internet affords rapid access to large numbers of potential subjects for a questionnaire-based study, I used my Web site for an investigation to determine if a personality testing tool would show any correlation to blood type. This was not a scientific study per se. Rather, it was an attempt to see if I would get results that were more or less consistent with other research.

I developed a small computer program that allowed any visitor to my Web site to take a test. I used a simpler, quicker version of a questionnaire called the Kiersey Temperament Sorter. This test, developed by psychologist David Kiersey, identifies personality characteristics based on Carl Jung's "extrovert-introvert" personality types.[11] By choosing between two columns on four screens, it was possible for subjects to determine which one of sixteen personality profiles they fit best.

> *Take the blood type personality test and learn more about the dynamics of blood type and identity at www.dadamo.com.*

From early June 1999, to December 1999, a total of 20,635 people took the test on my Web site. This represents such a significant sample that it deserves note. The testing group had the following demographics:

Total	20,635
Total Female	15,255
Total Male	5,380

The demographics by blood type:

A	AB	B	O
7187	1473	2809	9166
34.83%	7.14%	13.61%	44.42%

In addition, I asked subjects to characterize their somatypes. Most readers are familiar with the basic idea of somatypes, which is the connection between one's personality and one's body type. The theory was first advanced during the 1940s by William H. Sheldon, who constructed a precise measurement system that identified three basic body types and their correlation to personality characteristics. They are: **Ectomorphs:** Slender, often tall, people, with long arms and legs and finely drawn features. **Mesomorphs:** Stockier people, with broad shoulders and good musculature. **Endomorphs:** Chubby people, tending to "pear-shaped." Endomorphs are characterized by a preponderance of body fat.

A few trends could be observed from the personality/somatype questions:

BLOOD TYPE O.   Type Os most often described themselves in ways related to the following characteristics: responsible, decisive, organized, objective, rule-conscious, and practical. Both male and female Type Os reported a higher percentage of the mesomorphic body type when compared to controls. Type O women showed a statistically higher incidence of the endomorphic somatype. Type Os also had the lowest incidence of respondents reporting the ectomorphic type. Some of the traits associated with mesomorphism, such as zest for physical activity, indifference to what others think or want, competitiveness and a bold, assertive quality, consistently show up when the Type O personality is described.

BLOOD TYPE A.   Type As most often described themselves in ways related to the following characteristics: sensitive to the needs of others, listeners, detail-oriented, and analytical. Type As had a statistically significant percentage of individuals who described themselves as ectomorphs over mesomorphs. Interestingly, Type As also had a higher incidence of the endomorphic body type. This seems to indicate that Type A individuals have body types which tend towards the extremes. The percentages were even higher among male Type As. Some of the personality traits thought to be associated with ectomorphism, such as a preference for privacy, mental intensity and detail orientation, have been linked to Type A in the psychology literature.

BLOOD TYPE B.   Type Bs most often described themselves in ways related to the following characteristics: subjective, easygoing, creative, original, and flexible. Of all the blood types, Type Bs came closest to fitting the expected body type percentages of the controls.

BLOOD TYPE AB.   Type ABs most often described themselves in ways related to the following characteristics: emotional, independent, intuitive. Type ABs were the least likely to report that their body types were endomorphic. Unlike Type As, whose greater occurrence of the ectomorphic type was at the expense of a lowered incidence of meso-morphism, Type ABs appeared to be less endomorphic by virtue of be-ing more mesomorphic.

Taking both the data from other researchers and my own data, the following is a fairly reliable synthesis of personality characteristics by blood type:

TYPE O	TYPE A	TYPE B	TYPE AB
EXTROVERTED	INTROVERTED	INDEPENDENT	INTUITIVE
Strong	Intense	Free Thinking	Emotional
Leader	Inventive	Resilient	Passionate
Confident	Demanding	Creative	Friendly
Pragmatic	Perfectionist	Original	Trusting
Strategic	Sensitive	Subjective	Empathetic
Patient	Cooperative	Inveterate organizer	
Logical	Creative		

Putting It Together

BLOOD TYPE and personality offer a logical catalog of associations. Human nature seeks patterns, and our ultimate goal is to draw useful conclusions from the analysis. How does understanding your blood type–inspired personality tendencies help you?

Let's begin with the assumption that every characteristic has a basis in our genetic memory. Anthropological studies have proven irrefutably that certain archetypal personality and behavior traits throughout our evolutionary history are directly linked to survival. Proponents of socio-biology, a theory first advanced by E. O. Wilson, believe that the way we behave can be explained by examining our evolutionary patterns. Aggression, attraction, and cooperative behaviors all promote a continuation of the species. However, as we know, these behaviors are not automatic. They have been refined over time by shifting environments and cultural influences.

We might call this pattern of behaviors an example of intelligent evolution. As we will explain in the next chapter, these personality patterns have a strong correlation with chemical attributes that each blood type expresses. And these chemicals have important implications for your mental health.

THREE

Stress and Emotional Stability

Blood Type As a Mental Health Marker

UMANITY'S HARDSCRABBLE EXISTENCE ON PLANET Earth has always been fraught with peril. We may have risen to the top of the food chain because of our superior predatory instincts and intelligence, but we are fragile beings just the same. We are still vulnerable to the savage attack of microscopic predators. The increasingly volatile and changeable environment challenges our ability to survive. The evolving strains of antibiotic-resistant pathogens and the resurgence of diseases long thought routed pull at our mortality. The ravages of the aging process, the inevitable wearing down of our physical systems, remain life's end game.

Each and every encounter with our mortality is a trigger for stress. That's both good news and bad news. Even though most of us carry the proper mix of biochemical signals that help us respond to life's stressors appropriately, too much stress for too long causes psychological imbalance, physiologic breakdown, and disease. On the other hand, if we were without this series of signals, the hormonal/chemical alarm and response matrix that regulates our beings, the human race would have become extinct long before there was a language available to express such thoughts.

In modern times we face a dilemma: the very response mechanisms so elegantly designed to protect us have become dangerous to our health and well-being. One of the unfortunate consequences of our evolution has been the "piling-on" of stressors, which has placed an unnatural strain on our systems—a strain we were not designed to handle.

For our ancient ancestors, stress was an intense but intermittent reality, usually resulting from encounters with dangerous predators, territorial disputes with other creatures, and the ongoing hunt for sources of food.

Today's stressors are usually not life and death battles, but they aren't intermittent, either. They're constant. It's this "piling-on" factor that makes stress so dangerous. Yet, all of us know people who deal with similar levels of stress with what seems to be remarkable aplomb. In the madness of the morning rush hour, some people experience road rage while others take the delay in stride. The external circumstances may be exactly the same, but the responses are completely different. Why?

When I ask my patients about the levels of stress in their lives, what I'm hoping to discover is their subjective responses to external circumstances. What is their capability to adapt to stress? Are they producing large amounts of stress hormones or small amounts? Are they releasing these hormones when it's appropriate or is the rhythm off kilter? What is the relative balance of their nervous systems? What types of feelings are being produced? Are there safety valves, such as exercise, that relieve excess stress, or are the forms of exercise they've chosen adding to their stress? What is the total load of all the stressors? Are they close to their breaking points or have they already passed their breaking points and entered into a dangerous state known as maladaptation? Maladaptation occurs when an organism is pushed beyond its boundaries. Then, the adaptations it makes to survive don't always serve its best interests and can cause systemic breakdowns and disease, long after the actual stressor has passed.

Even though people have different capabilities for accommodating stress, we ultimately all have a breaking point. Given enough stressors of a high enough intensity for a long enough period of time, anyone will maladapt.

What does that have to do with your blood type? Quite a bit, it turns out. Some of the key elements that activate our particular reactions to stress are located in the same locus on our DNA as that of our blood type—9q34. You'll recall that there is an active interplay that takes place among various genes, especially those in proximity to one another. The blood type gene has this relationship with genes that control our stress responses.

When we examine the body of research on stress and blood type, we can see clear differences in the ways that humans respond to stress. Blood type plays a significant role in how much stress we carry around inside all the time, the way we respond to stress, and how quickly we recover from it.

The Mechanics of Stress

UNDER CIRCUMSTANCES of physiological or emotional stress, your body protects itself by reversing its polarities, shifting the relative balance of the autonomic (automatic) nervous system, which is actually two systems. In general, the sympathetic nervous system is responsible for the initial "fight or flight" response, while the parasympathetic branch is responsible for relaxing the nervous system after whatever set off the alarms indicating danger has passed. The proper functioning of both systems is a critical component of good health. Together, the two branches of the nervous system communicate with your endocrine system and internal organs to help you maintain proper function and respond to a wide range of potential challenges.

For the most part, the two branches of your nervous system are antagonists. They tend to work best in balanced opposition to one another. For example, sympathetic activity causes your heart to beat faster and more forcefully, while parasympathetic activity slows down your heart rate and unclenches the arterial muscle walls, allowing freer blood flow and oxygenation of the heart muscle.

The key to the proper functioning of your nervous system is balance. Problems occur when one of the two parts of this system has a continued dominance over the other for prolonged periods of time. Chronic stress acts like a weight on a scale—it tilts the scale in favor of the sympathetic branch at the expense of the parasympathetic branch. Since many of your body's activities associated with health and healing are driven by parasympathetic activity, prolonged time intervals with the scales out of balance will inevitably lead to a breakdown. The mechanics of a normal stress response involve the synchronized action of three endocrine glands: hypothalamus, pituitary, and adrenal. We refer to this interplay as the HPA axis. Here is a simplified description of the process:

Moment of Stress

- The hypothalamus gland in the brain, often called the "Master" gland, activates a messenger molecule called corticotropin-releasing hormone.
- The messenger hormone alerts the pituitary gland to release adrenocortropic hormone (ACTH).
- ACTH signals the adrenal gland to release its supply of stress hormones—adrenaline and cortisol.

End of Stress

- The hypothalamus gland is signaled to stop producing the messenger hormone.
- Homeostasis—balance—is restored.

Normally, the checks and balances built into this feedback loop will shut down the HPA axis when the stressor is removed. Unfortunately, chronic stress throws a wrench in the smooth operation of this axis and its feedback loops. The hypothalamus gland becomes less sensitive to the signal that tells it to stop producing the messenger hormone.[1]

Stress Hormones: The Vortex

THE CRITICAL moment in the stress response comes when the adrenal gland releases its supply of stress hormones. There are two types of stress hormones: catecholamines and cortisol, and these are the hormones that are most closely linked to blood type.

There are two catecholamines released from the adrenal gland in response to stress—*epinephrine*, more commonly recognized as *adrenaline;* and *norepinephrine*, also called *noradrenaline.* When these powerful chemicals are released into your blood stream, you experience an increase in heart rate, an increase in blood pressure, a decrease in digestive capability, an increase in arousal or alertness, and an overall shifting of your resources toward fight, flight, exercise, or some form of physical activity. The catecholamines can be thought of as the shock troops of the nervous system, acting as the immediate, short-term response to stress. Cortisol, on the other hand, is more like an occupying army, in for the long haul. Cortisol is a catabolic hormone; it will function to break down muscle tissue and convert the proteins from the tissue into energy. The adrenal glands will flood the system with cortisol in any traumatic situation. Exposure to cold, starvation, bleeding, surgery, infections, injuries, pain, and excessive amounts of exercise will be met by cortisol. Emotional and mental stress also influence the increase of this hormone. But cortisol also stimulates and marshals the powerful forces within our systems, all geared to survival.

Cortisol is essential for life. Since it enables us to get out of the way of danger, we would quickly die when exposed to stress if our adrenal glands stopped making this key hormone. However, cortisol is a double-edged sword. Excessive or prolonged release of cortisol disrupts the balance of a number of our internal systems. While the proper levels of cortisol will reduce inflammation, decrease our tendency to allergies, and help to heal tissue and wounds, inappropriate levels will create the opposite effect. Ulcers, autism, high blood pressure, heart disease, muscle loss, aging of the skin, increased risk of bone fractures, and insomnia are just some of the costs of cortisol intoxication. Chronic overproduction of cortisol also severely compromises the immune system, making us susceptible to viral infections. High cortisol levels can produce the daytime "brain fog" known as diurnal cognitive dysfunction. As a matter of fact, people with Alzheimer's Disease and senile dementia have chronically high cortisol levels.[2]

▪ FROM THE BLOOD TYPE OUTCOME REGISTRY ▪

Deborah P.
Type A
Middle-aged female
Improvement: Stress reduction and well-being

"I am a forty-six-year-old junior high school teacher in Oregon, and in June, I had completely had it. I was tired and *stressed* all of the time. I was asking questions of myself, like, 'What's wrong with you? You aren't that old to feel like you are eighty-seven' My girlfriend turned me on to your book. It made sense. I always knew that there was more to blood type than met the eye. I have been on the diet for Type A for about four weeks, as are my children, and we *all* feel *much better.* My nineteen-year-old has no more stomach ailments and I have more energy than I know what to do with. I am *not,* in any way shape or form, a 'weird, granola-type, bark-eating, health fanatic,' and that is why this is *so wonderful.*"

You may have heard at least some of this before. There is more awareness, through the popular media, of the costs of stress. What you may not have known, however, is that the action of the stress hormones has a direct connection to your blood type.

Blood Type and Stress

MOST OF THE STUDIES that record differences in a disease, hormones, or neurotransmitters according to blood type, show a continuum, with Type O at one end and Type A at the other. Usually, Type B and Type AB fall somewhere in the middle. This seems to represent a type of balance between opposing forces, or is the result of being a "later model" blood type that has been refined over time. So, too, with stress.

Type As tend to overrespond to even minor stress. This response can be measured by increases in cortisol. Type Os, at the opposite end of the continuum, produce the least amounts of cortisol and adrenaline in response to stress. This is one area where Type Bs fall closer to Type As than Type Os, while Type ABs are closer to Type Os. Of course, this simplistic description doesn't begin to tell the entire story—especially if you are Type B or AB. Each blood type has a very unique chemical profile.

Type A

While all of the blood types respond to stress by secreting more cortisol, Type As start with a higher basal level in their blood all the time. That means Type As are walking around with their physiology in a higher state of adrenal stress than the other blood types. They also don't benefit as much as the other blood types when they practice stress-reducing exercises.

Type A has to do much more, for far less return. This chemical discovery confirms my father's observations about Type A. His prescription of the need for Type A to "calm the nervous system" now makes sense on a real and measurable physiological level. Some of the effects of exercise observed in Type A, and probably the higher rates of cancer and heart disease, also begin to make more sense. In addition, Type A produces more adrenaline in response to stress than the other blood types, while also possessing the greatest ability to break down and eliminate adrenaline.[3]

Type O

Type Os require a lot more to knock them off kilter in the face of stress. However, once they are pushed to the point of dramatic response, it usually takes them longer to recover. In times of stress, Type Os tend to secrete higher levels of the catecholamines noradrenaline and adrenaline. This facility enables them to respond quickly and efficiently to danger.[4] Their recovery is more difficult because it takes them longer to break down catecholamines. An enzyme called monoamine oxidase (MAO) is responsible for, among other things, the breakdown or inactivation of adrenaline and noradrenaline. When measuring the activity of MAO in platelets, research has shown that even healthy Type Os have the lowest activity of this enzyme. This may explain their difficulty breaking down the catecholamines noradrenaline and adrenaline.

My colleague, Yuri Andriyashek, M.D., recently alerted me to a new study conducted by a Ukranian physiologist called "Methodological Recommendation for Selection of Sailors for Long Term Navigation." The research concluded that Blood Type O sailors were "not recommended for navigation duties for longer than one month" because their performance dropped significantly after that period. This research is consistent with other findings that prolonged stress seems to affect the levels of adrenaline clearance in Type Os, causing adrenal-neurological exhaustion.

It has been suggested that noradrenaline is more related to stress in-

---

▪ FROM THE BLOOD TYPE OUTCOME REGISTRY ▪

Jeff T.
Type O
Middle-aged male
Improved: Stress levels

"I started the Type O diet three months ago, thanks to my wife, also Type O, who stopped buying any 'avoid' foods. I've lost twenty-six pounds, and my wife has lost twenty-two pounds since we started eating this way. I'm also running again, which I haven't done since I was in my twenties, and I'm forty-one now. I feel better than I've felt in years, and I've completely stopped taking antacids, which I was addicted to. Several people at work have commented that I seem more mellow, and I don't let things get to me as much."

duced by anger and aggression, and, indeed, these characteristics are more typical of Type Os.[5] Type O is the classic example of the so-called "*Type A behavior.*" ("*Type A Behavior*" is not to be confused with Blood Type A. It will appear in quotes and be italicized.)

Type B

When it comes to stress hormones, Type B is closer to Type A, producing somewhat higher than normal levels of cortisol. This is something of an anomaly, since in most other areas, Type B tends to be closer to Type O. However, it is understandable when you consider the kinds of stress early Type Bs undoubtedly faced. Cortisol, you'll remember, is the "long-haul" stress hormone, breaking down muscle tissue and converting the proteins to energy. Type B would likely have inherited this adaptation from Type A, rather than from the early Type O hunter-gatherers.

This is not to say that Type Bs are A-like. The balancing forces always present in Type Bs give them a unique stress profile.[6] After many years of using the blood type system in practice, I have noticed on a fairly consistent basis that Type Bs tend to be very emotionally centered. Consequently, they are far more sensitive to stress-related imbalances, but they respond very quickly to stress-reducing techniques. In fact, Type Bs are inordinately gifted in harnessing the powers of visualization and relaxation, and therefore recover from stress much more quickly than Type As.

TYPE AB

We are not certain why, but research clearly shows that Type ABs are more like Type Os in their response to stress.[7] This, too, represents a departure, as in so many other crucial ways, Type ABs reflect A-like qualities.

Exercise and Stress

IN *EAT RIGHT 4 YOUR TYPE*, you learned about the symbiotic relationship between exercise and stress. The right kind of physical activity for your blood type can help you recover from stress and resist many of its harmful effects. Exercise is often described as a panacea when it comes to moderating against stress or helping to de-stress. However, this is not always the case. If you exert yourself beyond your level of tolerance, exercise can actually act as a stressor.

Many factors interact to determine your tolerance for exercise—such as proper nutrition, hydration, rest, prior training, level of fitness, and the stress in other parts of your life. An important factor influencing your level of tolerance is your blood type.[8]

To demonstrate the difference blood type makes, let's look at the effects of exercise on two polar opposites—a Type O and a Type A.

Oliver (Type O) and Adam (Type A) have decided to exercise together. They meet four days a week for a three-mile run. As their running program progresses, Oliver is experiencing many benefits. His energy level has increased and his fitness has improved. Best of all, running has provided the perfect antidote to his stressful profession. He feels more balanced and able to cope.

Adam's experience has been very different. Although he feels better immediately after running (running will release endorphins that cause this good feeling), within an hour or two, he feels sluggish and his concentration is poor.

If Oliver and Adam were to monitor their heart rates during the run, they would notice that Adam's is somewhat higher, and he is working harder to achieve the same level of performance as Oliver. After the run, it takes longer for Adam's heart rate to return to resting levels.

While Oliver marches off to work feeling energized and ready to take on the world, Adam continues to struggle. Sometimes, when he stands up abruptly, he feels lightheaded. He has trouble sleeping soundly at night. The longer he and Oliver run together, the more Adam experiences stress. If we could look inside to view his hormonal response, we'd see that he is releasing higher levels of cortisol, and his levels of DHEA are decreasing. Adam is now overtrained. Rather than helping him manage stress, his exercise program has pushed him into further maladaptation. If he stops exercising now, it might take days, weeks, or even longer for his hormone profile to return to normal.

Even trained athletes experience a rise in cortisol when they run, although conditioning will tend to offset some of the effects and keep cortisol levels in check. Since Adam, a Type A, is starting out with a higher level of basal cortisol to begin with, and he is not a regular runner, his cortisol levels spike high enough to interfere with his well-being. Running is making Adam sick.

Now let's say that Oliver and Adam's Type B friend Betty decides to join them in their runs. Like Adam, Betty is starting out with higher cortisol levels. However, after a few weeks, she is feeling well-conditioned and energized by the run. What's the difference between Betty and Adam? Twice a week, Betty is also taking a yoga class. With her remarkable Type B ability to recover from the effects of stress, Betty is able to get the best of both worlds.

When another friend, Abby, a Type AB, joins the run, she initially feels energized by the exercise, much like Oliver. But after a few weeks, Abby decides to cut back her runs to twice a week and takes a stretching class the other two days.

All physical activity, even when it is not exhaustive, usually leads to elevated blood levels of catecholamines and cortisol. However, following a period of training, most people will produce fewer stress hormones in response to exercise. In other words, once you get used to an exercise, it is not as stressful. That's what conditioning is all about. Generally speaking, trained athletes do not experience exercise internally as a stressful event, even if they slightly push past their normal training routine. In essence they have conditioned their physiology, their nervous system, and their endocrine system. For this reason, a well-conditioned Type A might have the same or greater tolerance than a poorly conditioned Type O. It's not a question of all or nothing. I've seen many Type Os who happily incorporate yoga into their exercise program, as well as athletic As who enjoy weight lifting and aerobics. You have to evaluate your relative capabilities before you exceed your point of stress. Normally, this point arrives sooner for Type As, but with proper conditioning, Type As can excel in more strenuous activities. At the same time, Type Os who are in the exhaustion stage because of accumulated stress should not continue with an intense exercise program.

A researcher I know of conducted a study of blood type and athletes and found the following: Generally, among good athletes, Type As could pull their resources together once or twice a year and do quite well in endurance events. However, they tended not to do as well when frequent competitions were involved. Type Os could compete constantly and have a balanced, sustained level of performance.

Mental Health Markers

I HAVE FOLLOWED the diet for sixteen months, I'd say thirteen-plus months quite rigorously. I'm forty-two, and had been a vegetarian for thirty years (absolutely no meat). I've always been athletic and lean, (no weight loss was needed) and into healthy eating. I can hardly describe the change I have experienced! It is very near the top of the list of most important things that have happened to me

in my life. I am in the same body, look about the same, but I feel completely dif-
ferent. I constantly have the thought, "This is amazing, so this is how (some)
other people feel. I wonder what I would have done in the last thirty years had I
felt like this." I recently visited a woman, now seventy-nine, who has known me
since I was twelve, when I became a vegetarian. She could definitely see the
change. She said I had been "the most ethereal person" she had ever known, and
she used to worry that I would "just float off." As the months go by I continue to
be amazed by the new territory in my psyche—grounded, firm, clear, able, with
lots of space to move around in and opportunity for choice. It's like having a
new brain or an expanded being. I wasn't at all a basket case before, but this is
a gift of extreme grace.

From the Outcome Registry, Leonore B., Type O

I have often come across people like Leonore in my practice. Although they appear to be functional, there is something missing, blocked, unbalanced, not quite right. Unable to identify its source or nature, they go through life never knowing how it feels to be content and grounded. Naturally, they're somewhat skeptical about the idea that the Blood Type Diet could help awaken a sense of mental well-being; this isn't a problem that's normally treated with food. Yet it makes perfect sense that eating the right diet for your blood type will have a positive impact on your psyche.

Many mental health problems have mechanisms that involve well-understood chemical imbalances, particularly with hormones and neurotransmitters, whose genetic controls lie very close to the genes that regulate blood type. Indeed, there are over ninety studies linking blood type and psychological dysfunction listed on MEDLINE, the National Institutes of Health's online medical database.[9] Many of these articles speculate that differences between the blood types and the occurrence of psychological disorders result from genetic linkages between blood type and genes that regulate the production of brain neurotransmitters or stress hormones. Let's track this continuum with each of the four blood types.

Type O: The Dopamine Factor

Type O's difficulty eliminating the catecholamines noradrenaline and adrenaline in conditions of stress has direct implications for mental disorders. Current research suggests that the problem is related to the activity of an enzyme called dopamine beta hydroxylase (DBH), which converts dopamine to noradrenaline. Remarkably, the gene for DBH is located at 9q34. It's literally sitting on top of the gene for blood type.[10]

What is the significance of this enzyme that converts dopamine to noradrenaline? Dopamine, like serotonin and norepinephrine, is one of a series of neurochemicals involved in higher thought. Dopamine is made deep inside the brain in an area called the substantia nigra. Unlike these other neurochemicals, dopamine does not project to all areas of the brain, but rather only to the brain's frontal lobes, where much of the higher, more abstract thought functions are initiated. Because of this, there is a very strong association between the release of dopamine and reward or reinforcement of behavior. For example, animals will push levers to deliver electric stimuli to their brains if those stimuli cause the release of dopamine. Cocaine, opiates, and alcohol produce rewarding effects, in part due to their abilities to promote the release of dopamine. Dopamine contributes to the feelings of bliss and regulates feelings of pain in the body.

There is a "sweet spot" with regard to dopamine levels and proper thought function: Too much dopamine in the parts of the brain that regulate feelings (the limbics) and not enough in the part that regulates thought (the cortex) may produce a personality given to bouts of paranoia or avoidance of social interactions. Normal to higher levels of dopamine in the cortex allow for improved ability to concentrate, feeling more relaxed, better control of stress, and having a more logical reaction to problems. Lower than average amounts of dopamine result in an inability to sustain attention, a tendency toward hyperactivity and temper tantrums, the ability to be easily angered, and a more emotional reaction to problems. A shortage of dopamine in the frontal lobe can also contribute to poor working memory.

Parkinson's Disease is accompanied by a selective destruction of dopamine neurons in the substantia nigra of the brain, which send stimulus to the part of the brain that is involved in the control of motor functions, such as our muscles. Parkinson's Disease is treated with L-dopa, which is a precursor for the production of dopamine in the brain.

On the other hand, schizophrenia, which is found in about 1 percent of the population, is related to an overabundance of dopamine and is treated with drugs that block the binding of dopamine to its receptor sites. The better the drug is at blocking dopamine, the better it is at reducing the schizophrenia. The dopamine hypothesis of schizophrenia is that there is excessive dopamine stimulation in the frontal lobe.

A simple way to visualize the whole working relationship is to envision happiness (dopamine) as a sink full of hot water. The water origi-

> **▪ FROM THE BLOOD TYPE OUTCOME REGISTRY ▪**
>
> *Lydia T.*
> *Type O*
> *Middle-aged female*
> *Improved: Depression*
>
> "I have been on antidepressants since 1991 (Prozac 50 mg daily, Wellbutrin 400 mg daily, most recently St.-John's wort 1600 mg). I had made numerous unsuccessful attempts to get off the antidepressants, only to dive into deep depression after five to ten days. My mental well-being started to improve after four to five days into the program. After one week I felt that I wanted to exercise (first time in three years). I have continually felt better and I have gradually tapered off of the St.-John's and stopped taking it. I no longer feel tired and groggy at work. I spend my breaks walking. I have been about thirty pounds overweight and I am losing weight without even trying."

nates in a well outside the house (tyrosine) then most of it gets pumped to the hot water heater (L-dopa); some gets diverted to water the lawn (used to make thyroid hormone). From the water heater (L-dopa), most of the hot water is sent through the faucet to the sink, although some is sent to the washing machine (melanin). Dopamine beta hydroxylase is like the plug at the base of the sink. When you pull it out, the hot water you wanted for your morning shave is sent down the waste pipe (converted to noradrenaline). Keep the plug in and you can have a nice sink full of hot water (normal dopamine levels).

Many of the disorders associated with variations in normal dopamine levels have been shown to be more common in Type Os. This includes schizophrenia, especially the recurrent type thought to be linked through family genetics. As we've said, schizophrenia is believed to be caused by too much dopamine activity. Its symptoms include: bizarre behavior, inappropriate laughter, strange posturing, low tolerance to irritation, excessive writing without apparent meaning, conversation that seems deep but is not logical or coherent, staring or vagueness, irrational statements or peculiar use of words or language structure. Schizophrenia is typically treated with drugs that are dopamine antagonists.

There is also an interesting association between Type Os and bipolar disease, or manic-depressive disorder, verified by several independent research studies. These studies have found a connection between blood type—particularly Type O—and a higher incidence of manic-depressive illness. Family studies have also demonstrated a higher occurrence of genetically transmitted bipolar disease. At least two studies showed a higher incidence of uni-polar, or deep depression, in Type Os as well.

Most investigators emphasize the importance of neurotransmitter substances, such as the catecholamines noradrenaline and adrenaline, in the pathogenesis of uni-polar and bipolar depressive states. According to this hypothesis, depression is associated with a deficit in brain catecholamines, while mania may be due to an excess of catecholamines.

Key Idea

Manic = High levels of dopamine hydroxylase = more enzyme activity = less dopamine and more adrenaline.

Depressive = Low levels of dopamine hydroxylase = less enzyme activity = more dopamine and less adrenaline.

Several other genes thought to be associated with affective disorder are also linked to the ABO gene locus. These may influence the role of dopamine beta hydroxylase and the effect of ABO genetics on dopamine beta hydroxylase.

From these studies we can see a picture developing: Type Os do not clear catecholamines when under stress as efficiently as the other blood types, and Type Os have a much higher rate of manic-depressive illness than the other blood types. This implies that the levels of dopamine beta hydroxylase activity, which is genetically linked to the ABO gene locus, oscillates much more dynamically in Type Os—a conclusion that would make perfect sense in an anthropological context. Since sourcing out wild prey would have placed a priority on aggressive instincts and a finely tuned fight or flight instinct, it would have been a very useful survival strategy in hunter-gatherer populations. Also, since periods of ease or stress would have been occasioned by huge sways in catecholamines, the ability to turn on or speed up dopamine beta hydroxylase, and then turn off or slow down its activity, would have served to make these early Type Os very effective hunters.

The oscillations in dopamine beta hydroxylase probably help explain both the tendency of Type Os to suffer more from bipolar illness

---

▪ FROM THE BLOOD TYPE OUTCOME REGISTRY ▪

Vera L.
Type O
Middle-aged woman
Improved: Depression

"I have long suffered from anxiety and depression, to the point that several years ago I lost the ability to work and was hospitalized for a short time. I was able to get back to work thanks to lithium and Wellbutrin, which I took for years. Although I was very grateful to be able to function again, I noticed that even on antidepressants I never really was happy to be alive, mostly just dreading the long, long life that I figured I'd probably have to 'get through, somehow.' I kept trying everything from homeopathy to supplements to feng shui. The only one of those that seemed to have some positive effect was flaxseed oil. Then I read your book and was very dismayed to discover, as a longtime vegetarian, that I was a Type O! It really rocked my world for a while, but I had so many of the other problems you mention Os usually have that I determined to try it and see, since I am nothing if not open-minded. The first thing I noticed was that I was not constipated in the morning if I'd eaten beef the day before (something loads of Metamucil could not even guarantee). To my surprise, the morning aching in my hands went away within weeks, as well as all my colon problems (gas, generalized abdominal pain). I'd always considered these things minor because it was the depression that affected my ability to earn a living. I now feel 'all the way back' from depression, and then some. I feel so much stronger, and enjoy physical exercise in a way I never did before. I actually feel exhilarated by it. I now look forward to the rest of my life—finally!"

---

and to exhibit "*Type A Behavior*" instincts. Since these attributes are partly the result of dopamine and the catecholamines, we can begin to see their expression as part of a trait linked to one of the few genes both variable and polymorphic in humans: the gene for your blood type.

This link may explain a curious circumstance that I've noticed over the years. Many Type Os crave either wheat or red meat. Wheat is one of the highest plant sources and red meat one of the highest animal sources of L-tyrosine, the building block of dopamine and the catecholamines. My Type O patients who choose to not eat red meat tell me, "I can eat rye and oat for a while, but every now and then I get an uncontrollable urge for a sandwich on whole wheat bread."

Other Type Os will say that they have always craved red meat. One Type O patient, who was a vegan for fourteen years, said, "I knew something was wrong with my diet when I was putting dog food in my dog's dish and began salivating!"

This stresses the importance of not only understanding your food urges, but making the correct choice between proper food urges and improper ones. If you are a Type O vegetarian who only feels good when you eat lots of wheat, you are feeling that way because you are using the tyrosine in the wheat to bolster your levels of dopamine and catecholamines. Since wheat is a poor choice for the Type O metabolic system, you would be much better off following the urge to use lean, high quality, free-range meats as a mood stabilizer instead.

Blood Type O and MAO

One other important aspect of the action of catecholamines in Type O is the role of the enzyme monoamine oxidase, or MAO. MAO is very important when it comes to emotions.

Indeed, until the newer class of seritonin uptake modifiers, such as Prozac, came along, the largest class of prescription antidepressants was a class of drugs called MAO-inhibitors (Iprozid, Neuralex). MAO comes in two variations: MAO-A and MAO-B. MAO-A is found throughout the body and especially in the GI tract, while MAO-B is found primarily in the brain. Both MAO-A and MAO-B metabolize dopamine into a variety of other compounds, so blocking this enzyme has the effect of increasing dopamine concentrations. Most MAO inhibitors block both MAO-A and MAO-B. Some block only one or the other. The drug selegiline, l-deprenyl (Eldeprine, Eldepryl, Eldapryl) blocks only MAO-B, which is made in the brain. This has the effect of increasing dopamine, which is why it is commonly prescribed for treating Parkinson's Disease. So, the effect of MAO is very much the opposite of dopamine beta hydroxylase—converting dopamine into other metabolites and having a profound effect on the pool of available dopamine for the brain.

As with the other influences on dopamine that we've discussed, MAO levels show some variability according to blood type, and again the consequences seem much more significant for Type Os. A 1983 study of seventy healthy young males showed that the platelet MAO activity of Type O subjects was substantially lower than that of other blood types—having the effect of making the control of catecholamines more difficult for Type Os.[11]

Platelet MAO is believed to be the peripheral marker for the central serotonin system. Low concentrations of this genetically determined marker may indicate vulnerability to psychopathology and certain behavioral disorders. In a 1996 Turkish study of delinquent boys at a reformatory, it was found that the group that contained sex crime offenders had the lowest platelet MAO of all groups studied, though the researchers had expected the group that contained other physically violent offenders to have the lowest platelet MAO activity.[12]

Low levels of platelet MAO have been linked to *"Type A Behavior"* traits, including ambitiousness, impatience, and competitiveness—all consistent with what we've observed in Type Os.[13] Variations in both platelet MAO and dopamine beta hydroxylase have been associated with bipolar (manic-depressive) illness, another Type O tendency.

Other personality characteristics linked to low platelet MAO include pathological gambling, negativism and verbal aggression, sensation seeking, impulsivity, and monotony avoidance. Individuals with low platelet MAO also tend to use more tobacco and alcohol products and are more likely to abuse alcohol and drugs.

Type A: The Cortisol Factor

The health costs of high cortisol levels can be devastating. There is a cortisol link to many killer diseases—cancer, hypertension, heart disease, and stroke, among others. High cortisol is often a factor in mental disorders, senility, and Alzheimer's disease.[14]

Scientists have long been aware that cortisol is elevated in many illnesses. However, until fairly recently, they thought high cortisol was the *result* of these diseases, not the cause.

That changed in 1984 with the publication of a landmark paper in the journal *Medical Hypothesis.*[15] In this study, the author presented strong evidence that high cortisol levels were a cause of disease, and not a result. This was especially true of subjects who were considered to have a *"Type C Personality,"* thought to be "cancer prone." This has important implications for Type As, since they have elevated resting levels of cortisol, and higher spikes in cortisol levels in response to stress.

In one imaginative study, the researchers decided to study the levels of cortisol made by the different blood types in response to a stress. The "stress" they chose was economical and imaginative—having blood drawn. Since getting blood drawn is stressful for most people, they figured they could stress subjects and test their blood levels in one step. The result: serum cortisol concentration was the highest in Type As (average 455 nmol/L), as opposed to Type Os (297 nmol/L). As we might expect, Types B and AB were somewhat in the middle, with Type B (364 nmol/L) closer to Type A, and Type AB (325 nmol/L) closer to Type O.[16]

▪ FROM THE BLOOD TYPE OUTCOME REGISTRY ▪

Jane I.
Type: Type A
Middle-aged female
Improved: Mood and energy

"It is the difference between night and day that people have noticed the change in me. I noticed my depression was gone and that I could learn better, not so fuzzy, happier, more energy, hormonal upsets were gone . . . smooth sailing ahead. I feel super! It is the best thing that ever happend to me!"

As we have seen, cortisol is an important part of the stress adaptation response. This higher resting level of cortisol may be responsible for the occurrence of a psychological disorder known to be much more common in Type As than in the other blood types: Obsessive-compulsive disorder, or OCD. [17]

Approximately five million people in the United States, or about one in every fifty Americans, suffer from OCD. It affects men, women, and children, as well as people of all races, religions, and socioeconomic backgrounds. There are two features to this disorder. Obsession involves recurrent and persistent thoughts, ideas, or images that involuntarily invade the conscious awareness. Common obsessive thoughts may center on violence, fear of contamination, or worry about a tragic event. Compulsion is usually a senseless, repetitive action taken in response to an obsessive thought. A great deal of anxiety is created if the compulsive action is not performed. A common example of a compulsion is repetitive hand washing by a person with obsessions about cleanliness or contamination. Usually the compulsive action temporarily relieves the anxiety; but the relief is short-lived, and the compulsion soon returns.

I have on occasion observed these traits in Type A patients. Most often they show up as excessive fears about getting sick, usually around cancer. The difference between someone who has a healthy understanding about risk factors and someone who is obsessive is quite clear.

I have seen people lose sleep, stop eating, and spend thousands of dollars on tests—becoming utterly consumed with the perceived danger lurking inside. OCD is very hard to treat and usually requires a multifaceted approach, involving therapy, medication, and behavior modification. However, you'd be surprised what a difference it can make when a person who is suffering learns that there is a genetic, biological explanation for the tendency.

I also think that much of the medical research on OCD is focused in the wrong direction. Current strategies are targeted toward a serotonin imbalance, using drugs like Luvox, which have not been that effective. Researchers should pay closer attention to the role of cortisol.

OCD patients have higher levels of cortisol and lower levels of melatonin than others, and have higher levels of free cortisol in their urine.[18] Indeed, it appears that the effect of using serotonin modulators to treat OCD may actually work in part by lowering cortisol.

Several independent studies in the literature clearly document an association between Type As and OCD. A Finnish study noted a prevalence of Type As in a small number of obsessive-compulsive subjects.[19] In a larger study of normal subjects using a tool called the Leyton Obsessional Inventory, Type Os were noticeably absent, which verified previous studies showing a low rate of OCD in Type Os as compared with Type As.[20] It's interesting to note that the catecholamines, which play such an important role in the stress response of Type Os, have no role in OCD.

In another large study of OCD sufferers done in 1983, Type As were again found to have a higher incidence of OCD over other blood types, as well as a higher incidence of hysteria. Finally, a 1986 study on two samples of psychiatric outpatients with Type A or Type O blood who completed a tool called the Brief Symptom Inventory showed that in both samples Type A patients scored significantly higher than Type Os on the "Obsessive-Compulsive" and "Psychoticism" factors.[21] The author concluded that "these findings are not attributable to differences in age, sex, or diagnosis, and are consistent with several previous studies. The influence of blood type on symptom expression may be mediated by cell membrane characteristics, influenced in part by blood type."

Type B and Type AB: The Nitric Oxide Factor

We noted earlier that Type B tends to exhibit neurochemical similarities to Type A, while Type AB is closer to Type O. However, it has become increasingly clear that these similarities are only part of the story. New research suggests that the mental processes of those who carry the B antigen may also be influenced by the nitric oxide molecule.

In recent years, nitric oxide has emerged as an important substance capable of modifying many biological processes—including the nervous system and immune functions. Typically, nitric oxide is released when the amino acid arginine is converted to the amino acid citrulline. Although it was only recently discovered in mammals, in 1998 alone there were already nearly 1,500 scientific papers dealing with this remarkable molecule, and a total of nearly 18,000 in the last five years.[22] From sunburn to anorexia, cancer to drug addiction, diabetes to hypertension, memory and learning disorders to septic shock, male impotence to tuberculosis—nitric oxide plays an important role.

Nitric oxide (NO) is a molecule with a very short life, somewhere around five seconds. Because it is manufactured and exhausted so quickly, NO is an important method of cross-system communication—between the nervous system and the immune system, or the cardiovascular system and the reproductive system. Much like our own language, which would be meaningless without commas, periods, and other forms of punctuation, nitric oxide contains many of the elements of language as well. As NO has a very short lifespan, it must be constantly synthesized. This is accomplished by the conversion of a precursor, the amino acid arginine.

In the late 1980s, scientists at the Johns Hopkins University School of Medicine showed that NO functions as a kind of mediator of certain types of neurons in the central nervous system. Unlike the other neurotransmitters, such as dopamine and serotonin, NO does not bind to specific sites on the nerve cell, but rather is diffused *into* the cell and works directly at the biochemic level, making it a "rapid response" neurotransmitter. NO also seems to be involved in the regulation of the opiates (endorphins) produced in the brain.[23]

Recently, two notations in the medical journal *Lancet* reported that patients who possessed a B antigen (Type B and Type AB) appeared to clear nitric oxide more rapidly than the other blood types when it was administered through inhalation therapy for certain pulmonary conditions.[25] The ability to rapidly clear nitric oxide can be highly beneficial to the cardiovascular system, but it also has implications for the activity of neurotransmitters, enabling faster recovery in conditions of stress. This discovery begins to explain a phenomenon my father first noticed and that I have repeatedly seen myself. Type Bs, in particular, have a remarkable ability to gain physiological relief and balance through the

> **▪ FROM THE BLOOD TYPE OUTCOME REGISTRY ▪**
>
> *Sherry N.*
> *Type B*
> *Middle-aged female*
> *Improved: Depression, addiction*
>
> "Within the first week of the diet, I went off antidepressants. Into the second week, I quit smoking. It scares me to feel this good! I had been depressed since childhood. I keep waiting for the other shoe to fall (so to speak), but it hasn't. It has to be a sin to feel this good. The sense of well-being has carried over into my marriage. People have noticed the change in my marriage, then they see the change in me, then my husband."

utilization of mental processes, such as meditation. And both Type Bs and Type ABs perform better when they achieve mental balance. The authors of the *Lancet* pieces had no clue as to why there might be a relationship between the B gene and the activity of nitric oxide, yet one of the possible answers lies right next to the ABO gene on 9q34. It is a gene for the enzyme arginosuccinate synthetase (ASS), which is critically responsible for the recycling of arginine. So the ability to modulate arginine conversion to nitric oxide is influenced by a gene lying immediately next to the gene for ABO blood type—and the efficacy of this gene is likely to be influenced by the activity of the allele for the Type B antigen.

It appears that the possession of a B antigen (Type B and Type AB) may enable a certain plasticity in the mind-body response. Type Bs, in particular, have a remarkable ability to gain physiological relief and balance through the utilization of mental processes. I have found that simple visualization techniques work well with Type Bs and Type ABs.

In Sickness and in Health

THE COMPELLING evidence of neurochemical differences among blood types leads seamlessly to the question: Is there a blood type personality? You can now see through the lens of science that blood type has something to do with the "self" you present to the world—the way you behave in relationships with others, how you perceive situations, and your emotional responses. In other words, it may help shape what kind of person you are.

We know there are developmental and chemical differences among the blood types, and these differences are capable of affecting our emotions and behavior. But how much of an effect do they really have? For this I return to Samuel Hahnemann, the creator of homeopathic medicine, and his theory of the *psora*. If you are in a state of health and balance, these factors might have no noticeable effect at all. They live in the background of your genetic makeup, but do not inform your daily life. If, however, you are in a state of high stress and maladaptation; if your immune system is compromised; if you're fighting chronic ill health; the blood type differences can become the *psora* or crack in your foundation. Living right for your type gives you control over your destiny and enables you to express your personality as a vital, positive characteristic of your human individuality. In the prescription section, you will see how these distinctions can be of practical value in achieving a healthy lifestyle that's right for your type.

FOUR

Digestive
Integrity

Blood Type's
Systemic Influence

I HAD AN OLD SAAB 900 ONCE, A CAR I LOVED. TROUBLE
was, the engine ran roughly, and the car stalled out at red lights. No me-
chanic could figure out what the problem was. Soon, I became quite
adept at braking with my left foot when the car was in neutral, while simultaneously gunning the accelerator pedal with my right foot. I'm sure
the sound of a car slowing down at a light with the engine roaring must
have startled a few pedestrians, but it worked. Eventually a good me-
chanic found the source of the problem.

The other mechanics had been using spark plugs for the sixteen-
valve engine Saab 900, while my car had the eight-valve engine. Once
this was corrected, I could stop my contortions.

I got to thinking about my Saab recently while talking with a Type A
woman who told me she had been "metabolically typed" as a "hunter-
gatherer." She insisted that her most beneficial eating plan was closer to
my recommendations for Type O. She even said that she felt so much
better on the high-protein diet than she had ever felt when she wasn't
eating meat.

I realized that this woman had, in effect, made the same contortion-istic adjustment to her diet that I had made in order to drive my Saab. Initially, I thought that the additional benefit of subtyping her for se-cretor status might help explain the problem. About 10 percent of Type As who are non-secretors can have genetically induced insulin resist-ance and some carbohydrate intolerance. Unfortunately, further studies showed that this woman was a secretor, which scotched that theory. Instead, it turned up over time that she suffered from extreme hypo-glycemia, which can make Type As feel terrible when they eat carbohy-drates. It didn't bother her, but she was just masking an underlying problem, not eating correctly. Since meats don't elicit the same insulin reaction as starches, hypoglycemics feel better on high protein—for the short term. However, it's just a matter of time until their engines begin stalling again, and this time there may be too much damage to fix the problem.

Not every digestive ailment manifests itself immediately or dramat-ically. It can take years for your body to sound a clear alarm. Regular maintenance—putting the right kind of fuel in your body, and keeping your digestive system tuned and balanced—will prevent problems down the road.

Nature provides us with all the mechanisms we need to convert the food on our plates into something biologically useful. The digestive sys-tem is designed with an intricate and beautiful logic. When you are eat-ing correctly, and there are no glitches, it's as efficient as the conveyor belt on an assembly line—only one that is devoted to disassembling. Before a morsel of food touches your mouth, a whole array of other senses have gone to work, and the assembly line is turned on and pre-pared to receive "product." Into the mouth it goes, where tongue, teeth, gums, lips, saliva, and mucus all go to work, preparing it to slide down the esophageal tube and into the waiting stomach and beyond, where a series of specialized processing stations—small intestine, the pancreas, the liver, the gallbladder—work in sync to process the product before sending the waste to the colon for disposal.

Your Blood Type at Work

YOUR BLOOD TYPE plays a key role in every step of the digestive process—from the moment the aroma of food hits your senses to the fi-nal absorption of nutrients and elimination of waste. These are the pri-mary actions of blood type in the digestive process:

1. SALIVA: Your blood type antigen is liberally distributed in saliva and mucus, providing a shield against bacterial invasion.
2. MUCINS: Blood type is the single most significant influence on the structure of mucins, the molecules found throughout the digestive tract, which offer protection against bacteria and food sensitivities. Mucin is the digestive gatekeeper.
3. STOMACH: There is more blood type antigen expressed in the lining of the stomach than in any other organ of the digestive tract. A considerable number of hormones and secretions are directly influenced by your blood type—including gastric juices, gastrin, pepsin, and histamine.
4. LIVER: Cells lining the liver's bile ducts express blood type antigens. Pancreatic juice and bile are heavily impregnated with blood type antigens. Blood type exerts an influence over the body's primary filter for nutrients and waste.
5. SMALL INTESTINE: Large amounts of blood type antigen are attached to the walls of the small intestine, interacting with nutrients and enzymes to control assimilation.
6. LARGE INTESTINE: Blood type antigens are extensively expressed in the large intestine, influencing intestinal flora.

Blood Type and Saliva: The Secretor Connection

BLOOD TYPE antigens are copiously produced by the submaxillary-sublingual salivary glands and extensively distributed in human saliva. Studies have linked certain illnesses with the inability to secrete blood type antigens into saliva. For example, there is a significantly higher number of non-secretors than secretors who suffer from Graves' disease, a common form of hyperthyroidism.[1]

As food is masticated, enzymes in the saliva start the process of breaking down sugars and starches, and a small amount of these are actually passed through the tissues of the mouth.

If you are a non-secretor, you're at a distinct disadvantage. The saliva of secretors contains substantially more diversity and total carbohydrate than that of non-secretors. The salivary carbohydrate structures found in mucins can clump and kill some oral bacteria, and also constituents of pellicle and plaque. Regardless of blood type, the average amount of cavities is lower for secretors than for non-secretors.[2] This difference is most significant for smooth surface areas of the teeth.

• FROM THE BLOOD TYPE OUTCOME REGISTRY •

Beverly B.
Type O
Young female
Improved: Dental

"About one month after I started following the diet for Type O, I visited my dentist about a chipped tooth. He announced to me that the lichens planus, which had chronically affected the inside of my right jaw, had almost disappeared. I had discovered that the alfalfa in the cholorphyll capsules and the aloe in my digestive enzymes were toxic for Type O and so found alternatives. The diagnosis was initially given at Indiana University Medical Center a year ago. My dentist who sent me to the medical center related to me that he could only see a tiny line as evidence that lichens planus was still present."

Your secretor status also influences the activity of lectins. If you are a secretor, you have a greater genetically endowed barrier against bacteria and lectins. Many lectins stimulate the production of mucus.[3] This is either a protective function or an allergic response and was for a time thought to be a positive action of certain lectins, as it promised some therapeutic benefit when applied to patients with cystic fibrosis. Normally, however, excess mucus caused by lectins may bind to the antigen-rich saliva and be eliminated. Production contributes to many ailments, including allergies, respiratory problems, and ear infections.

The Stomach's Delicate Balance

BLOOD TYPE is an important factor in the activity of stomach acids and enzymes. It controls the environment of your stomach—the practical consequence being that protein digestion is made easier or more difficult, depending on your blood type. Here's how it works:

As food enters your stomach, nervous stimulation causes the secretion of a liquid called gastric juice. Gastric juice is composed of water, hydrochloric acid, and enzymes. Abundant amounts of blood type antigens are secreted in gastric juice, more than in any other digestive secretion. The hydrochloric acid destroys germs in food, protecting the

---

▪ FROM THE BLOOD TYPE OUTCOME REGISTRY ▪

Camilla D.
Type O
Young female
Improved: Asthma, sinusitis

"I had no sense of taste or smell for eight years, unless I took steroids, which I did once or twice a year. I had asthma and chronic sinusitus, and often could breathe only through my mouth. I tried all the conventional strategies—surgery for nasal polyps, antihistamines, asthma medications, OTC remedies, allergy shots, and probably every antibiotic known to medical science for the chronic sinusitus. Then by accident I noticed *ER4YT* in our local bookstore last August. I tried it a little bit, and it seemed to help. A month later, I was talking to my family doctor, and it turned out he was enthusiastic about *ER4YT* too! When I followed the Type O recommendations to the letter—no more wheat products, no more potatoes, soy products, and all the other little no-no's like brussels sprouts—voila!!! For the last three weeks my sense of taste and smell has been perfect! The asthma is all gone, and I can breathe like a normal person. I love it! Best of all, no more medicine!"

---

gut from infection. However, this is also the acid that can reflux and cause heartburn in the esophagus.

Gastric juice becomes more alkaline when the food enters your stomach, because proteins in food tend to buffer the existing acid in the stomach. This rise in alkalinity stimulates the release of more gastrin, and therefore the release of more acid. As proteins are digested, the acidity of the stomach contents increases, and that action shuts off gastrin release to halt the secretion of more stomach acid. The enzyme pepsin helps break down the protein. Pepsin is very sensitive to the level of acidity of the stomach, so in the absence of sufficient amounts of hydrochloric acid, pepsin will not become active.

Your blood type and secretor status have a direct influence on the activation of pepsin. Most high-quality protein in the diet is derived from animal sources, though vegetables do contain significant amounts. Type Os typically manufacture more hydrochloric acid in their stomachs than the other blood types. After a meal, they also secrete greater amounts of pepsin, pepsinogen, and gastrin more quickly.[4] These are all necessary components for the proper breakdown of animal protein. There is also evidence that the Type A antigen, normally secreted in the gastric juice, binds to pepsin and inactivates it. This may account for Type A having low stomach acid.[5]

In addition to digesting proteins, the acid in the stomach serves as a barrier to most bacteria. This is an important function. The mixture of food and saliva you swallow is not sterile, and since the upper small intestine is designed for absorption of nutrients from the food, it would not be desirable for there to be large amounts of bacteria in this part of the gut. One of the major problems with having low stomach acidity—Type A and Type AB—is excessive bacterial overgrowth in the stomach and in the upper small intestine. This bacterial growth tends to be a chronic problem, which recurs within days or weeks after antibiotics are discontinued.

The Problem with Lectins

Among the greatest barriers to digestive health are the lectins in foods that interact with your blood type. There is a chemical interaction between your blood type and the foods you eat. In particular, lectins, which are proteins found in foods, interact in different ways according to blood type. When you eat a food containing lectins that are incompatible with your blood type, they can interfere with digestion, metabolism, and your immune system.

Many lectins are blood type specific, in that they show a clear preference for one kind of sugar over another, and mechanically fit the antigen of one blood type or another.[6] This blood type specificity results in their attaching to the glyco-conjugate antigen of a preferred blood type, while leaving other blood type antigens completely undisturbed. At the cellular level, a common effect of lectins is to cause the sugars on the surface of one cell to cross-link with those of another, effectively causing the cells to stick together and agglutinate, perhaps their most well-known effect. Not all lectins cause agglutination; many bacteria have lectinlike receptors that they use to attach to the cells of their host. Other lectins, called mitogens, cause a proliferation (or mitosis) of certain cells of the immune system.[7] But, in the most basic sense, lectins make things stick to other things. The word lectin was coined by William Boyd in 1954, to describe a class of blood type specific agglutinins that had been found in certain plants. The word is somewhat allegorical, being of Latin derivation meaning "to choose."[8] The degree that lectins "choose" the cells they stick to is primarily determined by the amount of glyco-conjugates, or degree of glycosylation, that a particular tissue has. For example, the cells lining the small intestine wall are usually very well glycosylated, and so have many sites for lectin binding. Even lectins that are not specific to a particular blood type can make an impact, by virtue of secondary effects that have blood type specific consequences. They can cause the inhibition of digestive hormones, as well as the production of toxins. As the eminent immunologist David Freed once wrote, "Lectins are causes in search of diseases."[9]

The digestive impact of lectins is pervasive. They can attack your system in various ways—well beyond what we normally think of as digestive problems:

LECTINS INTERFERE WITH THE IMMUNE SYSTEM OF THE GUT.   Many food lectins, including the common legume and cereal lectins, provoke the immune system to manufacture antibodies against them.[10] Since foods that contain these lectins are often thought of as "highly allergic," it's likely that some of these suspected food allergies are actually immune system reactions to the lectins contained in the foods.

LECTINS INTERFERE WITH PROTEIN DIGESTION.   Researchers observed that wheat germ agglutinin (WGA) dramatically enhanced the activity of membrane-bound maltase—an enzyme that helps to break down complex sugars into simple sugars in the small intestine. Under the same conditions, aminopeptidase—an enzyme that breaks down polypeptides into amino acids—was inhibited by wheat germ lectin.[11]

LECTINS ACTIVATE AUTOANTIBODIES IN INFLAMMATORY AND AUTOIMMUNE DISEASES.   Almost everyone has antibodies to dietary lectins in their bloodstream. Some of these have been linked to immune damage to the kidneys in nephropathy (kidney disease) patients. It has been suggested that the antibody produced in rheumatoid arthritis may in fact require activation by wheat germ lectin.[12]

I believe that many cases of fibromyalgia, a common, painful inflammatory disorder of the muscle tissue, may in fact stem from intolerance to wheat. Fibromyalgia sufferers might try avoiding wheat products for a period of time, to discover whether or not it has any positive effects on their condition. Interestingly, the amino sugar glucosamine, prescribed in combination with chondritin and now being used by so many arthritis sufferers, specifically binds wheat germ lectin.

DIETARY LECTINS DAMAGE THE INTESTINAL LINING.   It has been known for over fifteen years that several legume lectins damage the felt-like cover (microvilla) of intestinal absorptive cells in the small intestine. In one study, test animals were given red kidney bean lectin. Within two to four hours, the microvilli of test animals showed extensive vesiculation—bubbling—along the length of the villi, which returned to near normal within twenty hours. The individual length of the microvilli were also reduced significantly, but again returned to normal within twenty hours. The authors wrote: "We speculate that microvilli may be repeatedly damaged and repaired after ingestion of specific dietary lectins."[13]

▪ FROM THE BLOOD TYPE OUTCOME REGISTRY ▪

Ellen I.
Type A
Middle-aged female
Improved: Digestion/mucus

"I developed asthmatic responses two to three years ago. I always felt as if the build up of mucus had to do with something going on in my stomach. The doctor literally waved away that suggestion and prescribed an inhaler and the deadly Prednisone. Prednisone quickly caused muscle and vision problems, so I waved away the doctor's protocol, relying on an OTC inhaler, which works without the mouth irritation of the prescription. When I first heard about a blood type diet, I ignored it, but when I saw the book in my whole foods market I took a look. I eliminated wheat, potatoes, and pasta (which were a great part of my diet, often to the exclusion of fruits and fresh vegetables). I was amazed at the overwhelming presence of wheat in products (even my Tamari sauce!). I added peanuts as a snack, and they relieved that crawling feeling in my stomach I had previously thought to be excess acid. I was breathing and feeling better in less than a week. Lack of preparation and snacks from the vending machine bring it all back. Regular consumption of any flour product (even one spelt cookie a day) is a problem. *ER4YT* is of valuable assistance in this Type A's quest for freedom from mucus."

LECTINS INFLUENCE GUT PERMEABILITY.   Our intestines are very selective about the size and quality of what is absorbed through their lining. Food lectins have been shown to increase gut permeability, which may predispose those already on their way to developing an allergy or intolerance to other proteins also.

In one study, animals fed diets containing kidney beans showed increased intestinal permeability to serum proteins that had been injected into their bloodstreams. Then they were given an even bigger dose of kidney bean protein. The protein, again injected into the animals' blood streams, "leaked" into the open space of the inner body and was also detected in the walls of the small intestine. This showed that dietary lectins may be at least partially responsible for the loss of serum proteins, and they may also contribute to other food intolerances, as a consequence of the loss of gut integrity.[14]

LECTINS BLOCK DIGESTIVE HORMONES.   Cholecystokinin (CCK), a hormone that helps digest fat, protein, and carbohydrates by stimulating the secretion of digestive enzymes, is affected by several dietary lectins, especially wheat germ. The lectins bind to CCK receptors and inhibit their action. Since CCK is also present in the brain in relatively high concentrations, it is thought to play a role in appetite control, so these lectins also may contribute to weight problems.[15] So, when CCK is suppressed, appetite is increased. According to a working hypothesis, when lectins block the CCK receptor they inhibit the secretion of amylase, an enzyme necessary for the digestion of carbohydrates. The activity of amylase is typically higher in Type As, which makes perfect sense, as Type As are more suited to metabolizing complex carbohydrates than the other blood types.[16]

LECTINS IMPAIR ABSORPTION.   Test animals fed a diet composed mostly of raw navy bean flour were smaller and had 50 percent less ability to absorb glucose and utilize dietary protein than a control group that was fed navy beans with inactivated lectin. Lectins from wheat germ (*Triticum aestivum*), thorn apple (*Datura stramonium*), or nettle root (*Urtica dioica*) added to the diet of test animals reduced the digestibility and utilization of dietary proteins and stunted their growth. Wheat germ lectin did the most damage. The researchers were quite certain that the lectins had been bound and actively transported across the intestinal membrane. The three lectins acted as growth factors for the gut and interfered with its metabolism and function to varying degrees. The study also found: ". . . an appreciable portion of the absorbed wheat germ lectin was transported across the gut wall into the systemic circulation, where it was deposited in the walls of the blood and lymphatic vessels." Wheat germ lectin also stimulated the growth of the pancreas, while causing the thymus, a gland linked to immune system function, to shrink. The study concluded: "Although the transfer of the gene of wheat germ lectin into crop plants has been advocated to increase their insect resistance, the presence of this lectin in the diet may harm higher animals at the concentrations required to be effective against most pests. Its use in plants as natural insecticide is not without health risks for man."[17]

LECTINS STIMULATE ORGAN GROWTH.   Dietary lectins can cause growth in the size of the digestive organs. They do this by amplifying other growth stimulants through the release of a class of chemicals called *polyamines*. A number of studies have shown that increases in the size of the intestines, liver, and pancreas can occur as a result of feeding test animals dietary lectins. One study put the consequences quite blunty: "Lectins are essential and omnipresent plant constituents and are ingested daily in appreciable amounts by both humans and animals. As they are biologically highly active, their consumption may have serious consequences for metabolism and health. Lectins, by virtue of their stability and specific recognition and binding by gut brush border epithelial cells, are potent exogenous (external) metabolic growth signals for the gut and the body."[18]

> *Learn more about polyamines, page 100.*

Know Your Lectins

Certain lectins are more widespread and also more troublesome than others.

Wheat

"Man does not live by bread alone," stands as a profound philosophical statement. But, it appears that the majority of mankind never lived by bread at all, or at least bread as we know it today. Many people are wheat intolerant, though many don't realize it because the effects of this intolerance don't always reveal themselves in easily recognizable symptoms. Wheat contains considerable amounts of gluten and gliandins among its proteins. Although many other grains contain them as well, the immune system's cross reactivity with wheat gliandins is higher than in other grains. Gluten and gliandin sensitivity are major secondary influences in digestive health.

Fully *one half—50 percent—*of all people complaining of digestive problems have demonstrable antibodies to gliandin in their serum. The majority—as many as *9 to 1*—of gluten intolerant subjects, identified by family or population screening, don't manifest any complaints at all, although they are shown to lack protective intestinal mucosa.

The lectin in wheat, called wheat germ agglutinin, or WGA, is an important, though largely unrecognized dietary problem for many people. Like most dietary lectins, WGA resists digestion. It also exerts metabolic and hormonal effects. Wheat germ lectin mimics the effect of insulin on the insulin receptor. Consequently, it is one of the most commonly employed molecules used to study the dynamics of insulin metabolism. Though an accepted fact in molecular biology, it appears odd to me that no one seems to contemplate the real-world significance of such a phenomenon. For example, there is a study that showed that about 20 percent of the patients with insulin-dependent diabetes mellitus (IDDM) had antibodies to wheat germ lectin in their blood.[19]

Your susceptibility to the negative effects of WGA is dependent on your blood type. There is some evidence that the Type A antigen in the gut binds to wheat germ agglutinin in a somewhat modest manner, giving Type A and Type AB secretors an ability to dampen the effects of wheat germ lectin. They do this by binding the lectin to their free blood type antigen in digestive juice before it gets a chance to do any damage. This would not be the case for non-secretors.

Tomato

A frequent issue tossed around on the Message Board of my Web site is why some common foods are "avoids" on the Blood Type Diet, but highly recommended by nutritionists in general. Topping the list is the tomato—an avoid for Type A and Type B. However, many people want to know how this squares with the news that tomatoes might be an important antioxidant.

Tomatoes have recently been the object of considerable news coverage because they have been found to contain high concentrations of lycopene, a naturally occuring pigment that gives tomatoes, watermelon, and red grapefruit their characteristic red color, and which possesses antioxidant properties. Studies have shown that lycopene can decrease the risk of certain cancers, such as prostate, and help lower the rate of heart disease.[20]

Why then, would this food not be a great choice for all blood types?

The reason is simple. Tomatoes also contain a potent lectin called *Lycopersicon esculentum agglutinin*. This is one of a few lectins capable of agglutinating all blood types and is termed a *panhemmaglutinin*. (Rice also contains a panhemmaglutinin, but I've never seen it cause any problems. Perhaps it is destroyed by digestion.)

The lectin in tomato is far from innocuous. Tomato lectin lowers the concentration of mucin, an enzyme that protects the lining of your gut. This is probably why many people with food intolerances don't tolerate tomatoes well.

Tomato lectin does other damage as well. There is some evidence that it shows a preference for binding to nerve tissue. Tomato lectin also binds to one of the subunits of the "proton-pump," the cellular mechanism by which gastrin induces stomach acid production. That's probably why so many people complain of hyperacidity after eating tomato sauce.[21]

So, what about lycopene? First, you should realize that tossing a tomato into your salad is not going to give you very much lycopene. Tomatoes have a very high water content, so you'd only find greater concentrations in tomato paste—which, unfortunately, is also where you'll find the most tomato lectin.

Now for the good news: Lycopene is found in a number of other foods in addition to tomatoes.

FOOD	MICROGRAMS LYCOPENE PER 100 GRAMS
Tomato paste (canned)	8,580
Guava	6,500
Watermelon (raw)	5,400
Grapefruit (red)	4,100
Papaya	3,500
Tomato (raw)	3,100
Apricot (dried)	864
Rosehip puree	780

There is some evidence that Texas Red Grapefruit has the highest lycopene content of all commercially available grapefruit. As you can see from the chart, raw tomato does not place very high. Another interesting aspect of lycopene is that like all carotenoids, its absorption is greatly enhanced by the addition of fat.

Peanut

In medical school, I was taught not to recommend peanuts to my patients, because there is a small, but significant, number of people who are allergic to them. It is difficult to accurately define the incidence of peanut allergy, because many people who are allergic to peanuts are also allergic to other tree nuts, such as walnuts, almonds, and cashews. One estimate pegs the number of peanut and/or tree nut allergies at about 1.1 percent of American children, and about .3 percent of adults. One study, which evaluated 12,032 people, found peanut or tree nut allergy in 164 individuals.[22]

Peanut allergy is a classic allergy, in the sense that the afflicted individual has antibodies to proteins in the peanut that can result in the life-threatening allergic reaction called anaphylaxis. This is independent of blood type, and if you know that you are classically allergic to peanuts (as well as the other common food allergens, such as soy or wheat) you should, of course, avoid them.

There is growing evidence that the lectin in peanuts may be protective against several cancers, including cancers of the stomach, colon, and breast.[23] How does this square with the recent concerns that peanuts are a source of aflatoxin, which has been linked to the development of liver cancer in test animals? (No direct evidence has implicated aflatoxins as the causal agents for human cancer.)

It should be emphasized here that it is not the peanuts (or corn or sorghum or Brazil nuts or pecans or pistachios or cottonseed oil or walnuts) that contain aflatoxin. It is a contaminant produced by a fungus that develops on them in situations of poor storage or bad growing conditions. Levels of aflatoxin contamination vary from year to year, depending on the commodity, weather conditions, and other factors.

How big a problem is aflatoxicosis? There are no reported incidences of aflatoxicosis in the United States, and only a few isolated instances in Third World countries (Uganda 1971, India 1975, and Malaysia 1991), where methods of storage and identification are suspect. Indeed, in even these reported "outbreaks," none were associated with peanut consumption! In Uganda and India the cause was contaminated corn, and, in Malaysia, a type of noodle.

In the United States the Food and Drug Administration regulates aflatoxin, and it can be avoided or minimized with proper agricultural and manufacturing practices. Aflatoxins are highly controlled in food products for consumption, and the concern for safety has been reduced drastically. The FDA's efforts to ensure the safety and quality of foods and feeds are complemented by control programs carried out by USDA, state departments of agriculture, and various industrial trade associations.

If you are concerned about aflatoxins in peanuts, just purchase your peanut butter from a reputable manufacturer. All commercially manufactured peanut preparations are regulated.

The Protein Debate

UNDOUBTEDLY, one of the most controversial aspects of the Blood Type Diet is the assertion that Type Os and Type Bs require red meat for optimum health. Conventional nutritional thinking holds red meat responsible for, among other ills, high cholesterol, heart disease, and osteoporosis. Yet, our understanding of the role of intestinal alkaline phosphatase belies this thinking. Intestinal alkaline phosphatase is an enzyme manufactured in the small intestine, which, among its functions, aids the digestion of animal proteins and fats.

Recent studies clearly show that Type Os—and to a lesser degree, Type Bs—have high levels of intestinal alkaline phosphatase, which protect them from the harmful effects of high protein diets. However, Type As secrete almost no intestinal alkaline phosphatase, and whatever little they do secrete is inactivated by their own A antigen. This is a convincing reason why Type As should stick to low-protein diets. The serum alkaline phosphatase activity of non-secretors is also only about 20 percent that of secretors. If you are a Type A non-secretor, you may have dangerously low levels of this important enzyme.[24]

Evidence suggests that intestinal alkaline phosphatase, in addition to enhancing fat breakdown, also enhances the absorption of calcium. Perhaps this explains why Type Os have less incidence of bone fractures than the other blood types.

Although proponents of veganism promote plant-based diets as helping to prevent osteoporosis, the basis is very weak. While it's true that calcium excretion increases in some individuals on high-protein diets, this is at best a selective reading of the literature. Many studies clearly show the opposite to be true.

It has been known for years that alkaline phosphatase levels rise after a meal containing fat, but more recent research shows that the levels of the enzyme also rise markedly after a high-protein meal.

There is growing evidence that the extreme anti-animal protein position is scientifically unsupportable. A recent news report on the MD-Consult Web site reported research from Johns Hopkins, the University of Minnesota, and the Chicago Center for Clinical Research, which indicates that six ounces of red meat, five or more times weekly, may lower the individual risk of coronary disease by as much as 10 percent.

In particular, women consuming the most protein (about 24 percent of their calories), faced just three quarters of the heart disease risk seen in women deriving a mere 15 percent of their calories from protein. What's more, animal protein appeared as protective as protein derived from plants.

The Miracle of Digestive Health

DURING THE LAST few years, I have given dozens of talks all over the country—in bookstores, in health food stores, at medical conferences, and in front of various community groups. Usually, my talks are followed by at least an hour of conversation with individuals who gather around the podium to ask questions or share their experiences. I enjoy these personal discussions, as I always learn something new from them. Sometimes people complain that they don't have anything approaching the expected result. This always piques my curiosity, and I search for clues that will illuminate the discrepancy. If that doesn't work, I take the problem back to the lab and pursue it further. I am totally aware that I don't have all the answers, and it would be arrogant to claim I did. If we embark on the investigation of blood type science in the spirit of open curiosity, there are always puzzles to solve.

Often, though, I come away from my conversations with blood type dieters with fresh confirmation of the fundamental plausibility of the science. I've stopped counting the number of times I encounter people whose lives have been dramatically turned around when they began to eat right for their type. I can assure you, there is not a doctor alive who would not feel moved and gratified by these stories.

Recently, after giving a talk at a bookstore in Connecticut, I was approached by Robin, a fifty-two-year-old Type O woman who had been engaged in a sixteen-year battle with ulcerative colitis. This is a particularly gruesome, chronic condition in which the intestinal lining becomes raw and inflamed. The symptoms include cramps, diarrhea, and bloody stools; sometimes the hemorrhaging is severe. In the worst case scenario, you can experience extensive blood loss or suffer a ruptured bowel. Ulcerative colitis can even lead to cancer. The most debilitating aspect of ulcerative colitis is its tenacity. People who have suffered its long-term effects often give up hope of ever being completely well.

Robin approached me with a wide smile that brightened her wan features. After sixteen years of regular bouts of ulcerative colitis, she was at the beginning stages of her road to recovery, but her health had been compromised. "I hope you don't mind if I ramble," she said. "I am just so relieved." She went on to tell me her history of ulcerative colitis and wearily recounted the various anti-inflammatory drugs that were tried, and that failed to help her. At one point, she was so sick that she was in the hospital for six weeks, being fed through a tube.

Robin told me that her problem started after the birth of her son. At that time, she radically changed her diet, hoping to be as healthful as possible while she was breast-feeding her baby. She stopped eating meat and adopted a strict vegetarian diet, which included lots of grains, beans, and vegetables.

"Isn't it funny?" she said. "That's when I started having the colitis."

Robin heard about the Blood Type Diet just when she was trying to decide whether or not to have an intestinal resection—a relatively drastic surgical procedure that would involve the removal of part of her intestine and would necessitate wearing a colostomy bag for elimination. She decided she had nothing to lose by trying the diet.

"I have been on the Type O diet now for four months," she told me. "I am walking four miles every morning without fail. I am weaning myself from all my medications, and I am feeling better than I have in years. I am optimistic I'll never have to face surgery."

As pleased as I was to hear Robin's outcome, I couldn't help being infuriated by her story. Sixteen years of pain and suffering, and it never occurred to a single doctor to change her diet! Think about it. Imagine that you were given food every day and told it was good for you, but you were actually being fed poison. How long would it take for you to question how healthful the food could be if it was making you so deathly ill?

PART TWO

Keeping a Healthy Balance

Metabolic Synchrony

Blood Type's Biochemical Influence

N̲OW THAT YOU UNDERSTAND HOW YOUR BLOOD TYPE functions and have seen how it shapes a multitude of individual responses, let's examine some of the behind-the-scenes dynamics of metabolism and the immune system that are powerfully influenced by your blood type.

When *Eat Right 4 Your Type* was first published, the TV news program *Inside Edition* profiled the book by putting it to a test. Under the supervision of a nutritionist from New York's Equinox Health Club, two volunteers were put on the prescribed diet for their blood types. Loren, a Type O pastry chef, began the trial at 164 pounds. Miguel, a Type A producer at *Inside Edition*, started the trial at 199 pounds. After two weeks, the results were recorded. Loren had lost seven pounds. Miguel had lost eight pounds.

Deborah Norville, the show's anchor expressed amazement that two people on completely opposite diets could both lose so much weight. Her verdict: "We're convinced. Sign us up!"

Healthy weight loss is a welcome result for the majority of people who try the Blood Type Diet. However, the metabolic change that occurs with this weight loss is far more significant than the cosmetic effects you see in the mirror. Obesity results in a hormonal derangement that ultimately upsets the metabolic equation. Metabolic imbalance often involves insulin resistance—a condition where fat cells are no longer responsive to insulin.

Insulin resistance means that your body needs to produce more and more insulin to do less of its job, and you have a problem regulating sugar in your blood. At the same time, it hijacks your metabolism, shutting off the engine that burns fat for fuel and storing excess sugar and starch as body fat.

Insulin resistance is often triggered by the overconsumption of lectin-containing foods that react badly with your blood type. Some lectins actually have insulinlike effects on the fat cell receptors. Once they bind to the receptors, they signal fat cells to stop burning fat and to store extra calories as fat. Consuming large amounts of insulin-mimicking lectins wrong for your blood type has the effect of increasing body fat and decreasing active tissue mass.[1]

Many non-secretors have insulin resistance syndrome, which can cause impairment of triglyceride conversion, resulting in a lowered metabolic rate.[2] Low metabolism also promotes the storage of excess fluid as extracellular water, leading to edema.

> If you try to lose weight by restricting calories, you'll lose muscle tissue, even if you also exercise regularly. While exercise can offset some of the loss in muscle tissue, low-calorie dieting for more than ten to fourteen days in a row is deterimental to your overall body composition. This is the prime reason why I think that eating and exercising by blood type is the most rational method of balanced weight loss. If you eat correctly for your type, you gain active tissue mass, which increases your basal metabolic rate, which then allows the excess fat to be burned off, without loss of muscle tissue.

Once you are overweight, it becomes even more difficult to restore a normal balance. Your metabolic hardwiring has changed. Obesity is *always* accompanied by insulin resistance; resulting in higher insulin levels, in direct proportion to the fat content of the internal organs. When it comes to body fat and insulin resistance, the easiest way to think of this problem is in terms of a sliding scale: more body fat equals more insulin resistance. So, to some extent, this metabolic challenge faces virtually any person attempting to shed weight. A key concept to remember as we discuss this and the other metabolic derangements is that they all tend to occur in proportion to the amount of body fat and they tend to move toward normalization as body fat is lost.

In a review of obesity in children, investigators have reported metabolic stumbling blocks in a variety of endocrine systems including thyroid hormone activation, stress hormone production, androgen levels,

---

Eat right for your blood type ➡ Higher active tissue mass ➡ Higher BMR ➡ Excess fat burned without losing muscle.

---

growth hormone, and insulin levels. In these children, both basal and stimulated (by sugar or starch) insulin concentrations were high.[3] The condition most certainly exists in adults, as well. The regulation of energy metabolism in obesity is different from normal conditions in important ways:

BEING OVERWEIGHT PRODUCES LEPTIN RESISTANCE. Leptin (not lectin!), a hormone associated with the obesity gene, has been receiving a lot of research attention in recent years. Leptin acts on the hypothalamus to regulate the extent of body fat, the ability to burn fat for energy, and satiety. When you're overweight, your leptin levels increase, but its action is stifled. In obesity, leptin levels increase in concert with insulin levels, leading some researchers to conclude that this condition is the gateway to diabetes, cardiovascular disease, and stroke.

BEING OVERWEIGHT PROMOTES CORTISOL RESISTANCE. As a general rule, when you are overweight, you will have chronically higher levels of cortisol production.[4] Fat tissue accelerates the turnover of cortisol, facilitating cortisone production, which stimulates ACTH secretion and maintains stimulation of the adrenal cortex. Furthermore, high levels of cortisol in themselves promote weight gain. It's a vicious cycle. Cortisol differs from other steroid hormones, such as your sex hormones, in that it is classified as a glucocorticoid. That means its primary action involves increasing blood sugar levels at the expense of muscle tissue. While this is the desired effect in a fight-or-flight situation, on a chronic basis it will lead to insulin resistance and an alteration in body composition from muscle to fat. There's more. Experts believe that high cortisol tends to increase your appetite, due to an association with leptin. In animal studies, it was shown that cortisol is the primary factor that prevents leptin from decreasing appetite, increasing metabolism, and decreasing body fat. Similar findings have been shown with humans. This has special relevance to Type As and Type Bs, whose basal levels of cortisol are high to begin with.

Syndrome X

WHEN YOUR metabolic "symphony" is off-key, you will viscerally experience the jarring sensation that all is not well. Pay attention. Al-

---

Fitness Biomarkers

How do you measure metabolic fitness? The best way is to improve certain markers of function. In 1991, William Evans and Irwin Rosenberg coined the term "biomarker" to describe the modifiable aspects of function that were associated with healthier aging. As it turned out, many of these biomarkers were directly or indirectly a reflection of metabolic fitness. They are: muscle mass, strength, basal metabolic rate, body fat percentage, aerobic capacity, blood sugar tolerance, and bone density. These biomarkers provide a very useful portrait of your biological age, which can be much more relevant than your chronological age.

Muscle mass affects a critical aspect of your metabolism and is known as basal metabolic rate (BMR). BMR is the amount of calories that you would burn during the course of a day while at rest. A low BMR indicates that you're not burning calories efficiently. BMR tends to decrease with age, mostly due to the loss of muscle mass. In other words, most people have less metabolically active tissue as they get older.

Metabolically active tissue, often called active tissue mass, includes muscle tissue as well as organ tissues like your liver, brain, and heart, which actively burn fuel. Increased active tissue mass gives you more strength, a higher BMR, and better aerobic capacity. It also vastly improves your health profile: cardiovascular health, better utilization of sugar, improved maintenance of good cholesterol, and higher bone density.

A greater body percentage of active tissue mass translates into a more aggressive antifat metabolism, because more muscle tissue actually increases the rate and amount of fat you use for fuel while you are at rest.

though in our weight-obsessed culture, we tend to think of being over-weight as a cosmetic issue, it is actually the harbinger of a systemic breakdown, with far-reaching consequences for overall health.

Perhaps you've noticed that certain metabolic conditions often occur simultaneously. That is, a person with diabetes may also be overweight and have high blood pressure; or someone with heart disease may also have high triglycerides, obesity, and diabetic symptoms.

In recent years, medical researchers have given increasing attention to a condition they've dubbed Syndrome X. Syndrome X is a clustering of metabolic problems comprised of insulin resistance, high blood sugar, elevated triglycerides, high LDL (small low-density lipoproteins) cho-lesterol, low HDL (high-density lipoproteins) cholesterol, high blood pressure, and obesity (especially abdominal fat).

This cluster of metabolic disorders, with insulin resistance at the core, seem to interact to promote the development of diabetes (adult onset, or type 2), atherosclerosis, and cardiovascular disease.[5] This is where blood type comes in. Depending on your blood type, your car-diovascular risk profile will be different.

The Cardiovascular Connection

KNOWING YOUR blood type will change your beliefs and behaviors about avoiding heart disease. Groundbreaking research has led to an ex-planation for the seeming paradox of the Blood Type Diet—how meat can be beneficial for one blood type and poisonous for another. Perhaps it will finally allow us to put the "meat issue" to rest. While each blood type can develop elements of cardiovascular disease, they appear to do so for different reasons. It makes good sense to look for different causes of action in different people, since the evidence is so strong that there are substantial variations among heart disease sufferers.

There is a very distinct difference among the blood types with re-gard to their incidence of heart disease. Type O and Type B are less likely to get heart disease as a result of high cholesterol. Their pathway is carbohydrate intolerance. Type A and Type AB follow a more con-ventional path, through high cholesterol. Each of these pathways lead to a very different lifestyle plan and diet in order to stay heart healthy.

▪ FROM THE BLOOD TYPE OUTCOME REGISTRY ▪

Jack J.
Type O
Middle-aged male
Improved: Cardiovascular, blood sugar, well-being

"I began the *ER4YT* regime in September '98. At fifty-six years, 6'5",
and a mesomorphic body type, I weighed 340 pounds, had a BP of
160/96, a pulse of 92, and suffered full time lethargy and blood
sugar issues. My first observation was clearheadedness and improved thinking. I noticed weight loss in less than a month. Energy
returned in three to four months. I began walking because I wanted
to and it felt good to do so, where before I just couldn't muster the
energy. I now walk twenty miles a week, work out at a gym three
times a week for 2.5 hours. The muscular and athletic build of my
youth has returned, and I have incredible strength. I now weigh
238, have a BP of 130/68 with a resting pulse of 68. I was diagnosed two years ago with a left axis cardiac condition and suffered
mild angina. It is gone now, with no symptons visible in over nine
months. In addition, almost *all* of my lifetime allergies are gone and
I have not taken an antihistamine in a year. Also gone is my chronic
arthitis. My attitude is optimistic, I am charged with energy and I
have *never* felt better in my life. I expect to live another thirty to
forty years of vital and active living. My cardiologist told me that
this regime was a lifesaver and that the American Diet killed more
people than any other cause of death. I assure you that if I had been
armed with this information in my youth, I would never have become sedentary. I further assure you that I will never return to that
condition again if I have anything to do with it. Thank you for giving me back my life."

Type A and Type AB:
The Blood Type-Cholesterol Factor

A number of studies show that Type As and Type ABs are more likely to
be at risk of heart disease and death by virtue of elevated cholesterol:

- The relationship between blood type and total serum cholesterol
  level was examined in a Japanese population to determine
  whether elevated cholesterol levels are associated with Type A, as
  has been demonstrated in many West European populations. The
  results showed that cholesterol levels were very significantly elevated in the Type A group compared to other blood groups.[6]

- A study examining a total of 380 marker/risk factor combinations found associations between Type A and both total serum cholesterol and LDL cholesterol, while a negative association was found between Type B and total serum cholesterol.[7]
- A Hungarian study measured the cholesterol of 653 patients who underwent coronary angiography between 1980 and 1985 at the Hungarian Institute of Cardiology. The results showed that Type A was more frequent and Type O was less frequent than normally seen in the Hungarian population, and that there were differences between the blood types as to the areas of the vessels where the narrowing of the coronary arteries had occurred.[8]

■ **FROM THE BLOOD TYPE OUTCOME REGISTRY** ■

Barry F.
Type A
Middle-aged male
Improved: Cardiovascular

"Lab tests indicate dramatic decrease in blood cholesterol and triglycerides, lost twenty-plus pounds, digestion working much better, energy more stable throughout the day, clearer thinking. Everything got better on the plan. I practice acupuncture and herbal medicine and regularly recommend this to my patients."

Several forms of elevated lipoproteins are inherited. One of the more common forms of hyperlipoproteinemia is called Type IIB, and it is characterized by increased LDL and VLDL (*really* bad cholesterol). Type IIB hyperlipoproteinemia results in premature hardening of the arteries, obstruction of the carotid artery (the artery that supplies blood to the head and brain), peripheral artery disease, heart attack, and stroke. Since all of these disorders show higher rates of occurrence in Type As, it is not surprising that studies have found a significant connection between a hyperlipoproteinemia IIb and Type A in both newborns and in patients who have suffered heart attacks.

• FROM THE BLOOD TYPE OUTCOME REGISTRY •

Susan D.
Type A
Middle-aged female
Improved: Cardiovascular

"My LDL cholesterol has been over 250 for years. No diet that I tried reduced it—in fact the diet that the doctors and nutritionists suggested always raised it! After a few short months on your diet, my LDL cholesterol had lowered over 100 points! I am going back in a month for another test, because the doctor was skeptical. (PS: I'm *not* skeptical, because I know!)"

Type O and Type B: The Blood Type–Carbohydrate Intolerance Factor

For Type Os and Type Bs, the leading risk factor for heart disease is not so much the fat in the food as the fat on the person. In other words, carbohydrate intolerance. When Type Os and Type Bs adopt low-fat diets rich in metabolically inactivating lectins, they gain weight. This particular kind of weight gain is a major risk factor for heart disease.

For many years, heart experts have been saying that high triglycerides are not an independent risk for heart disease—only in combination with other factors. However, increasing evidence is pointing to elevated triglycerides as a risk factor on their own, and this partially explains the anomaly of the Type O and Type B pathway to heart disease.

Triglycerides are formed by three fatty chains linked to one another. Most fat in food and the human body exists in this form. Diabetics often have high triglyceride levels, and diabetes is believed to be the leading cause of hypertriglyceridemia. In other words, insulin resistance, caused by carbohydrate intolerance, leads to high triglycerides.

In one recent study, men with the highest fasting triglyceride concentrations were more than twice as likely to have a heart attack than men with the lowest levels, even after diabetes, smoking, and sedentary living were factored in. People with triglyceride levels as low as 142 mg/dL were still at risk of having heart attacks, which was surprising, because levels below 200 mg/dL were considered normal. Borderline high triglyceride levels are between 200 and 400 mg/dL; high triglyc-

---

▪ FROM THE BLOOD TYPE OUTCOME REGISTRY ▪

Karen T.
Type O
Geriatric female
Improved: Cardiovascular/ well-being

"The crushing fatigue that followed almost every meal disappeared, and along with it the need for No-Doz. My blood pressure dropped from 155/85 to 120/80. I no longer take Tums all day long. I am no longer constantly hungry. My weight is going down even though I don't weigh, measure, or count calories with my food. People have commented that I seem brighter. My doctor loves the results."

---

eride levels are between 400 and 1,000 mg/dL; and very high levels are over 1,000 mg/dL.[9]

A classic sign of insulin resistance in Type O and Type B is the apple-shaped figure, characterized by a broad girth at the mid-section. Fat cells located in the abdomen release fat into the blood more easily than fat cells found elsewhere. For example, pear-shaped individuals, with fat located in the hips and thighs, do not have the same health risks. The release of fat from the abdomen begins within three to four hours after a meal is consumed, compared to many more hours for other fat cells. This easy release shows up as higher triglycerides and free fatty acid levels. Free fatty acids themselves cause insulin resistance, and elevated triglycerides usually coincide with low HDL, or "good" cholesterol. Overproduction of insulin as a result of insulin resistance syndrome has also been shown to increase the "very bad" cholesterol, VLDL.

The link between obesity, triglycerides, and "bad" lipoproteins has been evidenced in Type Os. In a French study of blood donors, serum triglycerides and lipoproteins were shown to correlate with both obesity and Blood Type O in a study screening for cardio- or cerebro-vascular disease. There is also a connection between non-secretors and high triglyceride levels, as well as insulin resistance.[10]

At long last the medical establishment is beginning to recognize the need to step outside of its narrow box and expand its thinking regarding cardiovascular risk factors. Although there is ample evidence that for some people cholesterol plays an important role in atherosclerosis and heart disease, we must address the large number of people who do not fit this limited profile.

The Secret Weapon of
Type O and Type B

Nature has provided Type O and Type B with an additional secret weapon to allow them to benefit from those higher protein levels.

In chapter 4 we introduced intestinal alkaline phosphatase, an enzyme manufactured in the small intestine, which has the primary function of splitting dietary cholesterol and fats. Numerous studies since the mid-1960s have shown that Type O and Type B have higher levels of this enzyme—especially Type O and Type B secretors. Conversely, Type A and Type AB have lower levels of this enzyme. Recent studies suggest that it is the inability to break down dietary fat that in part predisposed Type A and Type AB to higher cholesterol and more heart attacks; while the opposite is true for Type O and Type B, who are aided in the breakdown of dietary fat by high amounts of intestinal alkaline phosphatase.

Pathways to Cardiovascular Disease

TYPE O = Carbohydrate intolerance, high triglycerides, insulin
resistance, "*Type A*" behavior
TYPE A = High LDL and total cholesterol, oxidative stress, clotting
excesses, high cortisol
TYPE B = Nitric oxide imbalance (high blood pressure),
carbohydrate intolerance, high cortisol
TYPE AB = High LDL and total cholesterol, oxidative stress,
clotting excesses
NON-SECRETOR = Insulin resistance, low intestinal alkaline
phosphatase, clotting irregularities

Intestinal alkaline phosphatase activity rises following the ingestion of a fat-containing meal, especially if the triglycerides in the meal are long-chain fatty acids. In a study of volunteers given different test meals, the after-meal rise in serum intestinal alkaline phosphatase activity was significantly greater following the long-chain fatty acid meal than following the medium chain fatty acid meal, and significantly higher in Type O and Type B over Type A and Type AB. Paradoxically, it appears that intestinal alkaline phosphatase gives Type O and Type B metabolic advantages when they eat high-protein meals. Studies show that the consumption of protein further increases the levels of alkaline phosphatase in the

---

▪ FROM THE BLOOD TYPE OUTCOME REGISTRY ▪

Mary N., Paul N.
Type O
Middle-aged male and middle-aged female
Improved: Cardiovascular, allergies

"My husband and I are both Type Os. My husband, fifty-nine years old, has a history of high blood pressure, borderline high cholesterol, sleep problems, and the start of varicose veins from standing all day at his job. He also has severe allergies to everything, asthma, a chronic ear infection, back sensitivity, and favoritism from a surgically corrected slipped disk twenty-five years ago. He experienced results right away on the Type O diet. His blood pressure, which was being controlled with three different prescription medications and a water pill, started to plummet. Snoring and sleep problems that have plagued him since forever have further been alleviated from being on your program. In fact, within the first few days, he stopped snoring. He's gradually reducing his blood pressure medications and is now down to one prescription and a water pill once a week—although I believe we didn't see complete results until just recently when we stopped using soy sauce (a necessity for Asians) that included wheat. In the past few years, Jay has avoided doing yard work due to his allergies, and there was a specific shrub that he hated because of the welts that it would leave on his body after pruning (photinia). We were out last weekend pruning these same shrubs, and his body was spotless afterward, not one sign of allergy. This is a miracle, and he's given up the allergy shots that he's been having for five years. He's still puffing on his inhaler for his asthma but many fewer puffs now. His breathing is remarkably improved, and he is sleeping through the night and feeling fully rested in the morning. I had moderate allergies and eczema on my scalp and skin. I was taking one regular over-the-counter Actifed each night for the allergies, but since starting this program, I'd only had to take it every other night, and using wheat-free soy sauce and eating fish allowed me to eliminate them altogether. My skin is much improved also. We'd been on a no-fat diet for the past two years, and with your program, we're eating more fat with the nuts and meat.

---

intestines of Type Os and Type Bs. Without protein in their diets, Type Os and Type Bs do not gain the benefits of the specialized fat-busting enzymes in their intestines. This explains why these blood types can lower their cholesterol by adopting high-protein diets.

Recently, an intriguing study helped cast some light on why Type As and Type ABs have such low levels of alkaline phosphatase activity. In an article entitled "Intestinal alkaline phosphatase and the ABO blood group system—a new aspect," researchers presented evidence that the Blood Type A antigen may itself inactivate alkaline phosphatase. It may be the case that the lower levels of this enzyme, and the subsequent inability to break down dietary fats, may not be genetically linked to blood type. Instead, this reaction is to the physical expression of the A antigen. The authors found that the red cells of Type A and Type AB bind almost all intestinal alkaline phosphatase, while the red cells of Type O and Type B did so to a much lesser degree.[11]

There is also a lectin connection. Additional research showed that the acid phenylalanine was almost 100 percent effective in inhibiting alkaline phosphatase, and indeed our research has shown that many common sources of phenylalanine, including yams and sweet potatoes, cause a marked increase in the production of the bowel toxin indican in our Type A patients.

▪ FROM THE BLOOD TYPE OUTCOME REGISTRY ▪

Harry T.
Type A
Middle-aged male
Improved: Cardiovascular

"In February 98 I had my cholesterol checked at Kaiser Permanente Hospital in Los Angeles, California, and found the total to be 274, with the Triglycerides at 226, the HDL at 43, the LDL at 186, and the ratio at 6.4. After three months on the Type A diet, I returned to Kaiser, had my cholesterol checked, and the results were total cholesterol 203, Triglycerides 127, HDL 38, LDL 40, and Ratio 5.3. Overall, my emotional swings have seemed to even out and things don't get under my skin as easily. I am due to go back in for another test in about 1½ months, can't wait to see what's up then. Most of the credit must go to my wife as she found interesting ways of combining the food on the A list and made some very good-tasting dishes. Thanks for all the research and perseverance toward this food-intake theory, now becoming a reality. Till the next time I get good results to share, I am one happy Type A+"

I'd like to share one story in particular because it demonstrates so clearly how the right diet for your type can combat heart disease—even when the diet is high in animal protein. The respondent is a forty-seven-year-old Type O male. Here is his report:

"I am currently a commander in the United States Navy, stationed at Naval Air Station in Patuxent River, Maryland. I was diagnosed as a type 1 diabetic in November 1998. I was put on four insulin shots a day. By January 1, my blood sugars were under control and I was taking thirty units of insulin a day—five units of regular for breakfast, lunch and supper, and fifteen units of NPH at night for my bedtime snack. I was exercising regularly, working with my dietician, and eating a well-balanced diet every day. I kept myself on a very rigid routine for seven weeks. I was doing very well, losing weight—ten pounds in ten weeks—and feeling great. I started your diet for Type Os on February 19, because of the high recommendations of a fellow worker. I was very skeptical of his claims, but because of my respect for him and his enthusiasm, I tried it. The day after I started your diet, my blood sugar levels started dropping off, and I had to start decreasing my insulin levels on the second day. This continued for four weeks. I am now down to twenty units a day and holding—one unit for breakfast and lunch, three units for supper, and thirteen units for my snack at night. That's a 33 percent decrease in my insulin shots in four weeks.

I also noticed a significant increase in my energy level after the first week, and it continues today, four weeks later. I've lost eleven more pounds in the last four weeks. I'm working out two hours a night, four to five nights a week, and I feel better than I have in twenty years. I feel like I'm on a constant energy high.

I also have a history of high cholesterol—of 300 or higher—which is now down to 188. I just had a medical checkup with my endocrinologist three days ago and needless to say, he was very happy with my progress. My glycosylated hemoglobin test was down to 6.4 percent. He is now anticipating taking me down from four insulin shots a day to two shots a day. I plan to stay on your Type O diet for the rest of my life."

The Immune
Battleground

*Blood Type as a Weapon
for Survival*

*I*MMUNITY IS OUR BASIC SURVIVAL MECHANISM. WE SURVIVE by virtue of the distinctions we make between friend and foe, "self" and "non-self." These distinctions are embedded in our cellular makeup and are ruthlessly supervised by our immune systems. Our blood type antigen is a powerful marker of self to our immune system. It is a guardian at nature's gate, allowing access to friends and preventing entry to foes.

Access is prevented through antigens, which are extremely powerful chemical markers on our cells that can effectively block foreign substances, such as dangerous bacteria, from entering our systems. Blood type's immune function is arguably its most important. It was this function, after all, that was responsible for the survival of the species.

Each blood type possesses a different antigen with its own special chemical structure. Your blood type is named for the blood type antigen you possess on your red blood cells. There is nothing special about the use of letters to name the blood types, other than the fact that the O antigen was given the letter O to indicate the number zero. As we will see, the immune systems of all the blood types view Type O as "self," so technically Type O has zero antigen. This distinction persists in Europe, where Type O individuals typically refer to themselves as "Type Zero." Here is a simple way to visualize the chemical structure of the blood type antigens. Think of antennae projecting out from each cell. These antennae are made from long chains of a repeating sugar, which terminate in a sugar called fucose. Fucose, by itself, forms the simplest of the blood types—Type O.

- The Blood Type O antigen serves as the base for the other more complex blood types.
- The Blood Type A antigen is formed by adding a second sugar, N-acetyl-galactosamine, to fucose.
- Blood Type B is formed by adding a second (different) sugar to fucose, called D-galactose.
- Blood Type AB is formed by adding both sugars—N-acetyl-galactosamine and D-galactosamine—to fucose; possesses both A and B antigens.

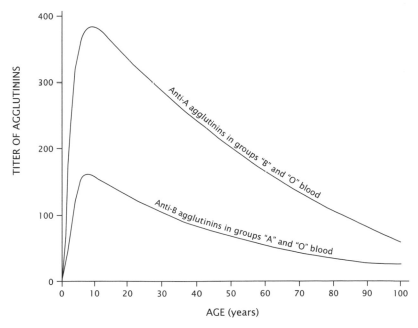

AGGLUTINATION AND THE PROCESS OF AGING   *As we age the amount of anti-blood type agglutinins in our blood diminishes, making us more susceptible to disease. A key factor in healthy aging is to maintain high levels of anti-blood type agglutinins.*

Your immune system creates antibodies to reject foreign antigens, including blood type antigens foreign to you. Your own blood type antigen prevents you from making antibodies to your own blood type antigen. People with Type A blood have an antibody to Type B in their blood plasma. This anti-B antibody helps the body destroy any Type B blood cells that might enter the system. Likewise, people with Type B blood have an antibody to Type A in their blood plasma, which helps destroy any Type A blood cells that might enter the system. Blood Type O has both anti-A and anti-B antibodies, and Blood Type AB does not carry any opposing blood group antibodies.

Our blood type antigen views other blood types as non-self to such an extent that we are genetically programmed to produce an extremely powerful antibody to opposing blood types—or, rather, to the microorganisms and foods that have other blood type antigens. No other immune mechanism is as powerful as our blood type. We do not start out in life with antibodies to opposing blood types coursing through our systems. However, we create them very quickly. Within two weeks of life, most infants are already becoming sensitized to opposing blood type antigens in their environment.

> Learn more about blood type and the history of disease page 359.

S. Breanndan Moore, M.D., a hematologist at the Mayo Clinic in Rochester, Minnesota, describes the formation of these naturally occurring antibodies in a very clear way: "Let's say a child is born with Type O red cells. The child will begin forming antibodies to Type A and B red cell antigens as soon as she starts eating food, because the A and B antigens are actually found in some plants. So, as soon as the child starts eating plant food, she'll be exposed to those antigens and start making antibodies against them. Later, if the child is transfused with blood that's not Type O, she'll destroy the new red blood cells in a process called hemolytic transfusion reaction."[1]

This is a very provocative statement. Take a moment to contemplate the fact that one of the major immune reactions against non-self, one of the few that is genetically programmed, is the result of hundreds, if not thousands, of tiny innoculations over the course of a child's early life, with substances in the diet that are chemically identical with getting the wrong blood type in a transfusion!

A recent study of 644 Taiwanese subjects showed that synthesis of anti-A and anti-B antibodies could be demonstrated in most Taiwanese infants by two to four months of age, increasing progressively to reach adult levels at around one year of age. Peak levels were reached at between three and ten years of age, and then declined with advancing years. Individuals eighty years and older showed reduced levels similar to those seen in six- to twelve-month-old infants.[2]

In this way your blood type offers a clear road map for the process of aging—and provides vital clues about how to slow the process. Here's a simple way to look at it. Consider your life in three stages. The first stage is education; your immune system is exposed to antigens and begins to learn which are friend and which are foe, creating antibodies against the foes. The second stage is maintenance; if your immune system has learned well, it will remain strong and healthy. The third stage is decay; a weakening of your defenses occurs and fewer antibodies against enemies are created. If viewed in this way, clearly the goal is to perform the education stage well enough so that the maintenance stage is healthy, and so that the decay stage is delayed. Living right for your blood type can be a vital key to health and longevity.

A disturbing trend that has serious consequences for our immune protection is the rate at which levels of anti–blood type isohemagglutinins are rising in the population. A French study showed that they are about 50 percent higher in children today than in 1929. The authors suggest that this increased immune reactivity of children may be due to the increased use of prophylactic vaccinations.[3]

Secretor Status: An Immune Factor

SINCE YOUR BLOOD TYPE antigen is the key to immune defense, what are the implications of being unable to secrete your blood type antigens in your bodily fluids? Quite dramatic, according to an impressive body of scientific research.

In general, non-secretors are far more likely to suffer from an immune disease than secretors, especially when it is provoked by an infectious organism. Non-secretors also have genetically induced difficulties removing immune complexes from their tissues, which increases their risk of attacking tissue that contains them. In other words, non-secretors are a bit more predisposed to view their own tissue as unfriendly.

Non-secretors are dominant in virtually every immune system disorder:

- Non-secretors are more prone to generalized inflammation than secretors.
- Non-secretors are more prone to both type 1 and type 2 diabetes than are secretors.

- Non-secretors who were type 1 diabetics have much more consistent problems with the yeast *Candida albicans*, especially in their mouths and upper GI tracts.
- Non-secretors account for 80 percent of all fibromyalgia sufferers, irrespective of blood type.
- Non-secretors have an increased prevalence of a variety of autoimmune diseases, including ankylosing spondylitis, reactive arthritis, psoriatic arthropathy, Sjogren's syndrome, multiple sclerosis, and Grave's disease.
- Non-secretors have an extra risk for recurrent urinary tract infections, and between 55 and 60 percent of non-secretors have been found to develop renal scarring even with the regular use of antibiotic treatment for UTIs.
- Non-secretors comprise 20 percent of the population, but 80 percent of people doctors categorize as "complex" patients. They're hard to diagnose properly and slow to cure.

You can see why it is so essential that you be tested for your secretor status. If you are among the 20 percent of the population that comprise non-secretors, you will need to factor that in to your prescriptive plan. Here is an example of relevancy: Blood Type Bs have a very high risk for developing urinary tract infections. If you are a Type B non-secretor, the likelihood that you will have chronic UTIs is more than doubled. Your best strategy is a long-term preventive program to avoid bacterial infections. On the other hand, Type As have a relatively low risk of UTIs. However, if you are a Type A non-secretor, your risk is increased by about 25 percent—which is not insubstantial.

Cancer: Surveillance Derailed

ALTHOUGH THERE are probably over a thousand publications on the associations of blood groups and disease, including cancer, many are based totally on statistical analysis. While statistical calculations alone do not provide definitive scientific proof, at some point it's impossible to ignore the sheer weight of the data on malignancy, coagulation, and infection. Clear patterns are revealed in this data. Some of the findings on microbe receptors, and the association with important immune proteins, are most convincing and suggest that blood type antigens do play an important biological role in cancer.

Blood Type and Cancer:
In Search of Answers

Our growing access to groundbreaking genetic information has allowed us to connect some of the dots—to pursue valid inquiries. It can be said at the outset, that cancers in general tend to be associated with Type A and Type AB, and slightly less strongly with Type B and Type O.[4] Perhaps the greatest focus of current research on the ABO blood type antigens is in the field of molecular oncology. Recent findings in membrane chemistry, tumor immunology, and infectious disease add a scientific rationale for several blood type associations, and there is an increasingly compelling rationale for some of the earlier statistical findings.

The huge interest in blood type stems from the developing awareness that blood type antigens are incredibly important components in the process of cell maturation and control. Of particular note is the fact that the appearance or disappearance of blood type antigens is a hallmark of malignancy in many common cancers.

Characteristics of a cancer cell

- Cancer cells have a typically round instead of the normal flat appearance.
- Cancer cells do not adhere to one another as normal cells do. This is due to the reduction in surface adhesion molecules on the cancer cell's surface. As we will see, one of the major adhesion molecules lost is the ABO antigen.
- There is limited contact inhibition of movement. Normal cells terminate movement when in contact with one another; cancer cells don't.
- Cancer cells are less anchored. Thus, they are free to invade other tissues and enter the blood and lymph systems (metastasis).
- Cancer cells are not inhibited by the density of surrounding tissues; cells are able to pile up on top of one another.
- Extracellular growth.

Several tumor antigens, called "tumor markers," are the known product of certain blood type precursors. Many of these tumor antigens are A-like, which helps to explain the striking number of cancer associations with Type A and Type AB. In essence, the tumor antigens would appear to be friendly to these blood types, and they wouldn't make antibodies to fight them. On the other hand, autoimmune disorders, characterized by an overproduction of antibodies, are associated with Type O—supporting the view of early immunologists that there is a fundamental antithesis between the two classes of disease. Heightened surveillance and overactive immune activity (Type O) results in less malignancy, and overly tolerant immune activity (Type A) encourages it. These observations suggest a more general hypothesis: In the tissues of all people, both normal and cancerous, there are A-like antigens present at a biochemical level that are usually inaccessible to the immune system. However, in the course of an autoimmune process, or during the immune response to a growing cancer, the antigens become accessible. At that point, a Type A person who cannot make anti-A antibodies will be more likely than a Type O person to tolerate the cancer, but less likely than a Type O person to attack their own tissues.[5]

However, the link between cancer and Type A is far from universal. A few tumors show strong associations with Type O and Type B. This implies that cancer is a condition associated with derangement of blood type activity in general, and the expression of A-like antigens on the surface of tumors is simply the most common of these derangements.

Blood Type Antigens and Metastasis

The spreading of cancer to distant parts of the body is called metastasis, a complex phenomenon consisting of several sequential steps:

- Invasion of primary sites
- Entry into blood or lymphatic vessels
- Transport
- Migration from the blood vessel into the tissues, and growth at the target sites

Studies have shown that certain types of carbohydrate antigen expressions in cancer cells are profoundly related to not only the mode of metastatic spread and the organ distribution pattern of metastasis, but also to the prognosis of cancer patients. Lymphatic metastasis was related to the expression of mucin core–type carbohydrates (Tn antigen and Tn-like antigens) in common, whereas there were no conspicuous similarities in the hematogenous metastasis–related carbohydrates among the cancers. The expression of blood type antigens appeared to be strong prognostic indicators of these cancers, although the relation of these antigens to each cancer varied. These results suggest that, to some extent, adhesion molecules and/or carbohydrates are one of the determinants of cancer metastasis and prognosis.

The deletion or reduction of A or B antigens in tumors of Type A or Type B individuals correlates with malignancy and metastatic potential because there is a lack of adhesiveness that a cancer cell achieves when it loses blood type antigens. Findings in human colon cancer indicate that the degree of motility and proliferation of colon tumor cells are directly associated with the deletion or reduction of the Type A antigen. As cells lost the A-like antigen, they seemed to also lose the ability to express many of the cell adhesion proteins, such as the integrins, which normally express an A-like antigen on their receptors to control cell movement.

Since the blood type antigens are needed to make the integrin receptors that hold cells together, their loss results in the tumor cells gaining the ability to move and circulate through the body. This link between blood type and cell adherence is probably as elemental to the development of cancer as it is to life itself. A growing fetus needs the ability to spawn new organs and grow an effective blood supply to supply them; in these instances, the loss of blood type would allow for this migration of embryonic cells to the sites of future organs and blood vessels. In fact, many of the embryonic cell tumor markers (such as the

---

▪ FROM THE BLOOD TYPE OUTCOME REGISTRY ▪

Kay P.
Type O
Middle-aged female
Improved: Ovarian cancer

"I have ovarian cancer. Two weeks after starting the Type O diet, my CA125 dropped from 400 to 390. Eight weeks after starting the diet, my CA125 was 370. My energy level has improved tremendously, and pain that I had been having in my feet has greatly subsided. Another great benefit I'm experiencing is weight loss. I've been overweight most of my life. At the time I was diagnosed with cancer, I weighed over 200 pounds, and after my initial course of chemotherapy (and the Decadron I took along with it) I had gained another 75 pounds, putting me at 300 pounds. I thought I was doomed to being fat forever. However, after eight weeks on *ER4YT*, I lost twenty-one pounds."

CEA) are expressed almost in parallel with the loss of blood type—the greater the loss of blood type antigen, the greater the production of embryonic tumor antigens. In malignancy, the loss of blood type means migration of an uncontrolled sort, and that means metastasis.

Tissues and organs that do not normally manufacture blood type antigens will show the reverse effect. They will *gain* blood type antigens when they turn cancerous. Sometimes, such as in the case of the thyroid and colon, changes taking place in the blood type antigen expression in one organ will influence the expression of blood type antigens in another.

T and TN: Pan-Carcinogenic Antigens

Many malignant cells (such as those found in breast and stomach cancer) develop a tumor marker called the Thomsen-Friedenreich (T) antigen. This antigen is suppressed in normal healthy cells, much like a rock that is covered over by water at high tide. T antigen only becomes unsuppressed as a cell moves toward malignancy, much like the covered rock in our example becomes uncovered as the tide moves out. It is so rare to find the T antigen uncovered in healthy tissue that we actually have antibodies against it. It is even more rare to find a Tn antigen (a less well-developed T) on a healthy cell. The good news is that everyone has pre-existing anti-T and anti-Tn antibodies, or a built-in immune system response against cells with these markers. The blood type catch here is that your blood type will often influence the amount and activity of these antibodies against T and Tn antigens.

The T and Tn antigens show some structural similarity to the A antigen.[6] Not surprisingly, Type A individuals have the least aggressive antibody immune response against the T and Tn antigens. In fact, the T and Tn antigens and the Type A antigens are immunologically quite similar because of their shared terminal sugar (N-acetylgalactosamine). You can see how easily the Type A and Type AB immune systems could be fooled by an A-like invader. This has led researchers to conclude that the Tn antigen is, in a broad sense, an A-like antigen. The hypothesis continues: because of the lower level of antibody against T and Tn antigens or stumps, and because of this tendency for the immune system of Type As to be a bit confused or disinclined to attack Tn antigens, Type A is at an immunological disadvantage in attacking any cells bearing T and Tn antigenic markers.

In an ideal world, your immune system would be naturally predisposed to fight against cells with incomplete or abnormal structures, just as it would against an invading virus. Type A and Type AB start with an immune disadvantage, since they cannot clearly see the danger. Some of the most virulent cancers have shown depressed levels of anti-T antibody, a leading example being breast cancer.

T and Tn are exuberantly expressed in cancerous cells of the stomach. Curiously, about one-third of all Japanese express some T antigen in apparently normal stomach tissue, and this may help explain why stomach cancer rates in Japan are among the highest in the world. Since gastric juice is typically loaded with blood type antigens anyway, it is not unlikely that Type A and Type AB would be at a disadvantage at recognizing the T antigens as cancer markers—and even if they do, would not likely mount much of an antibody response against them.

The exuberant secretion of the A antigen in stomach cancer is not limited to Type As. Large amounts of Type A antigen have also been observed in the less common tumors of Type B and Type O. The age-related decline in anti–blood type antibodies may help account for increased cancer rates in the elderly. It appears that the progression of stomach cells to cancer involves a necessary mutation at the ABO gene, the result of which is the production of A antigen, even if this is not the person's blood type. Of course, having Type O or Type B antigens and being capable of attacking A-like things, such as cancer cells, gives these blood types a considerable advantage. It appears that stomach and intestinal precancerous and cancer cells tend to lose the Type O and Type B antigens, making immune system detection in these blood types more likely.

Blood Itself— Another Type A Susceptibility

The A-like cancer hypothesis is a strong one, well-supported in the medical literature. However, several other Type A biological traits appear to convey additional susceptibility to malignancy. Perhaps the second most potent pathway by which Type As are made vulnerable to severe complications from malignancy is their "thicker" blood and tendency toward clotting.[7] We discussed this in the last chapter, on cardiovascular disease. Now we see the connection again.

Here is the hypothesis:

VON WILLEBRAND FACTOR AND FACTOR VIII. It has been noted that cancer cells can often hitch a ride on circulating platelets as they begin to metastasize. This is due to an aberrant platelet glycoprotein receptor expressed by human tumor cells, which appears to participate in the adhesive interactions required for the metastatic process. Von

Willebrand factor (vWF) and factor VIII are serum proteins that are a sort of molecular glue that platelets use to attach to blood-clotting proteins along the lining of the blood vessels. It is also required for this aberrant platelet glycoprotein to bind to cancer cells. Plasma specimens from patients with disseminated metastases showed that their plasma levels of von Willebrand factor and factor VIII were elevated (vWF almost double) above those of normal subjects, apparently because they lack adequate amounts of an enzyme required to cleave vWF and factor VIII into their inactive forms. Because of this, cancer patients with widely disseminated metastasis have levels of platelet activity upwards of 150 percent greater than that of normal subjects.

FIBRINOGEN.   As with heart disease and diabetes, studies have shown that Type A patients have higher levels of blood viscosity than Type O patients. The reason is the higher levels of the clotting protein fibrinogen. Fibrinogen is an "acute phase" protein, important in the inflammatory response and in wound healing. It is elevated in cancer patients, where its presence has been suggested to shorten survival and contribute to weight loss. As with vWF and factor VIII, fibrinogen serves as part of the adherence cascade by which cancer cells can attach to platelets and the walls of the blood vessels as a prelude to metastatic spread.

This helps explain why older studies have shown that cancer patients on blood-thinning medications have less metastasis. Type As have higher levels of vWF and factor VIII over the other blood types, which probably accounts for their thicker blood. Type As also have a tendency toward higher levels of fibrinogen. These two blood-thickening factors make Type As even more vulnerable to cancer.[8]

The A-Friendly Growth Factor

One little-known and underappreciated effect of the Type A antigen is its ability to attach to the receptor for some growth factors.[9] These factors control the growth of cells. In the case of malignancy, that growth is out of control. Overproduction of these growth factors as a result of oncogene activity contributes to a loss of the body's ability to regulate growth—which can result in cancerous cell growth.

Epidermal Growth Factor (EGF), which is normally synthesized to help tissue repair itself, also has important effects on the growth of prostate, colon, breast, and several other forms of cancer. These cancers are characterized by cells that have an excessively high concentration of EGF receptors (EGF-R) on their surfaces. The larger number of

EGF-R on the cancer cell means that the cell can bind an excessive number of molecules of EGF. It may be that this excessive dose of growth factor is critical to tumor growth. In fact, it is now clear that the growth of breast cancer is regulated by growth factor receptors, and their upregulation is associated with impaired prognosis. Because of its deregulation in many cancers (bladder, breast, cervix, colon, esophagus, head and neck, lung, and prostate), the epidermal growth factor receptor (EGF-R) has been selected as a potential target for chemoprevention.

As we discussed in the digestion section, EGF-R bears an antigenic determinant that is closely related to the Type A carbohydrate structure. It is now very well-documented that the Type A antigen can also bind to EGF receptors. It is not unlikely that free A antigen in Type A and Type AB, especially secretors, can find its way onto these excess EGF receptors and act to simulate cancerous cell growth.

Let's look at the various cancers and their blood type relationships:

Breast Cancer

TYPE O	TYPE A	TYPE B	TYPE AB	SECRETOR STATUS
Slight degree of resistance, and lower risk of death.	Higher risk, worse outcomes, and more rapid progression.	Slight degree of resistance and lower risk of death, unless there is a family history. Higher risk of recurrence.	Higher risk, worse outcomes, and more rapid progression.	Slightly less risk for non-secretors.

Breast cancer is the most common cancer among women. And while the mortality rates are falling slightly for some subpopulations of women, it is still a potentially lethal adversary. Standard treatment can vary, but procedures, such as lumpectomy surgery (removal of the tumor and some surrounding tissue), mastectomy (removal of the whole breast), chemotherapy, radiation, and hormone-blocking therapy are the norm, with any combination of the above strategies potentially employed. Mammograms have been a major push within medicine as a means of early detection. However, many of my patients have actually discovered their tumors on self-examination of breast tissue, so I cannot overemphasize this self-help procedure. While many risk factors are associated with the development of breast cancer, it is seldom mentioned that blood type has an influence on susceptibility and outcomes. In fact, some researchers have even gone so far as to say that "blood groups were shown to possess a predictive value independent of other known prognostic factors" when discussing breast cancer. Other researchers have actually suggested that a degree of the susceptibility to breast cancer, from a gene perspective, might be a result of a breast cancer–susceptibility locus linked to the ABO locus located on band q34 of chromosome 9.

▪ FROM THE BLOOD TYPE OUTCOME REGISTRY ▪

Kay S.
Type A
Middle-aged female
Improved: Breast cancer

"My grandmother and my aunt both died of breast cancer before I was born, but this wasn't discussed much in my family, and we didn't know then about inherited risks. My cancer was discovered when I had my first mammogram, at age forty-two, on my left breast, and I had a lumpectomy. I had always been healthy before that, but I knew I had to get really serious. I started the Type A Diet two months after my surgery. I have followed it religiously for almost four years, and there has been no sign of cancer returning. My blood tests are all perfectly normal. Even my doctor is impressed. My daughter, who is sixteen and also Type A, loves the diet. I now have some confidence that she can escape our genetic fate."

My observation, and the observations of others in the medical literature, show that Type A women have a generalized tendency to worse outcomes and a more rapid progression with breast cancer. Research indicates that Type A women are overrepresented among breast cancer patients, and, remarkably, this trend occurs even among women thought to be at low risk for cancer. Being Type A is also one of the most significant risk factors for a rapidly progressing breast cancer, and Type A women have been observed to have poorer outcomes once they are diagnosed with breast cancer.[10]

Type ABs have a susceptibility closer to Type As. They, too, tend to have a more dramatic trend toward recurrence and shorter survival times.

In contrast, being Type O infers a slight degree of resistance against breast cancer, and even when Type Os contract the disease, they show a significantly lower risk of death. Type B generally acts a bit more like Type O, imparting a degree of reduced susceptibility. This is particularly evident among women who do not have a family history of breast cancer. However, there are two areas to consider if you are a Type B woman. If you have had a family member with breast cancer, the protection normally associated with being Type B no longer seems to exist. Furthermore, if you are a Type B woman and currently have or have had breast cancer, statistically speaking, your odds of a recurrence tend to be higher. Part of the reason is that you tend to survive the original cancer, but nevertheless, you might want to consider some of the long-term immune building and anticancer strategies we will discuss.

Breast cancer shows a weaker association with being a non-secretor.

Female Reproductive Cancer (Gynecological Tumors)

TYPE O	TYPE A	TYPE B	TYPE AB	SECRETOR STATUS
Better survival rate with all reproductive cancers.	Higher risk, worse outcomes for all reproductive cancers.	Least likely to have malignant ovarian tumor; better survival rate for endometrial cancer; slightly increased risk for cervical cancer.	Higher risk, worse outcomes for all reproductive cancers, especially ovarian cancer.	Increased expression of Lewis antigens.

As a general rule, gynecological tumors occur more frequently and are associated with worse prognoses in Type A women. As examples, endometrial cancer occurs more frequently in Type A, ovarian cancer occurs more frequently in As and ABs. For both of these cancers, Type A is associated with worse survival rates. Conversely, the best survival rate is seen among Type O women, followed by B women. Type B women are also the least likely to have an ovarian tumor that is malignant. With regard to cervical cancer, analysis also shows a strong trend toward a higher frequency of cancer and poor outcomes among Type A women, a slight trend toward increased risk for Type Bs, and a better survival rate for Type Os.[11]

Normal endometrial tissue does not contain blood type antigens. However, over one-half of endometrial cancers have detectable blood type antigens. An increased rate of expression of Lewis group antigens, particularly Lewis(b) antigen, is also observed in endometrial cancers compared with its expression in normal endometria.

Bladder Cancer

TYPE O	TYPE A	TYPE B	TYPE AB	SECRETOR STATUS
Higher risk, higher tumor grade, increased aggressiveness, and more relapses.	Less risk and fewer relapses.	Higher risk, higher tumor grade, increased aggressiveness, and more relapses.	Less risk and fewer relapses.	No known association

Bladder cancer appears to be an exception to the general rule of Type A and aggressive cancers. In one study, the researchers noticed that Blood Type O had a tendency to increased aggressiveness, higher tumor grade, and more relapses, followed by Type B. On the other hand, Type A and Type AB were less likely to have the more aggressive form of this cancer and were somewhat protected against relapses. Another study had a similar finding. Researchers found that among 141 patients with bladder cancer, Type As had lower grade tumors and lower mortality rates. Type Os generally had higher grade tumors and higher mortality rates. Other researchers have also observed similar trends, such as the Type O tendency to higher grade tumors, larger tumors, progression to advanced disease, and increased rates of mortality— especially after eight years. Like most cancers, bladder cancer is characterized by a dissappearance of normal ABO antigen expression and the appearance of specialized adherence molecules.[12]

Lung Cancer

TYPE O	TYPE A	TYPE B	TYPE AB	SECRETOR STATUS
Slightly lower overall risk. (when other factors, such as smoking, are involved).	Slightly higher overall risk (when other factors, such as smoking, are involved).	Slightly lower overall risk (when other factors, such as smoking, are involved).	Slightly lower overall risk (when other factors, such as smoking, are involved).	No known association

ONLY A SLIGHT BLOOD TYPE CORRELATION. Lung cancer continues to be one of the leading causes of cancer deaths in the United States. It is expected that about 180,000 new cases will be diagnosed this year, and of these, about 160,000 people will die. While the incidence of lung cancer has been declining in men since the 1980s, it is still rising in women. The most well-known risk factor for lung cancer is cigarette smoking, which has been linked to 85 to 90 percent of all cases. Other well-known risk factors include exposure in the workplace to certain substances (such as asbestos and some organic chemicals), radiation exposure, radon exposure (especially in smokers), and even second-hand environmental tobacco smoke.

Because of the causal link between lung cancer with cigarette smoking, we would expect this strong risk factor to possibly overwhelm any blood type differences. However, we still see a higher number of Type As and a lower number of Type Os with lung cancer. This trend is even greater among individuals younger than fifty (where it is especially high). This suggests that smoking, which increases the risk for lung cancer with each decade of exposure, somewhat mutes the blood type connection in a population that has had many decades of smoking history, but still cannot camouflage the Type A connection.

Digestive System Cancers: Stomach Cancer

TYPE O	TYPE A	TYPE B	TYPE AB	SECRETOR STATUS
Very low risk.	Increased risk and poorer survival.	Lower overall risk.	Increased risk and poorer survival.	Slightly lower risk for non-secretors.

It has been consistently observed that Blood Type A is associated with an increased risk for stomach cancer and poorer survival rates. Type O, with a more robust response, is able to exert a protective effect that limits the growth and spread of the tumor. Type Os have much better survival rates than do Type As.

Because of this strong relationship between stomach cancer and Type A, some researchers have hypothesized that gastric cancer cells produce an antigen immunologically related to the A antigen—meaning the Type A antigen sees it as friendly and does not reject it. This appears to be the case to a degree, with stomach cancer cells expressing the A-like Thompsen-Friedenreich (T) antigen. Type As have a naturally lower anti–Thompsen-Friedenreich immune response.

Stomach cancer is also often characterized by exuberant secretion of Type A antigens. This characteristic is not limited to Type A. Large amounts of A antigen have also been observed in the less common tumors of Type B and Type O. It appears that the progression of stomach cells to stomach cancer involves a necessary mutation at the ABO gene, the result of which is the production of A antigen, even if this is not the person's blood type. Of course, being Type O or Type B and capable of attacking A-like things, such as cancer cells, gives these blood types a considerable advantage. Falling into the category of the slightly mysterious, being a non-secretor is associated with a slight decrease in the prevalence of stomach cancer.

Digestive System Cancers: Pancreatic Cancer, Liver Cancer, Gallbladder Cancer

TYPE O	TYPE A	TYPE B	TYPE AB	SECRETOR STATUS
Lower overall risk.	Higher risk for pancreatic, liver, and gallbladder cancers.	Higher risk for pancreatic and gallbladder cancers.	Higher risk for pancreatic, liver, and gallbladder cancers.	No known association

Pancreatic cancer carries an increased risk for both Type A and Type B, while Type O has a degree of protection.

Like many other cancers, blood type antigen structures on pancreatic cancerous cells are prevalent and capable of alteration. There is also a capability for inappropriate expression of blood type antigens with pancreatic cancer. In all reported cases, this has been manifested by either a Type A or Type O individual expressing B antigens on the pancreatic cancer. Perhaps this is indicative of a B-like nature to this cancer (at least in some individuals) and partly explains the increase in risk for Type Bs.[13]

Cancers of the liver show a slight association with Type A. Cancers of the gallbladder and bile ducts show a strong association with Type A and Type B.

Digestive System Cancers: Colon Cancer

TYPE O	TYPE A	TYPE B	TYPE AB	RH STATUS
No known association	No known association	No known association	No known association	Differences in disease spread: Rh− more localized; Rh+ metastatic.

ONLY A SLIGHT BLOOD TYPE CORRELATION; SOME RH CORRELATION. Colorectal cancer is among the most frequent cancers in the United States, with an estimated 133,000 new cases predicted (94,000 for colon and 39,000 for rectum). About 55,000 deaths from colorectal cancer are expected this year.

Some of the most common risk factors include a family history of colorectal cancer, colon polyps, and inflammatory bowel disease. Other risk factors can include physical inactivity, exposure to certain chemicals, and a high-fat or low-fiber diet.

Blood type itself is not a primary risk factor for colon cancer, but colon cancer is one of the relatively few diseases with a significant association to an individual's Rh blood type. Although Rh+ and Rh- individuals are about equally likely to have colon cancer, Rh- individuals are more likely to have a localized form of the disease, while Rh+ individuals are more likely to have metastatic disease. This suggests that Rh+ patients with colorectal cancer are less protected against tumor spread than Rh- patients, especially with regard to regional lymph node metastases.[14]

Early studies showed an association of cancers of the large intestine with Blood Type A. However, this association is weaker than that found with stomach cancer. Perhaps the largest link to blood type and colon cancer is found with respect to the appearance or disappearance of blood type antigens. It is commonly recognized that altered blood group antigen expression is a hallmark of malignancy in this form of cancer.

Some researchers have suggested that specific lectins (such as amaranth lectin) might provide a useful tool for early detection of colon cancer (in fact they might also be potentially useful therapeutically as well). The lectins under scrutiny have been specific for Type A. This would take advantage of the changed structural glycoconjugates, which tend to have a more A-like alteration. All of this would depend upon primary ABO type, secretor status, and Lewis phenotype.

Vicia faba agglutinin, the dietary lectin found in broad beans (fava beans), has also been suggested as a possibility to slow the progression of colon cancer. Basically, it appears that *Vicia faba agglutinin* can stimulate an undifferentiated colon cancer cell line to differentiate into glandlike structures. In other words, this lectin can make malignant colon cancer cells transform back to healthy, purposeful cells. The same researchers also found that this lectin, as well as the lectin in the common edible mushroom, inhibit proliferation of colon cancer cell lines.[15]

Digestive System Cancers: Oral Cavity and Esophagus

TYPE O	TYPE A	TYPE B	TYPE AB	SECRETOR STATUS
Relatively low risk.	Highest risk of oral and esophageal cancers.	Higher risk of oral and esophageal cancers.	Share Type A highest risk of oral and esophageal cancers.	*Secretor:* Higher risk of cancer of the salivary glands. *Non-Secretor:* Higher overall risk of oral and esophageal cancers.

Cancer of the lip is significantly associated with Type A. Cancers of the tongue, gums, and cheeks also have a Type A association. Cancers of the salivary glands are strongly associated with Type A, and weakly with Type B. Type Os seem to have substantial protection against this type of cancer. The salivary glands also appear to have an association with being a secretor.

In the chapter on digestion, we discussed the Type A association with Barrett's esophagus—a pre-neoplastic change to the tissue of the esophagus. So, it is not surprising to find Type As having a much higher incidence of esophageal cancer. Non-secretors (and Lewis(a+b-) also have an association with this cancer. Blood Type B also has a tendency to more cancers of the esophagus, while Type O has a definite degree of protection.[16]

As a general rule, a higher intensity of oral disease is found among non-secretors. When it comes to precancerous or cancerous changes to tissue of the mouth and esophagus, non-secretors seem to do worse than secretors. This oral disease susceptibility is reflected in the occurrence of epithelial dysplasia, which is found almost exclusively in the non-secretor group.

Cancers of the larynx and hypopharynx are associated with Type A, Type AB, and Type B.[17]

Structural changes to squamous cell cancers of the head and neck are quite common. In normal tissue of this region, your blood type is expressed. However, once squamous cell cancer develops, the A antigen disappears in about one-third of Type As and Type ABs, and the O antigen is expressed in carcinoma cells from all the blood types. These cancers generally have a poor prognosis. The T and Tn antigens we discussed earlier also become commonly expressed in these cancers.

Brain and Nervous System Cancers

TYPE O	TYPE A	TYPE B	TYPE AB	SECRETOR STATUS
Relatively low risk.	Highest risk of brain and nervous system tumors.	Somewhat high risk of brain and nervous system tumors.	Highest risk of brain and nervous system tumors.	No known association

A consistent association has been found between Type A and brain and nervous system tumors. A weaker association for these forms of cancer exists for Type B. Conversely, Type O has a favorable prognosis for brain and nervous system cancers.

Researchers investigating the use and efficacy of postoperative poly- and immunochemotherapy for malignant gliomas decided to examine the results according to blood type. When the efficacy of polychemotherapeutic and antibiotic intervention was analyzed according to survival time, it was a promising intervention for Type A and Type AB patients. However, it was ineffective in Type O patients. Based on their results, the researchers concluded that a schedule of chemo- and immuno-chemotherapy should be selected by blood type. While this is currently an isolated finding, it does draw attention to the possibility that medical interventions for cancer and many other diseases could be improved if blood type were factored into decisions about treatment.[18]

Thyroid Cancer

TYPE O	TYPE A	TYPE B	TYPE AB	SECRETOR STATUS
Relatively low risk.	Highest risk of thyroid cancer.	Moderate risk of thyroid cancer.	Highest risk of thyroid cancer.	No known association

Blood Type A has a propensity for thyroid cancer. Although Type O suffers from certain thyroid conditions, cancer is not one of them. Type O appears to be protected. Similar to many other cancers, the fine structure of various antigens is altered between healthy and cancerous cells. As a general rule, loss of A and B antigens, and the appearance of greater numbers of Tn antigens is a characteristic of thyroid cancers and is associated with a tendency for malignancy.[19]

Melanoma

TYPE O	TYPE A	TYPE B	TYPE AB	SECRETOR STATUS
Highest risk of skin cancer and malignant melanoma; lowest survival.	Best survival, especially women.	No known association	No known association	No known association

Only two studies have been conducted on blood type and skin cancer. In general, cancer of the skin appears to be strongly associated with Type O. Type O has also been found to have the highest frequency of malignant melanoma, and the lowest average time of survival after diagnosis. Type A tends to have the longest survival times, with this trend particularly strong in Type A women.[20]

Bone Cancers

TYPE O	TYPE A	TYPE B	TYPE AB	SECRETOR STATUS
Relatively low risk of bone cancer.	Slight risk of bone cancer.	Highest risk of bone cancer.	No known association	No known association

Bone cancers show the strongest association with Type B, and a weaker association with Type A.[21]

Leukemia and Hodgkin's Disease

TYPE O	TYPE A	TYPE B	TYPE AB	SECRETOR STATUS
Lower risk of leukemia, especially for women; higher risk of Hodgkin's disease.	Higher risk of leukemia, especially for A2.	No known association	No known association	No known association

Type As are more predisposed to leukemia. This trend is particularly strong for Type A2s. Being Type O appears to grant a degree of resistance, especially in acute leukemia. This protection is most noted among female Type Os. Because of this, some researchers have suggested that there might be a "sex-responsive" gene near the ABO gene locus on chromosome 9, which protects Type O women against acute leukemia. However, Hodgkin's disease has shown an association with Type O.[22]

Leukemia is usually characterized by a loss of blood type antigens. After complete remission, it is not uncommon for blood type to revert to normal and reappear on cells.

Your blood type is the key to healthy immune function. More than that, it is the key to survival, and always has been. When you live according to the genetic code your blood type writes into every cell of your body, you increase the chance that you—and your offspring—will be selected for survival.

SEVEN

Restoring Balance

Biological Harmony
and Detoxification

A T ITS MOST EFFECTIVE, THE BLOOD TYPE DIET AND Prescription produces deep, permanent changes in people, and its benefits can accrue for many years to come. But how do you know that a diet is working properly? Can you base a decision on how good (or bad) you feel by the second week? I've learned that very often what can appear to work in the short term might be completely ineffective, or even disastrous, in the long run. On the other hand, rapid change can be unsettling to the body and produce some uncomfortable side effects, but does that mean the program is not working? To take it one step further, how do you know when good things are going on inside you, and how do you know when bad things are going on inside you?

Most naturopaths would agree that those "bad things" are toxic in some form, although conventional medicine dismisses the idea of toxicity, other than the type of toxins that kill you in twenty-four hours or less. To most, the idea that a person's interior ecosystem could be toxic is remote. Yet in my own probably conservative estimate, 70 percent of all the inflammatory, digestive, or stress-related illnesses I see in my practice involve some sort of toxic imbalance.

So, that raises another question: How do you know—before it is too late—that something is toxic? Well, actually, most of the time you don't. I remember once hearing a story about miners in the early part of the century. Since they lacked a means of measuring toxic gases, they didn't know when the gases were starting to build to a dangerous level. Many men were overcome before they even knew what was happening to them. The miners began taking a caged canary into the mines with them to give a forewarning that dangerous toxic gases were building up as they worked. If the bird keeled over, it was time to get out of the mine and head for the surface.

This is why, for two generations, the D'Adamos have viewed the Blood Type Diet as a tool for detoxification and have always been interested in studying its effects in that regard.

How Are You Doing?
The Indican Test

BY MATCHING your dietary protein sources to your blood type physiology you can cut down on the level of unabsorbed proteins left in the digestive tract and their toxic byproducts. Also, by cutting back on lectin-containing foods reactive with your blood type antigen and developing a proper balance of flora in the intestinal tract, you're paving the path to greater vitality and better immune system response. By the end of this chapter, I think you will agree that the long-term results of factoring these choices into a life plan can be nothing short of miraculous—limiting your chances of developing a wide variety of chronic diseases and disabilities.

For years I've used a procedure called the urinary indican, or Obermeyer Test, to measure the level of certain proteins linked to bowel toxicity.[1] I run the test, at some time or another, on virtually all of my patients. It is one of several ways to chart whether or not the patient's diet is working properly. The test measures the amount of indican in a sample drawn from the first urine passed in the morning. Elevated levels of indican in the urine usually result from the unwanted conversion of tryptophan into indol by bacteria in the upper intestines. In a healthy system, the residual levels of acid in the stomach act as a barrier to bacteria entering the upper intestines, though some forms are thought to pass quite easily. Bacteria may also enter the lower intestines from the colon, but they do not typically inhabit the upper intestines.

In a sick system, low stomach acid does not serve as an effective bar-

> **• FROM THE BLOOD TYPE OUTCOME REGISTRY •**
>
> *Marie L.*
> *Type A*
> *Middle-aged female*
> *Improved: Digestive/immune problems*
>
> "I was a patient of yours about eight years ago. After a year of coming to you and following your diet, I left thinking you were the craziest person with the craziest ideas I ever heard. At the time, I was premenopausal, a little hysterical, and not resigned to following orders or being scared to death of cancer. I have since seen two other holistic physicans, and finally, on my own accord, decided that I was meant to be a vegetarian (I am an A+, secretor, A2 blood type). I follow your diet fairly religiously. Somehow, at age fifty-five, with half of the females I know having breast cancer (I'm fine) or the other half looking like fat bloated cows on Premarin, I'm proud to say that I am not taking hormones. I'm doing okay with a vegetarian diet, soy products, lots of vegetables, fruits, and hardly any animal protein, except three or four fish meals a week. I don't have any more allergies, and I am no longer depressed from hormones out of whack. I apologize for thinking you were a crazy man."

rier to bacteria, which can pass through and colonize the upper intestine. The low stomach acid also does not completely break down proteins, which serve as a food source for the bacteria. The incomplete proteins attract more bacteria from the lower intestines. The putrefaction of these undigested protein residues produce the indoles, which are then absorbed through the bloodstream and eliminated as indican, excreted with the urine.

So, from the level of indican in the urine we can gauge the levels of indols in the intestines, which is the real problem. Because of this, the indican count is an indirect measurement of one type of intestinal toxicity.

Why is the urinary indican measurement so closely related to the Blood Type Diet? When you eat right for your type, you better match the grade of fuel you are burning in your specific engine. Think of a car's carburetor. If there is too much fuel and not enough air, the mix burns "dirty" leaving soot and other sludge behind. In the same way, if we don't efficiently absorb and metabolize our food, we leave behind incompletely digested fats and proteins. Eventually, they will be eliminated, but not before they disrupt the balance of good bacteria in the intestines. The fallout of malabsorption shows up on your indican. If you had a high urinary indican count, you'd find that following the Blood Type Diet would effectively lower it, much like a detergent gasoline will gradually clean out a fouled carburetor.

At my clinic we routinely run a urinary indican on all new patients. About one in three have elevated levels indicating bowel toxicity. Many Type O vegetarians with high-starch diets show high indican levels because there are so many lectins found in grains. Type As who favor high-protein diets will often have high indican levels as a result of an incomplete breakdown of animal protein. I often see Type Bs, with lectin-heavy diets that include chicken, corn, and buckwheat, also showing high indican levels.

It has become clear at my clinic, and with the other physicians who use the Blood Type program in their practices, that diligent adherence to the correct diet for a patient's blood type soon drops the level of indicans to indiscernible amounts, which is good, because high indole levels can be very bad for you. Left unchecked, high levels of indicans can contribute to significant health issues in both direct and indirect ways. Perhaps that explains why of all the aphorisms of Hippocrates, his primary advice to all physicians was "First, cleanse the bowels."

For example, indols and indican have proven to be a carcinogenic enabler, enhancing the carcinogenic qualities of cancer-causing chemicals. High levels of urinary indican also reveal that sizable quantities of protein are being lost in the intestinal tract, instead of being broken down and metabolized properly.

Polyamines:
A New Twist on Toxicity

WHILE I WAS A STUDENT at Bastyr University in the 1980s, I discussed the concept of detoxification with one of my teachers, Edward Madison. Dr. Madison felt that if we were to begin to scientifically quantify a concept as broad as toxicity, we would have to identify the chemicals that were responsible for producing a toxic state. In Dr. Madison's opinion, indoles qualified as a viable toxin, in addition to other chemicals commonly found in the intestines, such as putrescine, spermidine, and cadaverine.

A few years ago, as I was scanning the literature for data on dietary lectins, I once again came upon those descriptive titles. They belonged to a class of chemicals called polyamines. The polyamines are proteins called biogenic amines and are present in low concentrations in all human, animal, and plant cells. Your body's organs require polyamines for their growth, renewal, and metabolism. Proper cell development depends on polyamines, which have a profound stabilizing effect on a cell's DNA. They are also critical to the healthy function of the nervous system. Young children need polyamines for growth, and they manufacture enormous amounts of polyamines—far more than adults.

Many dietary lectins, in addition to being blood type specific, have also been shown to be potent inducers of polyamine production in the gut. This is probably the result of the intestinal cells synthesizing large amounts of polyamines in an effort to repair the damage to the microvilli caused by the lectins.[2]

Paradoxically, lectins can actually lower the total levels of polyamines in the body, producing enough disturbance to the gut wall to cause the cells of the intestinal lining to begin sequestering any and all polyamines they can find, to speed repair, thereby lowering the total level of polyamines available for use by other tissues in the body. This is one possible reason why vegan-raised children tend to be smaller on average than comparable omnivores. The high lectin content of a typical grain-based vegan diet can cause the intestinal cells to sequester enough polyamines to actually deprive other tissues of needed polyamines, thereby stunting growth of tissues like the child's bones and muscles.

Many lectins cause unhealthy growth in the size of certain organs, including the liver, pancreas, and spleen. These organ enlargements are the result of a huge influx of polyamines into the organs. For example, wheat germ lectin induces significant polyamine production. Incorporating wheat germ lectin into the diet of lab animals reduced the digestibility and utilization of dietary proteins and significantly slowed the growth of the test animals. It also induced extensive polyamine-dependent growth in the pancreas and the small bowel tissue.[3] These same effects have been shown to occur with several bean and legume lectins as well. It is not unrealistic to assume that the stimulatory effects of wheat germ lectin on polyamine synthesis, coupled with the lectin's ability to mimic the actions of insulin, account for undesirable weight gain in many Type Os and Type Bs who overconsume it.

Polyamine control through diet is one more issue of balance in nature: We need enough polyamines to help growth and healing, but not so much as to slow down our immune systems and change the metabolism of our tissues. Following the Blood Type Diet allows you to control the intake of food lectins that would otherwise increase levels of polyamines in your intestines.

• FROM THE BLOOD TYPE OUTCOME REGISTRY •

Amelia K.
Type B
Middle-aged female
Improved: Digestive/immunity/energy

"I've followed the Blood Type B program in its broadest outlines for more than a year now. Principally, I've eliminated chicken, corn products, and most legumes from my diet, and have done what I can to avoid the 'avoid list' foods for my type. The most exciting result is an improvement in my immunity. I haven't had a cold or even a sniffle since I started the diet. In the past, I would have had at least three serious colds in this length of time. I've begun to feel like Wonder Woman when it comes to fending off the little bugs that go around! Secondly, I've seen a tremendous upsurge in energy and sense of well-being. I didn't realize until I started getting enough protein, how protein-deprived I must have been from years of trying to do the 'healthy' thing and avoid meat. Finally, I credit the diet with an overall change in my body chemistry that has allowed me to moderate my disordered eating and slowly begin to lose weight."

Polyamines in Your Food

Biochemistry textbooks often refer to polyamines as "dead flesh" proteins. When living tissue is shocked, or dies, its protein structure cracks open. Bacteria or enzymes contained in the food itself subsequently convert many of the protein fragments into polyamines. This is why polyamines are found in very high amounts in the tissues of severely injured trauma patients and in food products whose texture and taste has been permanently altered—shocked by excessive processing such as rapid freezing. Though some advocates of universal vegetarianism use polyamines as a justification for avoiding meat and seafood, polyamines are found as abundantly in vegetables, grains, fruits, and sprouts as they are in animal foods. And often, if they're not found in plant foods per se, they are produced by the body in response to the lectins contained in many plants, grains, and legumes.

Polyamines are typically found in fermented foods like cheese beer, sauerkraut, and yeast extracts. They are also found in processed foods, where canning or freezing has "shocked" the structural integrity of the tissues. Most aged or sharp cheeses are very high in putrescine. Vegetables such as potatoes, canned and frozen vegetables (other than green vegetables), and certain fruit, such as oranges and tangerines, can have very high concentrations of putrescine. Fermented soy sauce (containing wheat) is also a rich source of polyamines, particularly putrescine. Shrimp, especially the packaged and frozen kind, has high levels of putrescine. Mature cheeses, fermented soybeans, fermented tea, Japanese sake, domestic mushrooms, potatoes, and fresh bread are high sources

---

▪ **FROM THE BLOOD TYPE OUTCOME REGISTRY** ▪

Phillip N.
Type B
Middle-aged male
Improved: Digestive/immune

"For the past couple of years I had been struggling with what I felt was an immune deficiency, constantly battling recurring bouts of bronchitis, colds, flu, etc. Things finally reached a head when I was diagnosed with a hiatal hernia, and was told that the only way to control it was through medication. Seeking alternative methods of control, I visited an acupuncturist who recommended that I try this diet, if nothing else than to aid my digestion. Before reading this book, I was eating chicken about four to five times a week—roast chicken, chicken soup, chicken sandwiches . . . well, you get the idea. I thought it would be difficult to cut chicken out of my diet, but I started eating lamb in its place. While I didn't start this diet to lose weight, I lost about ten pounds in two weeks, and this is without following the recommended portion size. The best thing, however, is that my overall health has improved. I no longer go through the day feeling like a slug and people tell me that they can see the difference in my energy level. I am now down to a weight of 142 pounds, the same as when I graduated from college. This is without even attempting to cut back on calories. While I was never really considered 'fat,' people tell me that they can see a big difference in my weight. The most amazing part is that now my body feels that it can fight off common ailments. Used to be that when I started getting a cold, there was no way to avoid it. Then I'd be in bed for a couple of days. The last couple of times that I've started getting sick, I expected to wake up the next day feeling terrible. Amazingly, I would wake up and my symptoms had all but disappeared. Even with the results that I've gotten, people are still skeptical. But who cares, I say. I feel great and I won't have to worry about my belly hanging out when we go to Hawaii."

of spermidine. Cereals, canned or frozen vegetables, meat products, red meat, and poultry are high sources of spermine.

Are Your Polyamine Levels Too High?

There is no convenient direct method to assess polyamine levels, although you can use several other indirect measures as barometers of polyamine levels:

HIGH OR HIGH NORMAL SERUM ALBUMIN.   The liver manufactures albumin, an important protein used to rapidly transport other nutrients; it decreases production in times of environmental, nutritional, toxic, and trauma stress. Polaymine synthesis has a positive effect on albumin levels. Albumin is used to assess the long term nutritional status of patients since it reflects body protein stores for the last month. The reference range: 3.5 to 5.2 G/dL. Levels above 4.8 probably indicate higher polyamine levels, levels below 4 safe levels.

HIGH URINARY INDICAN.   The indican test gauges the level of indoles in the intestine by looking for the product of their metabolite, indican, in the urine. Large amounts of indican are usually a sign of high bacteria counts in the upper intestine. Large amounts of bacteria in the upper intestines produce large amounts of polyamines.

HALITOSIS (BAD BREATH).   If despite your best efforts (cleaning, flossing, etc.), you suffer with persistent bad breath, there is a good chance your polyamine levels are too high. Putrescene and one of the secondary polyamines, cadaverine, are responsible for much of the odor characteristic of halitosis. In addition, high levels of polyamines in the mouth inhibit the migration of white blood cells to areas of infection and inflammation.

GET A HEADACHE FROM FERMENTED FOOD.   Polyamines enhance the effect of histamine, usually present in histadine-containing foods, such as red wine. A common symptom of high levels of polyamines are headaches resulting from eating fermented foods such as wine, beer, or sauerkraut.

Signs of possible indican or polyamine excess by blood type:

TYPE O.   If you are Type O, monitor your intake of grain lectins; they will increase the production of polyamines by the cells of the intestines, pancreas, and liver. Grain lectins will also mimic the growth effects of insulin, which amplifies the growth-enhancing actions of polyamines.

Signs of toxicity in Type Os

1. Excess inflammation, such as joint problems and pains of a nonspecific nature, such as fibromyalgia; menstrual difficulties
2. Difficulties losing weight, excess water retention (especially in Type O non-secretors)
3. Bowel problems: cramping, flatulence, and elimination difficulties
4. Fatigue, mental hyperactivity
5. Carbohydrate intolerance. Fatigue and "spacing out" after high-carb meals
6. High triglycerides

TYPE A.   If you are a Type A and overconsume animal products, the malabsorption that results from the incomplete breakdown of animal protein will serve as a very tempting source of amino acids for the intestinal bacteria. In gratitude for this free meal they will synthesize huge amounts of polyamines.

Signs of toxicity in Type As:

1. Skin problems, such as psoriasis, eczema, or acne
2. Headaches, typically dull frontal types that don't respond well to aspirin or acetaminophen
3. Cystic breasts
4. Mental agitation, poor stress-coping abilities
5. Stomach fermentation leading to halitosis (especially true of Type A non-secretors)
6. Hypoglycemia (low blood sugar)
7. High cholesterol
8. Odiferous stools

TYPES B AND AB.   There is an interesting link between arginine and blood type. Ornithine is often made from a more common amino acid, arginine. The gene for the enzyme that manufactures arginosuccinic acid, the precursor to arginine, happens to lie adjacent to the ABO gene on 9q34, and studies have shown their linkage to strongly correlate. Thus genetic elements of blood type expression influence the amount of arginine available for conversion into ornithine and subsequently into polyamines. Nitric oxide is also derived from arginine.[4] These linkages help explain why Type B and Type AB who possess the B antigen handle nitric oxide differently than the other blood types. These blood types are fairly sensitive to changes in nitric oxide levels, and they are adversely affected when polyamines rob the arginine supply from nitric oxide production.

Signs of toxicity in Type Bs and Type ABs:
1. Lack of libido (sex drive)
2. Circulatory insufficiency, such as cold hands and feet, blood pressure differences when standing or lying (orthostatic hypotension), hemorrhoids, varicose veins, and fatigue
3. Sensitivity to light (photophobia) and many fragrances
4. Stomach fermentation, halitosis (AB non-secretors typically)
5. Feeling of fullness and discomfort in the lower intestinal tract
6. Cystic breasts

As you'll see by reviewing the polyamine-rich foods, many of them are avoids for every blood type. Interestingly, many of the foods that block ODC and lower polyamines are also neutral or beneficial for all blood types. If you follow your specific Blood Type Diet, you can further reduce the level of polyamines in your intestines with proper lectin avoidance. Also beware of going beyond your blood type's nutritional capabilities. This is a good reason to eat as many organically grown foods as possible; chemicals, improper storage, and pollutants "stress" foods and raise their polyamine content.

Foods that Lower Polyamines and Indols

- LARCH ARABINOGALACTAN (ARA6):   Larch helps promote better balance in the intestinal tract, while also lowering the end-products of protein digestion, such as ammonia. Usable by all blood types.
- WALNUTS: Research shows that walnuts inhibit ODC. Usable by all blood types.
- GREEN TEA: Research shows that polyphenols in green tea inhibit ODC. Usable by all blood types.
- DARK BLUE, PURPLE, OR RED PIGMENTED FRUITS: These foods contain anthrocyanidins, antioxidants that research has shown inhibit ODC. Examples are elderberries, cherries, and blueberries. Most are neutral or beneficial for all blood types.
- POMEGRANATES, PLANTAINS, AND GUAVA: Inhibit ODC. *Blood Type Note:* Pomegranates should be avoided by Types AB and B. Plantains should be avoided by Types A and O.
- ONIONS, DILL, TARRAGON, BROCCOLI LEAVES, AND GARLIC: Are mildly antibacterial against many of the polyamine producing strains, while also slight inhibitors of ODC. Usable by all types.

- CURCUMIN AND TURMERIC: Common spices in Indian cooking and long in use by Ayurvedic practitioners, curcumin is a potent inhibitor of polyamine synthesis. Usable by all blood types.

Fight Fire with Fire:
The Probiotic Lifeline

IN 1910, WHEN A Russian biologist named Élie Metchnikoff, proposed that the best way to improve health and prolong life was to eliminate gastrointestinal toxicity, many in the medical establishment regarded him as a quack. Intestinal "cleansing" was something of a fad at the time, with restorative clinics and spas a favorite upper-crust getaway, and elixirs flooding the market. The medical establishment, pathologically suspicious of any theory that did not bear its imprimatur, discounted Metchnikoff's idea along with all the rest—a real shame, since it happened to be valid.

Metchnikoff coined the word "probiotic," meaning "in favor of life," to explain his premise that aging is a process mediated by chronic exposure to putrefactive intoxication caused by imbalances in intestinal bacteria. This process, he suggested, could be halted by the routine ingestion of lactic acid bacteria and their "cultured" food products.

Today, nearly a century later, it is widely accepted that "friendly" intestinal bacteria protect your cells, improve immune function, and have a positive effect on your ability to fully utilize the nutrients in the foods you eat. What often escapes notice is the key fact that your blood type antigens orchestrate the proper balance of friendly bacteria.[5]

As we discussed earlier, blood type antigens are prominently expressed in any part of your body that interacts with the outside world. If you're a secretor, they are also expressed in the mucus secretions that line and protect your digestive tract. What role do these blood type antigens play in the balance of intestinal flora? Bluntly put, they serve as "bug chow."

Your blood type antigens are complex sugars, which bacteria happen to be very fond of. Different blood type antigens are composed of different combinations of sugars, and bacteria are choosy. Many of the friendly bacteria, in effect, eat right for their type all of the time, by using your blood type as their preferred food supply. When there are enough of them, they will compete for food much more effectively than the more harmful forms (after all, they happen to *like* you) and will eventually crowd bad bacteria out. Proper strains of colon bacteria, matched to blood type, will metabolize the blood type antigens into short-chain fatty acids, which are very beneficial for the health of the colon.

Where does this "preference" come from? It is based on a concept known as adherence. Much like a key will only click into its preferred lock, bacteria will only adhere to certain configurations of sugars that form complementary attachment sites. While not all of the attachment sites for bacteria in your intestines and digestive tract are blood type specific, the process of attachment for many friendly (and unfriendly) bacteria is dictated by your blood type. In fact, almost 50 percent of all bacterial strains tested show some blood type specificity.

To give you an idea of the magnitude of the blood type influence on intestinal microflora, it has been estimated that someone with Blood Type B will have up to 50,000 times more strains of friendly bacteria than either Type A or O individuals. *That's* preference! (I've recently designed a line of blood type-specific probiotic formulas. These "D'Adamo 4 Your Type" supplements are available through North American Pharmacal, Appendix E, or at your local health food store.)

Your blood type antigen is sprinkled throughout your intestinal tract to attract particular types of healthy bacteria, in the same way you might sprinkle bird seed in your yard to attract particular kinds of birds.

The bottom line: stick to your prescription to maintain a clean and healthy internal environment.

PART THREE

The Live Right Prescriptions

EIGHT

The Key to Living Right

Making the Most of Your Live Right Prescription

Dear Dr. D'Adamo,

I want to report incredible success for my Type O son Peter, who is nine months old. Peter was born with a diaphragmatic hernia corrected five days after birth and again at five months. He is otherwise mentally and physically normal. He is a twin, and the other boy is doing fine. However, Peter was suffering from severe reflux for which medication (Cissapride, Zantac) did nothing.

Peter's diet primarily consisted of baby cereal, mixed with fruit, and very thick, as instructed by the hospital dietician. Within three days of taking him off cereal and feeding him meats and vegetables, he has gone from vomiting each and every meal two and three times, to keeping more than 75 percent of them down, the other 25 percent with a small vomit and then a successful re-feed. The last two days have seen no vomiting. The improvement was visible immediately.

I was told that surgery (fundoplication) would be the only option. I now believe and hope surgery is not needed. Thank you for changing Peter's life. You cannot imagine the change in this baby. I am so grateful that I heard of your book and had the good sense to buy it.

Yours gratefully,
Anne T.

Here resides the true measure of success. What more could we have hoped from the publication and subsequent popularity of *Eat Right 4 Your Type* than outcomes such as Peter's? His mother's instinct to look beyond what was being offered, to do some investigative research, led a nine-month-old boy out of what could have been an increasingly drastic series of missteps. Most important, Peter has overcome what might have become a chronic medical condition. I've often imagined how different the lives of so many of my patients would have been had they eaten correctly for their blood types from an early age. Unfortunately, by the time the majority of people seek treatment, they've usually been fighting uphill battles for a long time.

Fighting an uphill battle is a military euphemism, used to describe a *losing* battle. It's a fair description of what I see with people who have been dealing with chronic or severe conditions for a long time. They're tired. They come to me with compromised immune systems, metabolic imbalances, long-term digestive irregularities, lifetime struggles with obesity and diabetes—all the result of following diet and health regimens that are genetically incompatible with their systems. At nine months old, Peter and his twin brother have a chance of reaping a lifetime of advantages by eating right from the very start.

The Blood Type Prescriptions will help you make the necessary connections for yourself and your family. From the moment *Eat Right 4 Your Type* was published in January 1997, readers have been clamoring for *more* information, and a deeper understanding of the blood type dynamic. And that's just what we plan to offer here. These Prescriptions, along with the substantial scientific support material, are your complete family resource guide to understanding your blood type and its relationships.

Making the Most of This Book

YOU MAY BE A healthy person who wants to optimize your potential and increase your longevity. Perhaps you've been trying to find the solution to a vexing problem—such as a recent weight gain, difficult or painful periods, digestive disorders, chronic infections, or debilitating migraines. You may be in deeper trouble—suffering from a more severe or life-threatening condition. Whatever brings you to an interest in the blood type connection, you will receive some benefit from the investigation. Information cannot hurt you; only the absence of information can.

I've developed several principles that are essential to the search. Keeping them in mind will help you make the most of this book.

1. BE OPEN AND FLEXIBLE. The science of blood type is not one-dimensional. By its very nature, it's the study of differences, so it stands to reason that everything isn't going to always fit neatly into one of four categories. Remain open; be cautious. Don't end up merely replacing one rigid construct with another. Instead, plan to grow into this program gradually, experimenting with what works for your unique situation. You may be very excited about the Blood Type Diet and other prescriptions, but the key is balance.

As the popularity of *Eat Right 4 Your Type* began mounting, I became inundated with mail from panic-stricken dieters. They were micromanaging every morsel of food they put into their mouths. They feared that any deviation—a pinch of cinnamon, a pickle, a dab of mustard—would send armies of lectins marching through their bloodstreams, strewing agglutinated clumps of cells everywhere. This is the classic dieter's mentality—and it's counterproductive. The point isn't to live in fear that an errant food will "get" you. The point is to work toward a more synchronous balance between your genetic propensities and your overall diet and health practices. If you're generally healthy, you can afford to be flexible when the occasion demands it. I am a Type A who happens to like tofu. I've eaten it my entire life. But, about once a year, I get a terrible craving for one of my wife Martha's old family recipe favorites: stuffed cabbage with ground meat. And I enjoy every bite of it.

I also get a great deal of mail from people who are having a problem with one or another of the recommended foods—Type As who can't tolerate peanuts, Type Os who won't eat red meat, Type Bs who can't live without chicken; pretty much what you'd expect. There are always variations; it's our ability to understand and deal with those variations that allows us to take some control. That is one thing we will attempt to do here.

2. BE SKEPTICAL OF REDUCTIONIST CONCLUSIONS. The association between blood type and disease, which we'll explore, is not a simple matter of cause and effect. Take heart disease as an example. You can have heart disease whether you're Type O, A, B, or AB. What alters is the road you travel to get there, and the method by which you become well. Most cases of chronic disease are multifactoral, meaning that there is more than one way to develop them. The priceless asset of using the blood type and disease correlations lie in their ability to help predict which factors present the greatest risk for you.

The question of what constitutes risk factors, and how seriously you should gauge them, is confusing to many people, and for good reason.

The language of conventional medicine seems to imply that there is a direct relationship between a risk factor and a disease. Cause and effect—such as "Smoking causes cancer," or "Stress causes high blood pressure."

When we talk about blood type–related risk factors, we are not saying that being a particular blood type *in itself* creates a higher risk factor for certain diseases. Only that, in combination with other factors, like the wrong diet, stress, or environmental conditions, there may be an increased risk for developing a certain disease. In immeasurable increments, this risk factor may increase a lot, or it may increase a little. Be wary of claims that "meat consumption increases toxicity," or "all carbohydrates turn into fat." They are overly simplistic, and a dieter's compliance is often based on fear, which is a terrible reason to do something.

Our knowledge of the mechanisms surrounding blood type also underscore another important keynote concerning risk factors. Risk factors may be genetic: they're not *generic*. Current medical science tends toward a "one-risk-factor-fits-all" mentality, which does not account for the variations that are in plain sight.

The science of blood type provides an opportunity to look at things from another perspective. When we apply the blood type connection to the physiology of a particular disease, we are able to open up a fresh investigation. We can examine risk factors in a new context, calculate the variations in human physiology, and formulate treatments that go right to the heart of the susceptibility.

To maximize the effectiveness of your blood type prescription, you need to educate yourself. Learn everything you can about the variables that make up your individual profile—blood type, secretor status, family history, medical conditions, and lifestyle. Always be suspicious about any declaration that is deemed to be true for everyone.

3. BE YOUR OWN INVESTIGATOR. How do you know something is true? What constitutes scientific proof? That's a question that has some urgency when you're embarking on a new course of diet and health. Not only do you need to know that blood type science has validity, but you may need to convince your primary care physician or other medical providers as well. To help you convince them, I've provided a substantial list of references, based on some 1,200 scientific study articles (40 percent of which were reported in the past three years.) These articles illuminate various pieces of the blood type puzzle,

> *Are you interested in participating in the Blood Type Registry? Go to www.dadamo.com.*

based on clinical and laboratory testing in animals and humans, as well as sophisticated analyses of predominant characteristics according to blood type. In addition, you will find throughout the book the results of my three-year Blood Type Outcome Registry, which has been developed through my Web site to measure the effects of the Blood Type Diet. The 2,330 respondents culled from the registry for use in this book are backed by medical records and other evidence. They are classified as:

Blood Type Diet Outcome Registry
Total: 2,330
Gender
Male: 546
Female: 1,784
Age
Pediatric: 85
Adolescent: 71
Young Adult: 666
Middle Aged: 1,411
Geriatric: 97
Blood Type
Type O: 1,209
Type A: 724
Type B: 318
Type AB: 79

Each of the respondent's outcomes fits into one of the following categories:

- Energy/well-being
- Weight loss
- Digestive/eliminative
- Immunologic/cancer
- Muscular/skeletal
- Cardiopulmonary
- Hormonal/reproductive
- Neuro/psychological

While this does not constitute an "official" study, it is clinical and anecdotal support for the premises of the Blood Type Diet. In addition, I think you'll find the stories of many of the participants fascinating, encouraging, and instructive.

As you absorb the information in this book, please employ your own rigorous truth detector. I still think the best starting point in determining the validity of a theory is to find out if it works for you. The science of blood type provides an opportunity to look at things from another perspective. When we apply the blood type connection to the physiology of a particular disease, or a certain lifestyle factor, we are able to open up a fresh investigation. We can examine risk factors in a new context, calculate the variations in human physiology, and formulate treatments that go right to the heart of the susceptibility.

4. GIVE IT TIME.   Chronic illness can take decades to develop. Any system that promises quick and effortless improvement should be regarded with suspicion. The Blood Type System is not just a diet. It is a blueprint for a lifestyle.

5. DON'T ASSUME BLOOD TYPE WILL DO ALL THE WORK. You can follow every blood type prescription in this book, but if you work in a carcinogenic environment, you might still get cancer. If you live in a situation where there's domestic violence, you will still suffer the physical and psychological consequences. If your shoes are too tight, your feet will hurt. The point is, take care of yourself—your *whole* self. There are practical strategies that make sense for everyone, regardless of blood type. The first step in any health program is to develop a screening schedule. The schedule on page 117 is the standard recommendation for all blood types. In addition, an annual checkup and regular dental exams and cleaning are fundamental to good health.

The Blood Type Prescriptions

IN THE NEXT four chapters, you will find detailed prescriptions for each blood type. Here is an explanation of the contents:

The Blood Type Profile

YOUR PROFILE: A summary of the primary identifying features of your blood type.

THE HEALTH RISK PROFILE: A demonstration of how your blood type characteristics are manifested in measurable tendencies, and how these tendencies can lead to disease.

Suggested Screening Schedule

TEST	PURPOSE	SCHEDULE
Salivary Secretor Test	Determine secretor status.	Once in a lifetime
Urinary Indican	Detect signs of toxicity-indicans and polyamines risk factors for all poor health conditions.	One to two times a year.
Blood Test	Screen for: blood count, serum albumin, serum cholesterol, triglycerides, blood sugar, iron, hormonal levels.	Once a year. More often if you have any of the following conditions: diabetes, thyroid disease, anemia, high cholesterol, high triglycerides, HIV, cancer.
Bioelectrical Impedence Analysis	Measures muscle mass vs. fat; Presence of intracellular water.	One to two times a year.
EKG	Measures heart activity.	Once a year. More often if you have a heart condition.
Blood Pressure	Measures systolic and diastolic pressure.	Once a year. More often (even daily, with a home monitor) if you have hypertension.
Breast Exam (women)	Detect abnormalities in breast tissue.	• Self exam once a month after menstrual period. • Physician exam once a year.
Mammography (women)	X-ray that detects abnormalities in the breast not otherwise detectable.	• Baseline between ages 35–40. • Every year or two between 40–50. • Annually after 50.
Sigmoidoscopy	Examination of the rectum and last part of the large intestine to check for benign growths or colorectal cancer.	Annually after age 40. Colonoscopy after 50.
Prostate (men)	Blood test and rectal exam to detect early signs of prostate cancer.	Annually after age 40.
Pelvic Exam and Pap Smear (women)	Detect abnormalities and signs of cervical cancer.	Once a year after the onset of menses.

The Blood Type Prescription

LIFESTYLE STRATEGIES: These strategies use what we know about the ways in which biological and chemical interactions differ according to blood type.

ADAPTED LIFESTYLE STRATEGIES: Practical advice for children, the elderly, and people in special circumstances, according to blood type.

EMOTIONAL EQUALIZERS: Strategies for stress management and avoiding the mind-body complications associated with your blood type.

THE TWO-TIER DIET: A more advanced diet plan than the one appearing in *Eat Right 4 Your Type*, this two-tier system offers a way to increase compliance according to your needs. It also provides special adjustments according to your secretor status.

> *Individualized Dietary Guidelines:* The basic blood type–specific guidelines for healthy individuals.

>> *Tier One: maximize health:* This level, along with neutral foods for general nutritional supplementation will suffice for most healthy individuals.
>> *Tier Two: overcome disease:* These adaptations are designed for those who are suffering from a chronic disease, or wish to follow the diet at a higher compliance level.

INDIVIDUALIZED THERAPIES FOR CHRONIC CONDITIONS: Depending on your blood type, you have an increased risk of certain medical conditions. Your Live Right Prescription will include many therapeutic recommendations for these conditions, in addition to the diet. Keep in mind, however, that just because your blood type places you at low risk for a condition, doesn't mean that lifestyle and genetic factors won't make you vulnerable. For that reason, I've supplied the index below, so you can easily find advice on any condition—even if it doesn't appear in your own blood type prescription.

Therapy Index

The risk profiles and disease therapies are organized by blood type. However, you may suffer from a condition that is less common for your blood type. Below is an index of Individualized Therapies for Chronic Conditions, which appear in the prescription sections, along with the page numbers.

Digestion
Barrett's Esophagus, 220
Crohn's Disease, 165
Dental Disease, 128
Gastro-Esophageal Reflux Disease (GERD), 161
Gallbladder and Liver Disease, 222
Lactose Intolerance, 252
Ulcers, 162

Metabolism
Blood-Clotting Disorders, 170, 231
Syndrome X, 166, 276
Heart Disease, 230
High Cholesterol, 228
Obesity/Low Metabolism, 225

Immunity
Autoimmune Diseases, 285
Autoimmune Thyroid Disease, 172
Bacterial Infections, 281
Cancer, 232
Candida Infection, 171
Chronic Fatigue Syndrome (CFS), 286
E. Coli Infection, 281
Ear Infections, 222
Fibromyalgia, 283
Inflammatory Conditions, 173
Influenza, 282
Menopausal Symptoms, 230
Streptococcal Disease, 283
Kidney and Urinary Tract Infections, 281
Viral/Nervous System Disorders, 283

Miscellaneous
ADD/ADHD, 133, 248
Autism, 224
Depression, 131
Osteoporosis, 225
Smoking Cessation, 126

Live Right 4 Type O

CONTENTS

THE TYPE O PROFILE

THE TYPE O PRESCRIPTION

The Type O Profile

CARRYING HUMANITY'S dominant blood type forward into a twenty-first–century environment is a mixed blessing. The Type O ancestral prototype was a canny, aggressive predator. It was instinctual for Type O to strive for position, to leave the weak and feeble behind, in order for the majority to survive. These were the pragmatic, unyielding qualities that enabled the human race to prevail over the savage elements that surrounded it. A hostile environment breeds a clever survivor. Aspects of the Type O profile remain essential in every society to this day—leadership, extroversion, energy, and focus. At their very best, Type Os can be powerful and productive. Conversely, a Type O under a great deal of stress may demonstrate the extremes of these qualities. Good leadership can be inspiring and reassuring. Leadership that goes awry turns governance into a deadly game of kill or be killed, creating conditions that play badly in modern societies.

Type O produces high levels of catecholamines and low levels of MAO when stressed. These characteristics reflect the legacy of the Type O ancestry, enabling an immediate "fight or flight" instinct to take charge in times of danger. However, this finely tuned response to stress, so vital to the early Type Os, is not always so beneficial in modern times. The Type O stress response can cause bouts of excessive anger, temper tantrums, hyperactivity, and even create a severe enough chemical imbalance to bring about a manic episode. Since there is a powerful, synergistic relationship between the release of dopamine and palpable feelings of reward, reinforcement, and bliss, Type O is also more vulnerable to destructive behaviors when overly tired, angry, depressed, or bored. These include pathological gambling, sensation-seeking, risk-taking, substance abuse, and impulsivity.

Your imperative, as a modern-day Type O, is to harness the remarkable physiological strengths that are part of your genetic heritage. You are "wired" for efficiency, with your digestive, metabolic, and immune systems acting in concert to promote strength and endurance. When that wiring gets crossed—as a result of a poor diet, lack of exercise, unhealthy behaviors, or elevated stress levels—you are vulnerable to a series of negative metabolic effects. These include insulin resistance, sluggish thyroid activity, edema, and weight gain. And while your Type O immune system is generally hardy, offering a natural aversion to cancer, a systemic imbalance can lead to inflammation, arthritis, and allergies.

When you customize your life to your Type O strengths, you can reap the benefits of the best of your ancestry. Your genetic inheritance offers you the opportunity to be strong, lean, productive, energized, long-lived, and optimistic.

The Type O Prescription

THE TYPE O Prescription is a combination of dietary, behavioral, and environmental therapies to help you live right for your type:

- LIFESTYLE STRATEGIES to structure your life for health and longevity
- ADAPTED LIFESTYLE STRATEGIES for children, the elderly, and non-secretors

continued on page 124

Type O Health Risk Profile

CHARACTERISTICS	MANIFESTATIONS
MIND/BODY Tendency to build-up higher levels of catecholamines (noradrenaline and adrenaline) during stress, due to low levels of the elimination enzyme MAO	• Imbalance of the neuro-chemical, dopamine • Monotony avoidance leads to risky behavior • Tendency to express anger and aggression during stress • Overly emotional and hyperactive • Tendency to be "moody"—up one minute and down the next • Extroverted and controlling
DIGESTION Overproduction of stomach acid, more rapid production of pepsinogen after meals	• Supports efficient digestion of animal protein • Can trigger gastrointestinal discomfort
High levels of the enzyme intestinal alkaline phosphatase	• Promotes easy breakdown of fats • Offers added protection against coronary artery disease • Strengthens bones
H. pylori bacterium favors Type O antigen sugar	• Susceptibility to *H. pylori* infection • Increased inflammation
METABOLISM Low levels of blood-clotting factors	• "Thinner" blood • Bleeding disorders
Metabolism designed for efficient use of calories	• Poor utilization of carbohydrates • High carb diet results in edema, and increase in body fat • High carb diet raises triglyceride levels and promotes insulin resistance • High carb diet leads to hypothyroidism
IMMUNITY Manufactures high levels of anti-blood type (A and B) antigens	• Increases risk of autoimmune disease
Type O antigen is fucose sugar	• Allows adherence of lectin-like molecules that allow white cell migration
High antibody IgE levels	• Increases sensitivity to pollens
High antibody IgA levels	• Overly aggressive immune response

INCREASED RISKS	VARIATIONS
• Bipolar (manic-depressive) disease • Depression • Heart disease (if *Type A* personality) • Parkinson's disease • Schizophrenia • Substance abuse	CHILDREN: High catecholamine levels and dopamine imbalance are associated with hyperactivity
• Ulcers • Gastritis • Duodenitis	NON-SECRETOR: Carries additional risk
	SECRETOR: The highest levels of intestinal alkaline phosphatase
• Ulcers	NON-SECRETOR: Risk even higher in Type O non-secretors
• Stroke (caused by bleeding in the brain)	
• Low risk factors for diabetes and heart disease when metabolism is in a balanced state • High carb diets promote Syndrome X, a condition leading to heart disease	NON-SECRETOR: Higher risk of Syndrome X
• Inflammatory Bowel Disease	NON-SECRETOR: Risk even higher in Type O non-secretors
• Inflammatory conditions • Ulcers	NON-SECRETOR: More prone to generalized inflammation
• Respiratory allergies	NON-SECRETOR: Greater risk of respiratory problems, especially allergies
• Autoimmune disease, especially of the thyroid • Denture inflammation and plaque	NON-SECRETOR: Lower risk of increased IgA, but increased risk of dental problems

- EMOTIONAL EQUALIZERS and stress relievers
- SPECIALIZED DIET PLAN: Tier One for maximum health
- TARGETED DIET PLAN: Tier Two to overcome disease
- INDIVIDUALIZED THERAPIES for chronic conditions
- THERAPEUTIC SUPPLEMENT PROGRAM for extra support

Lifestyle Strategies

Keys for Type O

🔑 Develop a clear plan for goals and tasks—annual, monthly, weekly, daily—to avoid impulsivity.

🔑 Make lifestyle changes gradually, rather than trying to tackle everything at once.

🔑 Eat all meals, even snacks, seated at a table.

🔑 Chew slowly, and put your fork down between bites of food.

🔑 Avoid making big decisions or spending money when you're stressed.

🔑 Do something physical when you feel anxious.

🔑 Engage in forty-five to sixty minutes of aerobic exercise at least three times a week.

🔑 When you crave a pleasure-releasing substance (alcohol, tobacco, narcotics, sugar), do something physical.

The following are guidelines for building a lifestyle plan that will maximize the Type O health and longevity.

1. Eat Right for Strength and Balance

In addition to eating right for Type O, pay special attention to these guidelines for keeping stress levels in balance:

- Avoid caffeine and alcohol, especially when you're in stressful situations. Caffeine can be particularly harmful, because of its tendency to raise adrenaline and noradrenaline—already high for Type Os.
- If you start to crave wheat, eat some protein; the craving will *usually* go away.
- Don't undereat or skip meals, especially if you're expending a lot of energy in exercise. Food deprivation is a huge stress.
- Plan ahead to have foods on hand for a quick energy snack. This is especially important if you're on the go during the day. It's very difficult to find fast food that doesn't contain wheat.

2. Exercise for Emotional Balance

Type O benefits tremendously from brisk regular exercise that taxes the cardiovascular and muscular skeletal system. But the benefit derived surpasses the goal of physical fitness. Type O also derives the benefit of a well-toned chemical release system. The act of physical exercise releases a swarm of neurotransmitter activity that acts as a tonic for the entire system. A Type O who regularly exercises also has a better emotional response. You are more emotionally balanced as a result of well-regulated, efficient chemical transport systems. More than any other blood type, Type O relies on physical exercise to maintain physical health and emotional balance. Below is a list of exercises that are recommended for Type O, along with some general tips for making the most of your exercise program.

EXERCISE	DURATION	FREQUENCY
AEROBICS	40–60 minutes	3–4 x week
WEIGHT TRAINING	30–45 minutes	3–4 x week
RUNNING	40–45 minutes	3–4 x week
CALISTHENICS	30–45 minutes	3 x week
TREADMILL	30 minutes	3 x week
KICKBOXING	30–45 minutes	3 x week
CYCLING	30 minutes	3 x week
CONTACT SPORTS	60 minutes	2–3 x week
IN-LINE / ROLLER SKATING	30 minutes	2–3 x week

Tips: Maximize your exercise program

- If you are easily bored, choose two or three different exercises, and vary your routine.
- For the best results, engage in an aerobic activity for thirty to forty-five minutes, at least four times a week.
- Be sure to warm up, with stretching and flexibility moves, before you start your aerobic exercise.
- To achieve maximum cardiovascular benefits, work toward an elevated heart rate that is about 70 percent of your capacity. Once you reach the elevated rate, continue exercising to maintain that rate for twenty to thirty minutes.
- Finish each aerobic session with at least a five minute cooldown of stretching and relaxation moves.

To calculate your maximum heart rate and performance level:

1. Subtract your age from 220.
2. Multiply the difference by .70 (or .60 if you are over age sixty.)
   This is the high end of your performance.
3. Multiply the remainder by .50. This is the low end of your
   performance.

3. Stop Smoking.

Obviously, anyone who smokes should try to quit, regardless of blood type. However, Type Os often need special help. Many of my Type O patients who are smokers have a particularly difficult time kicking the habit. I suspect this is related to a dopamine imbalance. Smoking releases a chemical response that mimics pleasure and reward. Maladapted Type Os tend to be vulnerable to addictive, pleasure-seeking behaviors. By keeping your stress levels in check, you will have an easier time overcoming this habit. Here are some additional suggestions, suited to Type Os:

- Keep a journal to record your progress on a stop-smoking program. Record the benefits you experience from not smoking.
- Exercise vigorously to cut down on cravings
- Avoid situations that normally trigger the desire to smoke. Be especially wary of situations that cause anger, boredom, or depression.
- If you typically smoke after eating a meal, get up from the table immediately and brush your teeth.
- When you have the urge to smoke, perform this deep-breathing exercise:

  1. Inhale deeply through your nose.
  2. Slowly exhale through your mouth.
  3. Repeat four times.

- Find alternative "rewards" for when you need a lift.
- Discuss with your physician whether you are a candidate for smoking cessation patches (Habitrol), the smoking cessation pill (Zyban), or the nicotine inhaler.

ADAPTED LIFESTYLE STRATEGIES	TYPE O CHILDREN

Structure your Type O child's life to include these essential strategies for healthy growth, wellness, and diminished risk for disease.

Young Children

- Encourage independence and flexibility within daily routine.
- Emphasize social interaction on the peer level. Type O children tend to be natural leaders, and they thrive in preschool, playgroups, and other organized social settings.
- Plan an hour of active time every day—running, climbing, swimming, biking.
- Start introducing Type O Diet elements at an early age—for example, replacing cow's milk with healthy juices and using spelt instead of whole wheat flours.
- Make a point of giving praise and affirmation when your child accomplishes a goal. All kids need this, but your Type O child really thrives on attention and praise.
- Establish firm rules to deal with temper tantrums—time-outs, consequences—while teaching more positive ways of dealing wih anger. If your Type O child can learn anger management at a young age, he or she will be less likely to develop stress-related problems later.

Older Children

- Allow your child to take on responsibilities in the household.
- Nurture natural leadership abilities, and emphasize teamwork and team building.
- Encourage physically challenging group sports activities.
- Educate your child about the dangers of alcohol, tobacco, and drugs, while modeling positive behavior yourself. Type O tendency toward monotony avoidance can lead to risky behavior.
- Stay out of fast food restaurants. It's almost impossible to find wheat-free foods.
- Teach problem-solving as a way to manage anger and frustration.

Type O Vaccination

TYPE O KIDS.   Proceed with special care when a vaccination is recommended for your Type O child. Because of Type O's hyperactive immune system, you need to monitor the necessity of each vaccination, the delivery system used, and the potential side effects. Your child should receive the oral form of the polio vaccine, not the injected form, which is more potent. After your child has been vaccinated, watch closely for complications. These include: inflammation, joint pain, and fever. Don't give him or her Acetominophen, the most commonly prescribed OTC medication (Tylenol). Instead, use the Herb feverfew, which is derived from the chrysanthemum flower. *Dosage: 4 to 8 drops of liquid tincture mixed with juice every four hours.*

TYPE O MOMS-TO-BE. Type O pregnant women should avoid the flu vaccine—especially if your baby's father is Type A or Type AB. The flu vaccine will boost the presence of anti-A antibodies in your system, which can attack your fetus. Also take 3–4 grams fish oil capsules (DHA) daily.

ADAPTED LIFESTYLE STRATEGIES | TYPE O SENIORS

Mobility is a primary issue for seniors, and this is especially true for Type Os, who thrive on physical activity. Pay careful attention to the following strategies:

- Maintain a high-protein diet, using protein shakes as supplements, if you need to. Protein is the key for preventing arthritis and inflammatory conditions, which are problems for Type Os. It is also the key for maintaining healthy bones and muscle mass.
- If you have painful rheumatoid arthritis or inflammation, avoid using nonsteroidal anti-inflammatory drugs, such as ibuprofen and naprosin. These are known to cause peptic ulcers in Type O patients. Here you'll want to be 100 percent wheat- and corn-free.
- Stay active. It's very important that you continue an exercise program, even if it only involves taking a walk every day. Above all, think twice about undergoing elective surgery that might keep you off your feet for a few days. Studies show that for the average elderly person, one week of hospitalization is equivalent to one year of lost activity.

Other Strategies for Type O Seniors:
- Denture stomatitis, an inflammation of the mouth that occurs in denture wearers, has been found to be most prevalent and severe in Type Os. One of the more common causes of dental stomatitis is infection with the parasite *Candida albicans*. If you wear den-

tures, be sure to follow the recommendations on page 171 for preventing *Candida*.
- Supplement your Type O Diet with:
  Folic acid—400 micrograms for prevention of gum disease
  Calcium—1,000–1,200 milligrams for healthy bones
  Valerian—400 mg or in tea to relieve irritable bowel condition
  Menopausal Women: 40 milligrams black cohosh and maca root, for relief of symptoms

Emotional Equalizers

Keys
- Practice anger management techniques.
- Plan your weeks and days to minimize monotony. When Type Os get bored they tend to take unreasonable risks.
- Break up your work day with physical activity, especially if your job is sedentary. You'll feel more energized.
- Set up small "rewards" you can give yourself when you accomplish tasks.
- Stop smoking and avoid stimulants.
- Avoid MAO-inhibiting antidepressants.

For emotional health and avoidance of Type O–related mind-body imbalances, incorporate the following behaviors into your daily life.

1. Identify Your Tendencies
Studies show that so-called *"Type A Behavior"* is much more common in Type Os than in the other blood types.[1] We know that many of the disorders linked to blood type, such as duodenal ulcer and heart attacks, have possible psychosomatic components. One study focused on the relationship between blood types and various indicators of behavior patterns (such as *"Type A Behavior"* scores and anger ratings) in young patients who'd suffered early heart attacks. Type O patients scored significantly higher on *"Type A Behavior"* scales and related anger indicators than did Type A patients. Type B and Type AB patients responded on several scales between Type O and Type A.

They described persons with *"Type A Behavior"* as having an intense, competitive desire for achievement; an exaggerated sense of urgency; afraid of the passage of time; always in a hurry; with frequent aggression or hostility toward others. These people often try to do two things at once and believe that the only way to get something done right is to do it themselves. They're often fast-talking, fast-thinking, and abrupt. They are typically too busy to notice the things around them, like the color of the wallpaper in the dining room, or to be interested in things of beauty, such as art, music, or sunsets.

Evaluate whether or not you fit any of the personality characteristics that researchers suggest are more typical for your blood type—in particular, the so-called *"Type A Behaviors,"* which Type Os have a tendency to manifest. In a state of emotional imbalance, your natural leadership qualities and extroverted personality can lead to a state of anger, frustration, and aggression. It is not my intention to label you. Your personality is quite individual, and genetic predispositions only form a small part of the picture. You might consider, though, what this data means to you. In my experience, these prototypical behaviors tend to emerge most strikingly when resistance is low and stress is high.

2. Employ Anger Management Strategies

If you have the Type O tendency toward *"Type A Behavior,"* these strategies can help you manage your anger:

- When you start to feel as if you can't control your anger in a situation, take a time-out. Go for a walk around the block, get a drink of water, do aerobic exercises, or pound a pillow. Wait for your anger to dissipate before you tackle the problem.
- Express yourself in writing. If you are angry with another person, don't confront him or her immediately. Instead, sit down and write a letter detailing your feelings. You'll find that it is impossible to stay in a physical state of anger when you are writing.
- Identify your anger triggers. Examine whether they result from unrealistic expectations, attitudes learned in childhood, or mistaken ideas about the motivations of others.
- Focus on how *you* feel, not on how the other person is behaving. Example: Instead of saying, "You ruined everything," say, "I am so disappointed." This will give you more power in a situation.
- Find an activity that is your personal equivalent of counting to ten.
- Learn problem-solving techniques. Anger is most often the result of feeling a loss of control. When you are intent on solving a problem, rather than exploding in a helpless rage, your stress hormones will remain steady.
- Make sure to have a person or persons you can talk to when you're frustrated or angry. The extroverted Type O releases stress by engaging in a supportive conversation.

3. Use Adaptogens to Improve Your Stress Response

The term "adaptogen" has been used to categorize plants that improve the nonspecific response to stress. Many of these plants have a bidirectional or normalizing influence on your physiology—if something is too low, they bring it up; too high, they bring it down. The following adaptogens are well-suited for Type O.

RHODIOLA ROSEA AND RHODIOLA SP.   In addition to its anti-stress activity, *Rhodiola* has a significant ability to prevent stress-induced catecholamine activity in the heart and promote stable heart contractility. *Rhodiola* can also prevent abnormalities in cardiopulmonary function when you're at high altitudes

PLANT STEROLS AND STEROLINS.   Plant sterols and sterolins are phytochemicals generally described as plant "fats," which are chemically very similar to cholesterol, but appear to have adaptogenic biological activity. They prevent immune system imbalances found during stress and help to normalize stress levels. The proprietary name of these plant "fats" is "Moducare." I have also found it to be very useful in preventing inflammatory conditions in Type Os.

B VITAMINS.   Type Os generally need an ample supply of B vitamins to promote a balanced stress response. Of particular importance are B_1, *pantethine*, and B_6. When you're dealing with stress, take them at levels several times the RDA.

LIPOIC ACID.   The antioxidant lipoic acid is important in catecholamine metabolism, making it beneficial for the Type O stress response.

The best action you can take to counter depression or manic-depressive illness is to follow the Type O diet, exercise, and lifestyle plans. Your goal is to balance your stress hormone levels, especially the catecholamines. In addition, several supplements can either help or hinder that process.

4. Avoid MAO Inhibitors/St. John's Wort

My Type O patients who take the herb St. John's wort (*Hypericum perforatum*) complain that it makes them feel very lethargic after one or two weeks, and they often report having "weird dreams." Although there has been some debate about whether St. John's wort is an MAO inhibitor, this debate stems from a poor reading of the available literature. The principle antidepressant part of St. John's wort probably doesn't inhibit MAO, although other components of the plant, principally the flavonols and xanthones, certainly do. These components specifically inhibit MAO-B, the type of MAO found on platelets. Since this enzyme is already low in Type Os, St. John's wort can worsen the condition. In addition, the anti-MAO effects of crude St. John's wort preparations can lower platelet MAO to a threshold where *"Type A Personality"* problems, such as impulsivity and sensation-seeking, worsen.

In addition, a little-known effect of St. John's wort is its ability to inhibit dopamine beta hydroxylase. Alcoholic extracts, which contain the whole plant and are probably the form most often purchased in health food stores, inhibit dopamine beta hydroxylase much more readily than pure hypericin. Inhibiting dopamine beta hydroxylase can have catastrophic effects for a Type O on the "high" dopamine cycle. There is a danger of increasing dopamine to levels of psychosis. (Remember, schizophrenia is associated with high dopamine levels).

Also avoid *kava-kava*—less well-known, but growing in popularity. Long used by native Pacific Islanders in a ritualistic drink, kava-kava is a tranquilizer that induces relaxation and promotes sleep. However, the kava-kava extracts commonly available in health food stores can significantly inhibit platelet MAO.

5. Use These Supplements for Neurochemical Balance

L-TYROSINE.   Boosting your levels of the amino acid L-tyrosine can increase dopamine concentrations in the brain. In one study, military cadets using a tyrosine-rich drink during a demanding military combat training course performed better on memory and tracking tasks than a comparable group supplied with a carbohydrate-rich drink. These findings suggest tyrosine may, in circumstances characterized by psychosocial and physical stress, reduce the effects of stress and fatigue on cognitive tasks. It has been my experience that L-tyrosine can be helpful for Type Os who suffer from depression.

5-HTP.   This serotonin precursor seems to work well for Type Os. It also raises dopamine levels. If you are depressed, have carbohydrate or food cravings, sleep problems, or are feeling generally sluggish, 5-HTP can be helpful—either alone, or in combination with L-tyrosine.

GLUTAMINE.   Glutamine is an amino acid that is transformed into the GABA class of neurotransmitters. It can be particularly helpful for Type Os with a sweet tooth. Mix 500 mg in a glass of water when you feel the need for a carbohydrate.

FOLIC ACID.   Most people will not respond well to pharmaceutical antidepressent drugs (Prozac, Zoloft) if they are deficient in this vitamin. Type Os who suffer from mood swings should always supplement with extra folic acid, along with other B-complex vitamins.

METHYLCOBALAMIN. 500 mg.

| SPECIAL STRATEGIES | YOUR TYPE O ADD/ADHD CHILD |

High catecholamine levels and dopamine imbalances have been associated with hyperactivity. In my clinic, I often treat Type O children who have been diagnosed with Attention Deficit Disorder (ADD) or Attention Deficit Hyperactivity Disorder (ADHD). Although these conditions are difficult to legitimately diagnose (and many physicians believe that they are overdiagnosed), the manifestations include overstimulation, inability to concentrate, mood swings, aggressive behavior, impulsivity, and periods of high energy followed by fatigue.

Traditionally, hyperactivity is treated with drugs such as Ritalin. However, drugs only treat the symptoms, not the problem, and they completely ignore the well-known underlying causes, including elevated stress hormones, autoimmune syndromes, and diet.

If your Type O child exhibits hyperactive behavior patterns, try these strategies:

- Feed your child according to the Type O diet. Emphasize high-quality protein foods over carbohydrates. Limit the amount of sugar your child eats and be more rigorous about eliminating "avoid" foods, such as wheat, potatoes, and corn.
- Make sure your child has the opportunity to develop athletic abilities. This is a piece of advice my father always gave to parents of Type O children, and it's consistent with what we know about the role exercise plays in stress reduction for Type Os. If team sports are difficult for your child, encourage solo activities, such as swimming, biking, running, or rope jumping.
- Research shows that many ADHD children also suffer from hypersensitivity and allergies, which are autoimmune problems. Typically, I find that Type Os with allergies are eating wheat-based diets. When wheat is replaced with high-protein alternatives, both the allergies and the hyperactivity improve dramatically.
- Give your child a supplement of folic acid and vitamin B_{12} (400 mcg daily). In conjunction with the Type O Diet and exercise program, I

have successfully treated hyperactivity in my young patients. These B vitamins are responsible for producing red and white blood cells. Feed your child these foods, which are rich in these vitamins:

> *Folic acid:* liver, green leafy vegetables, mushrooms, peas, beans, nuts
> B_{12}: beef, liver, lamb, poultry, fish

- Practice anger management strategies—time-out, pounding a pillow, playing a musical instrument—as alternatives to having a tantrum.
- Provide lots of positive reinforcement, which serves as a method of social reward and a self-esteem booster.
- Set manageable, short-term goals that provide frequent opportunities to experience success.

Type O Two-Tier Diet

The Two-Tier Diet is designed to offer a more individualized program. It has been my experience that some people do very well on the basic Tier One Diet—that is, a moderate degree of adherence to the primary beneficial and avoid foods, with heavy reliance on neutral foods for general nutritional supplementation. Others need a more rigid plan, especially if they suffer from chronic conditions. Adding the Tier Two Diet will increase the compliance to overcome disease and restore a state of well-being.

> SECRETOR or NON-SECRETOR?
> Before you start the diet, take the easy home saliva test to determine your secretor status. See page 358.

Your secretor status can influence your ability to fully digest and me-

---

BENEFICIAL: These foods possess components that enhance the metabolic, immune, or structural health of your blood type.

NEUTRAL: These foods usually have no direct benefit or harmful effect, based on your blood type, but many of them supply nutrients needed for a well-balanced diet.

AVOID: These foods contain components that are harmful for your blood type.

tabolize certain foods. For this reason, each food list contains a separate column of rankings for secretors and non-secretors. Although the majority of people are secretors and can safely follow the recommendations in the secretor column, the variations can make a big difference if you are among the approximately 20 percent who are non-secretors.

In rare cases, your Rh and MN status may influence a food ranking. Those distinctions are listed as variants in the appropriate chart.

The Blood Type Diet Tier System

Tier One: Maximize Health
Make these choices as soon as possible to maximize your health. Using Tier One choices in combination with neutral foods for general nutritional supplementation will suffice for most healthy individuals.

Tier Two: Overcome Disease
Add these choices if you are suffering from a chronic disease or wish to follow the diet at a higher compliance level. If you are adhering to the Tier Two Diet, use caution when you incorporate neutral foods for general nutritional supplementation.

Individualized Dietary Guidelines

If you are a healthy Type O, the Tier One Diet will provide the combination of foods you need for good health. To make the most of it, pay special attention to these guidelines:

Keys

- Eat small to moderate portions of high-quality, lean, organic meat several times a week for strength, energy, and efficient metabolism. Meat should be prepared medium to rare for the best health effects. If you charbroil or cook meat well-done, use a marinade composed of beneficial ingredients, such as cherry juice, lemon juice, spices, and herbs.
- Include regular portions of richly oiled cold-water fish. Fish oils can help counter inflammatory conditions, improve thyroid function, and boost your metabolism.
- Consume little or no dairy foods. They are difficult for you to digest.
- Eliminate wheat and wheat-based products from your diet. They usually cause more problems than any other food for Type Os. If you have digestive or weight problems, also eliminate oats.

🗝 Limit your intake of beans, as they are not a particularly good protein source for Type Os.

🗝 Eat lots of beneficial fruits and vegetables.

🗝 If you need a daily dose of caffeine, replace coffee with green tea. It isn't acidic and has substantially less caffeine than a cup of coffee.

🗝 Use beneficial and neutral nuts and dried fruits for snacks.

Type O Dietary Strategies

These strategies are designed to help the healthy Type O avoid the problems that can arise from your specific neurological, digestive, metabolic, and immune makeup.

Control High Stomach Acid Levels

TAKE DGL (DE-GLYCYRRHIZINATED) LICORICE. DGL increases secretin, a hormone that inhibits stomach acid production. Licorice can also inhibit the release of the hormone gastrin, which acts to stimulate stomach acid production. This form of licorice also has an ability to promote the healthy production of the mucus layer that protects your stomach cells from being damaged by acid. DGL licorice is widely available in health food stores as a pleasant tasting powder or in lozenge form. Avoid crude licorice preparations, as they contain a component of the plant that can cause elevated blood pressure. This component has been removed in DGL.

SUPPLEMENT WITH SLIPPERY ELM BARK (*Ulmus rubra*). It promotes the health of the membranes of the stomach, intestine, and urinary tract. Slippery elm bark is also soothing to intestinal tissue and encourages lactobacilli growth.

USE GINGER RHIZOME. It contains anti-inflamatory, anti-ulcer, and antioxidant compounds and promotes gastric motility.

USE CLOVE FRUIT. It is a rich source of eugenol, an anti-inflammatory and anti-ulcer compound. Clove fruit also helps prevent Candida infection.

SUPPLEMENT WITH TURMERIC ROOT. Turmeric has many beneficial properties. It contains powerful antioxidant, anticarcinogenic, and anti-inflammatory compounds, decreases ornithine decarboxylase activity, promotes gastric integrity, increases mucin production, offers gastroprotective effects, promotes secretion of digestive enzymes, and improves liver function.

USE CAYENNE FRUIT. It protects your digestive tract from toxins and contains anti-inflammatory, anti-ulcer, and antioxidant compounds.

DRINK CARBONATED MINERAL WATER.   A glass of lukewarm or room temperature carbonated mineral water can help decrease gastrin production and stomach acid production. It can also decrease appetite.

AVOID MILK, BEER, ALCOHOL, AND WHITE WINE.   These can increase gastrin production. Red wine is okay, in moderation, better for non-secretors.

AVOID COFFEE AND BLACK TEA.   All forms of roasted coffee (decaffeinated or not) have been shown to increase gastrin production. Black tea has been shown to increase stomach acid secretion.

AVOID ACID-STIMULATING FOODS,   such as oranges, tangerines, and strawberries. Drink vegetable juice in preference to fruit juice.

▪ FROM THE BLOOD TYPE OUTCOME REGISTRY ▪

Karen T.
Type O
Middle-aged female
Improved: Multiple food intolerances

"I had reached the point where it seemed that all food was poisonous to me. I was very ill at least twice a day, lived on Immodium to get through a day at work. Avoided activities away from my home. I was also being treated for several health problems with traditional medicine. My gallbladder was removed, my high blood pressure was out of control, and I had a minimally functioning thyroid. Within a week of changing to the Type O diet, I noticed significant improvement. All intestinal pain was eliminated. My high blood pressure and low thyroid activity were finally able to be regulated. I lost some weight, but the big change was in my general well-being and energy levels. People who had known me previously and had watched my daily struggle to find something to eat that wouldn't half kill me and were aware of my general weakness, fatigue, and extremely low energy levels were dumbfounded. I became like a teenager again. I am a believer in eating right for your type and the evidence in my own life of its benefits cannot be questioned. I have been fortunate to also have found a doctor and chiropractor who both believe that this diet is very beneficial to my health and support me in my endeavors. I am now placing my thirteen-year-old daughter on it and anticipate excellent results."

Prevent Lectin Damage

AVOID FOODS THAT ARE TYPE O RED FLAGS.   The worst are: wheat (wheat germ agglutinin)

corn
kidney beans
navy beans
lentils
peanuts
potatoes

Type Os can help block the actions of dietary lectins by using polysaccharide sacrificial molecules, such as those found in :

- NAG (N-Acetylglucosamine)
- Fucus vesiculosis—kelp
- Laminaria (seaweed)
- Larch arabinogalactan

Meat and Poultry

PROTEIN IS critical for Type Os. Inadequate protein intake can seriously interfere with your ability to metabolize fats, leading to diabetes and cardiovascular problems. For Type Os, high-quality protein is one of the best preventive measures to take against obesity. Protein increases active tissue mass, which increases the Basal Metabolic Rate, which allows for excess fat to be burned off. In general, Type O nonsecretors should lean even more toward a paleolithic, hunter-gatherer diet.

Choose only the best quality, chemical- and pesticide-free, low-fat meats.

BLOOD TYPE O: MEATS AND POULTRY			
Portion: 4–6 oz. (men); 2–5 oz. (women and children)			
	African	Caucasian	Asian
Secretor	6–9	6–9	6–9
Non-Secretor	7–12	7–12	7–11
Rh–	Increase by 1–2 servings weekly		
	Times per week		

Tier One

FOOD	TYPE O SECRETOR	TYPE O NON-SECRETOR
Bacon/ham/pork	Avoid	Avoid
Beef	Beneficial	Beneficial
Buffalo	Beneficial	Beneficial
Lamb	Beneficial	Neutral
Liver (calf)	Beneficial	Neutral
Mutton	Beneficial	Beneficial
Quail	Avoid	Neutral
Turtle	Avoid	Neutral
Veal	Beneficial	Beneficial
Venison	Beneficial	Beneficial

Tier Two

FOOD	TYPE O SECRETOR	TYPE O NON-SECRETOR
Heart/sweetbreads	Beneficial	Beneficial

Neutral: General Nutritional Supplementation

FOOD	TYPE O SECRETOR	TYPE O NON-SECRETOR
Chicken	Neutral	Neutral
Cornish hens	Neutral	Neutral
Duck	Neutral	Neutral
Goat	Neutral	Neutral
Goose	Neutral	Neutral
Grouse	Neutral	Neutral
Guinea hen	Neutral	Neutral
Horse	Neutral	Neutral
Ostrich	Neutral	Beneficial
Partridge	Neutral	Beneficial
Pheasant	Neutral	Beneficial
Rabbit	Neutral	Beneficial
Squab	Neutral	Beneficial
Squirrel	Neutral	Neutral
Turkey	Neutral	Neutral

Fish and Seafood

FISH AND SEAFOOD represent a secondary source of protein for Type Os. In general, many of the seafood avoids for Type O have to do with lectins or polyamines commonly found in the foods. Many of the lectin-containing fish and seafood appear to impact Type O non-secretors more than secretors, perhaps because of their lower levels of gut-protecting antibodies. Avoid using frozen fish, as the content of polyamines in it is much higher than fresh.

BLOOD TYPE O: FISH AND SEAFOOD			
Portion: 4–6 oz. (men); 2–5 oz. (women and children)			
	African	**Caucasian**	**Asian**
Secretor	2–4	3–5	2–5
Non-Secretor	2–5	4–5	4–5
Rh–	Increase by 2 servings weekly		
	Times per week		

Tier One

FOOD	TYPE O SECRETOR	TYPE O NON-SECRETOR
Abalone	Avoid	Avoid
Barracuda	Avoid	Avoid
Catfish	Avoid	Neutral
Cod	Beneficial	Beneficial
Conch	Avoid	Avoid
Frog	Avoid	Avoid
Muskellunge	Avoid	Avoid
Octopus	Avoid	Avoid
Perch (all types)	Beneficial	Beneficial
Pike	Beneficial	Beneficial
Pollack	Avoid	Avoid
Squid	Avoid	Avoid

Tier Two

FOOD	TYPE O SECRETOR	TYPE O NON-SECRETOR
Bass (all types)	Beneficial	Neutral
Halibut	Beneficial	Neutral
Red snapper	Beneficial	Neutral
Shad	Beneficial	Beneficial
Sole	Beneficial	Beneficial
Sturgeon	Beneficial	Beneficial
Swordfish	Beneficial	Beneficial
Tilefish	Beneficial	Beneficial
Trout (rainbow)	Beneficial	Beneficial
Yellowtail	Beneficial	Beneficial

Neutral: General Nutritional Supplementation

FOOD	TYPE O SECRETOR	TYPE O NON-SECRETOR
Anchovy	Neutral	Avoid
Beluga	Neutral	Neutral
Bluefish	Neutral	Neutral
Bullhead	Neutral	Neutral
Butterfish	Neutral	Neutral
Carp	Neutral	Neutral
Caviar	Neutral	Neutral
Chub	Neutral	Neutral
Clam	Neutral	Neutral
Crab	Neutral	Avoid
Croaker	Neutral	Neutral
Cusk	Neutral	Neutral
Drum	Neutral	Neutral
Eel	Neutral	Neutral
Flounder	Neutral	Neutral
Gray sole	Neutral	Neutral
Grouper	Neutral	Neutral
Haddock	Neutral	Neutral
Hake	Neutral	Beneficial
Halfmoon fish	Neutral	Neutral
Harvest fish	Neutral	Neutral
Herring	Neutral	Beneficial
Lobster	Neutral	Neutral

Mackerel	Neutral	Beneficial
Mahimahi	Neutral	Neutral
Monkfish	Neutral	Neutral
Mullet	Neutral	Neutral
Mussels	Neutral	Avoid
Opaleye fish	Neutral	Neutral
Orange roughy	Neutral	Neutral
Oyster	Neutral	Neutral
Parrot fish	Neutral	Neutral
Pickerel	Neutral	Neutral
Pompano	Neutral	Neutral
Porgy	Neutral	Neutral
Rosefish	Neutral	Neutral
Sailfish	Neutral	Neutral
Salmon	Neutral	Neutral
Sardine	Neutral	Beneficial
Scallop	Neutral	Neutral
Scrod	Neutral	Neutral
Scup	Neutral	Neutral
Shark	Neutral	Neutral
Shrimp	Neutral	Neutral
Smelt	Neutral	Neutral
Snail (*Helix pomatia*/escargot)	Neutral	Neutral
Sucker	Neutral	Neutral
Sunfish	Neutral	Neutral
Tilapia	Neutral	Neutral
Trout (brook)	Neutral	Neutral
Trout (sea)	Neutral	Neutral
Tuna	Neutral	Neutral
Weakfish	Neutral	Neutral
Whitefish	Neutral	Neutral
Whiting	Neutral	Neutral

Dairy and Eggs

DAIRY PRODUCTS should be avoided by Type O secretors and non-secretors. They can lead to undesirable weight gain, increased inflammation, and fatigue. Eggs can be consumed in moderation. They are a good source of DHA and can help Type Os build active tissue mass.

BLOOD TYPE O: EGGS			
Portion: 1 egg			
	African	**Caucasian**	**Asian**
Secretor	1–4	3–6	3–4
Non-Secretor	2–5	3–6	3–4
		Times per week	

BLOOD TYPE O: MILK AND YOGURT			
Portion: 4–6 oz. (men); 2–5 oz. (women and children)			
	African	**Caucasian**	**Asian**
Secretor	0–1	0–3	0–2
Non-Secretor	0	0–2	0–3
		Times per week	

BLOOD TYPE O: CHEESE			
Portion: 3 oz. (men); 2 oz. (women and children)			
	African	**Caucasian**	**Asian**
Secretor	0–1	0–2	0–1
Non-Secretor	0	0–1	0
MM	Decrease milk and yogurt by 2 servings weekly		
		Times per week	

Tier One

FOOD	TYPE O SECRETOR	TYPE O NON-SECRETOR
American cheese	Avoid	Avoid
Blue cheese	Avoid	Avoid
Brie	Avoid	Avoid
Buttermilk	Avoid	Avoid
Camembert	Avoid	Avoid
Casein	Avoid	Avoid
Cheddar cheese	Avoid	Avoid
Colby cheese	Avoid	Avoid
Cottage cheese	Avoid	Avoid
Cream cheese	Avoid	Avoid
Edam cheese	Avoid	Avoid
Emmenthal cheese	Avoid	Avoid
Gouda	Avoid	Avoid
Gruyère	Avoid	Avoid
Half & half	Avoid	Avoid

Ice cream	Avoid	Avoid
Jarlsberg cheese	Avoid	Avoid
Kefir	Avoid	Avoid
Milk (cow-skim or 2%)	Avoid	Avoid
Milk (cow-whole)	Avoid	Avoid
Monterey Jack cheese	Avoid	Avoid
Muenster cheese	Avoid	Avoid
Neufchatel cheese	Avoid	Avoid
Paneer	Avoid	Avoid
Parmesan cheese	Avoid	Avoid
Provolone cheese	Avoid	Avoid
Quark cheese	Avoid	Avoid
Ricotta cheese	Avoid	Avoid
Sherbet	Avoid	Avoid
Sour cream (low/non-fat)	Avoid	Avoid
String cheese	Avoid	Avoid
Swiss cheese	Avoid	Avoid
Yogurt	Avoid	Avoid

Tier Two

FOOD	TYPE O SECRETOR	TYPE O NON-SECRETOR
Goose egg	Avoid	Neutral
Milk (goat)	Avoid	Avoid
Quail egg	Avoid	Neutral
Salmon roe	Avoid	Neutral
Whey	Avoid	Avoid

Neutral: General Nutritional Supplementation

FOOD	TYPE O SECRETOR	TYPE O NON-SECRETOR
Butter	Neutral	Neutral
Duck egg	Neutral	Neutral
Egg (chicken)	Neutral	Neutral
Egg white (chicken)	Neutral	Neutral
Egg yolk (chicken)	Neutral	Neutral

Farmer cheese	Neutral	Avoid
Feta cheese	Neutral	Avoid
Ghee (clarified butter)	Neutral	Neutral
Goat cheese	Neutral	Avoid
Mozzarella cheese	Neutral	Avoid

Beans and Legumes

ESSENTIALLY carnivores when it comes to protein requirements, Type Os can do well on proteins found in many beans and legumes, although this food does contain more than a few foods with problematic lectins. Given the choice, get your protein from animal foods.

BLOOD TYPE O: BEANS AND LEGUMES			
Portion: 1 cup, dry			
	African	Caucasian	Asian
Secretor	1–3	1–3	2–4
Non-Secretor	0–2	0–3	2–4
			Times per week

Tier One

FOOD	TYPE O SECRETOR	TYPE O NON-SECRETOR
Copper bean	Avoid	Avoid
Kidney bean	Avoid	Avoid
Lentil (domestic)	Avoid	Neutral
Lentil (green)	Avoid	Neutral
Lentil (red)	Avoid	Neutral
Navy bean	Avoid	Avoid
Pinto bean	Avoid	Neutral

Tier Two

FOOD	TYPE O SECRETOR	TYPE O NON-SECRETOR
Adzuki beans	Beneficial	Neutral
Black-eyed pea	Beneficial	Neutral
Tamarind bean	Avoid	Avoid

Neutral: General Nutritional Supplementation

FOOD	TYPE O SECRETOR	TYPE O NON-SECRETOR
Black bean	Neutral	Neutral
Broad bean	Neutral	Neutral
Cannellini bean	Neutral	Neutral
Fava bean	Neutral	Avoid
Garbanzo bean	Neutral	Avoid
Green bean	Neutral	Neutral
Jicama	Neutral	Neutral
Lima bean	Neutral	Neutral
Mung beans (sprouts)	Neutral	Neutral
Northern bean	Neutral	Neutral
Red bean	Neutral	Avoid
Snap bean	Neutral	Neutral
Soy bean	Neutral	Avoid
Soy cheese	Neutral	Avoid
Soy flakes	Neutral	Avoid
Soy granules	Neutral	Avoid
Soy milk	Neutral	Avoid
Soy, miso	Neutral	Avoid
Soy, tempeh	Neutral	Avoid
Soy, tofu	Neutral	Avoid
White bean	Neutral	Neutral

Nuts and Seeds

NUTS AND SEEDS are a secondary source of protein for Type O. Walnuts are excellent detoxifiers, and flaxseeds are helpful for a strong immune system. However, use caution, because many nuts and seeds possess lectin activity for Type Os, including beechnut, sunflower seeds,* and chestnuts.*

*New rating

BLOOD TYPE O: NUTS AND SEEDS			
Portion: Seeds (handful) Nut Butters (1–2 tbsp)			
	African	Caucasian	Asian
Secretor	2–5	2–5	2–4
Non-Secretor	5–7	5–7	5–7
		Times per week	

Tier One

FOOD	TYPE O SECRETOR	TYPE O NON-SECRETOR
Beechnut	Avoid	Avoid
Brazil nut	Avoid	Avoid
Cashew/cashew butter	Avoid	Avoid
Chestnut	Avoid	Avoid
Peanut	Avoid	Avoid
Peanut butter	Avoid	Avoid
Pistachio	Avoid	Avoid
Pumpkin seed	Beneficial	Beneficial
Sunflower butter	Avoid	Avoid
Sunflower seed	Avoid	Avoid
Walnut (black)	Beneficial	Beneficial
Walnut (English)	Beneficial	Beneficial

Tier Two

FOOD	TYPE O SECRETOR	TYPE O NON-SECRETOR
Flaxseed	Beneficial	Neutral
Litchi	Avoid	Avoid
Poppy seed	Avoid	Avoid

Neutral: General Nutritional Supplementation

FOOD	TYPE O SECRETOR	TYPE O NON-SECRETOR
Almond	Neutral	Neutral
Almond butter	Neutral	Neutral
Almond cheese	Neutral	Avoid
Almond milk	Neutral	Avoid
Butternut	Neutral	Neutral
Filbert (hazelnut)	Neutral	Neutral

Hickory	Neutral	Neutral
Macadamia	Neutral	Neutral
Pecan/pecan butter	Neutral	Neutral
Pine nut (pignola)	Neutral	Neutral
Safflower seed	Neutral	Avoid
Sesame butter/tahini	Neutral	Neutral
Sesame seed	Neutral	Neutral

Grains and Starches

GRAINS AND STARCHES are the Achilles' heel of Type Os. All Type Os tend to do poorly on corn, wheat, sorghum, barley, and many of their byproducts (sweeteners, etc.). These common grains have a very pronounced effect on increasing body fat in Type Os. The agglutinin in whole wheat can also aggravate inflammatory conditions. This is especially true if you are a non-secretor, and even more significant if you are a male non-secretor. If you are a non-secretor, oats should be avoided, although they are neutral for secretors.

BLOOD TYPE O: GRAINS AND STARCHES			
Portion: 1/2 cup dry (grains or pastas); 1 muffin, 2 slices of bread			
	African	**Caucasian**	**Asian**
Secretor	1–6	1–6	1–6
Non-Secretor	0–3	0–3	0–3
Rh–	Decrease by 1 serving weekly		
	Times per week		

Tier One

FOOD	TYPE O SECRETOR	TYPE O NON-SECRETOR
Barley	Avoid	Avoid
Corn (white/ yellow/blue)	Avoid	Avoid
Cornmeal	Avoid	Avoid
Couscous (cracked wheat)	Avoid	Avoid
Gluten flour	Avoid	Avoid
Popcorn	Avoid	Avoid

Sorghum	Avoid	Avoid
Wheat (bran)	Avoid	Avoid
Wheat (germ)	Avoid	Avoid
Wheat (gluten flour products)	Avoid	Avoid
Wheat (refined unbleached)	Avoid	Avoid
Wheat (semolina flour products)	Avoid	Avoid
Wheat (white flour products)	Avoid	Avoid
Wheat (whole wheat products)	Avoid	Avoid
Wheat bread (sprouted commercial)	Avoid	Avoid except Essene and Ezekiel

Tier Two

FOOD	TYPE O SECRETOR	TYPE O NON-SECRETOR
Essene bread (manna bread)	Beneficial	Beneficial

Neutral: General Nutritional Supplementation

FOOD	TYPE O SECRETOR	TYPE O NON-SECRETOR
Amaranth	Neutral	Neutral
Artichoke pasta (pure)	Neutral	Avoid
Buckwheat/kasha	Neutral	Avoid
Ezekiel bread (commercial)	Neutral	Neutral
Gluten-free bread	Neutral	Avoid
Kamut	Neutral	Neutral
Millet	Neutral	Neutral
Oat flour	Neutral	Avoid
Oat/oat bran/ oatmeal	Neutral	Avoid
Quinoa	Neutral	Neutral

Rice (cream of)	Neutral	Neutral
Rice (puffed)/rice bran	Neutral	Neutral
Rice (white/brown/ basmati)/bread	Neutral	Neutral
Rice (wild)	Neutral	Neutral
Rice cake/flour	Neutral	Neutral
Rice milk	Neutral	Neutral
Rye flour	Neutral	Neutral
Rye/100% rye bread	Neutral	Neutral
Soba noodles (100% buckwheat)	Neutral	Avoid
Soy flour bread	Neutral	Avoid
Spelt	Neutral	Avoid
Spelt flour/products	Neutral	Avoid
Tapioca	Neutral	Avoid
Teff	Neutral	Neutral

Vegetables

VEGETABLES provide a rich source of antioxidants and fiber, in addition to helping to lower the production of polyamines in the digestive tract. Some vegetables, however, such as cauliflower, leeks, taro, yucca, potatoes, juniper, cucumber,* and bitter melon contain reactive lectins that may be blood type specific. Type Os should be careful not to substitute starches for vegetables. Many vegetables are rich in potassium, which helps lower extracellular water in the body, while raising intracellular water.

BLOOD TYPE O: VEGETABLES			
Portion: 1 cup, cooked or raw			
	African	**Caucasian**	**Asian**
Secretor Beneficials	Unlimited	Unlimited	Unlimited
Secretor Neutrals	2–5	2–5	2–5
Non-Secretor Neutrals	2–3	2–3	2–3
Non-Secretor Beneficials	Unlimited	Unlimited	Unlimited
MM	Try to use mostly Tier One Beneficials		
	Times per week		

*New value

Tier One

FOOD	TYPE O SECRETOR	TYPE O NON-SECRETOR
Alfalfa sprouts	Avoid	Avoid
Aloe/aloe tea/aloe juice	Avoid	Avoid
Beet greens	Beneficial	Beneficial
Cauliflower	Avoid	Avoid
Chicory	Beneficial	Beneficial
Collard greens	Beneficial	Beneficial
Cucumber	Avoid	Avoid
Cucumber juice	Avoid	Avoid
Dandelion	Beneficial	Beneficial
Ginger	Beneficial	Beneficial
Horseradish	Beneficial	Beneficial
Juniper	Avoid	Avoid
Kelp	Beneficial	Beneficial
Leek	Avoid	Avoid
Mushroom (silver-dollar)	Avoid	Neutral
Olive (black)	Avoid	Avoid
Onion (all kinds)	Beneficial	Beneficial
Pickle (in brine)	Avoid	Avoid
Pickle (in vinegar)	Avoid	Avoid
Rhubarb	Avoid	Avoid
Seaweed	Beneficial	Beneficial
Spinach/spinach juice	Beneficial	Beneficial
Taro	Avoid	Avoid
Yucca	Avoid	Avoid

Tier Two

FOOD	TYPE O SECRETOR	TYPE O NON-SECRETOR
Acacia (arabic gum)	Avoid	Avoid
Artichoke (domestic/ globe/Jerusalem)	Beneficial	Beneficial
Broccoli	Beneficial	Beneficial
Caper	Avoid	Avoid
Escarole	Beneficial	Beneficial
Kale	Beneficial	Beneficial

Kohlrabi	Beneficial	Beneficial
Lettuce (romaine)	Beneficial	Neutral
Mushroom (shiitake)	Avoid	Avoid
Mustard greens	Avoid	Neutral
Okra	Beneficial	Beneficial
Parsnip	Beneficial	Neutral
Pepper (red/cayenne)	Beneficial	Beneficial
Potato (sweet)	Beneficial	Neutral
Potato (white/red/ blue/yellow)	Avoid	Avoid
Pumpkin	Beneficial	Beneficial
Swiss chard	Beneficial	Beneficial
Turnip	Beneficial	Neutral

Neutral: General Nutritional Supplementation

FOOD	TYPE O SECRETOR	TYPE O NON-SECRETOR
Agar	Neutral	Avoid
Arugula	Neutral	Neutral
Asparagus	Neutral	Neutral
Bamboo shoot	Neutral	Neutral
Beet	Neutral	Neutral
Beet/beet greens juice	Neutral	Neutral
Bok choy	Neutral	Neutral
Brussel sprout	Neutral	Avoid
Cabbage (Chinese/ red/white)	Neutral	Avoid
Cabbage juice	Neutral	Avoid
Carrot	Neutral	Beneficial
Carrot juice	Neutral	Neutral
Celeriac	Neutral	Neutral
Celery	Neutral	Neutral
Celery juice	Neutral	Neutral
Chervil	Neutral	Neutral
Chili pepper	Neutral	Neutral
Cilantro	Neutral	Neutral
Daikon radish	Neutral	Neutral

Eggplant	Neutral	Avoid
Endive	Neutral	Neutral
Fennel	Neutral	Neutral
Fiddlehead fern	Neutral	Beneficial
Garlic	Neutral	Beneficial
Lettuce (bibb/Boston/ iceberg/mesclun)	Neutral	Neutral
Mushroom (abalone)	Neutral	Neutral
Mushroom (enoki)	Neutral	Neutral
Mushroom (maitake)	Neutral	Neutral
Mushroom (oyster)	Neutral	Neutral
Mushroom (portobello)	Neutral	Neutral
Mushroom (straw)	Neutral	Neutral
Olive (Greek/Spanish)	Neutral	Avoid
Olive (green)	Neutral	Avoid
Pea (green/pod/ snow)	Neutral	Neutral
Pepper (green/ yellow/jalapeño)	Neutral	Neutral
Pimento	Neutral	Neutral
Poi	Neutral	Avoid
Radicchio	Neutral	Neutral
Radish	Neutral	Neutral
Radish sprouts	Neutral	Neutral
Rappini	Neutral	Neutral
Rutabaga	Neutral	Neutral
Sauerkraut	Neutral	Avoid
Scallion	Neutral	Neutral
Senna	Neutral	Neutral
Shallots	Neutral	Neutral
Squash (summer/ winter)	Neutral	Neutral
String bean	Neutral	Neutral
Tomato/tomato juice	Neutral	Neutral
Water chestnut	Neutral	Neutral
Watercress	Neutral	Neutral
Yam	Neutral	Neutral
Zucchini	Neutral	Neutral

Fruits and Fruit Juices

FRUITS ARE RICH in antioxidants, and many, such as blueberries, elderberries, cherries, and blackberries, contain pigments that block the liver enzyme ornithine decarboxylase. This has the effect of lowering the production of polyamines, chemicals that act with insulin to encourage tissue growth and weight gain. Thus a diet rich in proper fruits and vegetables can help weight loss by tempering the effects of insulin. Also, fruits can help shift the balance of water in the body from high extracellular concentrations to high intracellular concentrations. Many fruits, such as pineapple, are rich in enzymes which can help reduce inflammation and encourage proper water balance. Oranges should be used sparingly: they are high in the polyamine putrescine. Several fruits, such as kiwi,* contain Type O reactive lectins.

BLOOD TYPE O: FRUITS			
Portion: 1 cup or 1 piece			
	African	Caucasian	Asian
Secretor	2–4	3–5	3–5
Non-Secretor	1–3	1–3	1–3
MM	Try to use mostly Tier One Beneficials		
	Times per week		

Tier One

FOOD	TYPE O SECRETOR	TYPE O NON-SECRETOR
Asian pear	Avoid	Avoid
Avocado	Avoid	Beneficial
Banana	Beneficial	Beneficial
Bitter melon	Avoid	Avoid
Blackberry/ blackberry juice	Avoid	Avoid
Blueberry	Beneficial	Beneficial
Cantaloupe	Avoid	Avoid
Cherry (all)	Beneficial	Beneficial
Cherry juice (black)	Beneficial	Beneficial
Coconut milk	Avoid	Avoid

*New Value

Fig (fresh/dried)	Beneficial	Beneficial
Guava	Beneficial	Beneficial
Guava juice	Beneficial	Beneficial
Honeydew	Avoid	Avoid
Kiwi	Avoid	Avoid
Mango/mango juice	Beneficial	Beneficial
Orange/orange juice	Avoid	Avoid
Plum (dark/green/ red)	Beneficial	Beneficial
Prune/prune juice	Beneficial	Beneficial
Tangerine/tangerine juice	Avoid	Avoid

Tier Two

FOOD	TYPE O SECRETOR	TYPE O NON-SECRETOR
Pineapple juice	Beneficial	Beneficial
Plantain	Avoid	Avoid

Neutral: General Nutritional Supplementation

FOOD	TYPE O SECRETOR	TYPE O NON-SECRETOR
Apple	Neutral	Avoid
Apple cider/apple juice	Neutral	Avoid
Apricot/apricot juice	Neutral	Avoid
Boysenberry	Neutral	Neutral
Breadfruit	Neutral	Neutral
Canang melon	Neutral	Neutral
Casaba melon	Neutral	Neutral
Christmas melon	Neutral	Neutral
Cranberry/cranberry juice	Neutral	Neutral
Crenshaw melon	Neutral	Neutral
Currants (black/red)	Neutral	Neutral
Date (all types)	Neutral	Avoid
Dewberry	Neutral	Neutral
Elderberry (dark blue/purple)	Neutral	Neutral

Gooseberry	Neutral	Neutral
Grape (all types)	Neutral	Neutral
Grapefruit/grapefruit juice	Neutral	Neutral
Kumquat	Neutral	Neutral
Lemon/lemon juice	Neutral	Neutral
Lime/lime juice	Neutral	Neutral
Loganberry	Neutral	Neutral
Mulberry	Neutral	Neutral
Musk melon	Neutral	Neutral
Nectarine/nectarine juice	Neutral	Neutral
Papaya/papaya juice	Neutral	Neutral
Peach	Neutral	Neutral
Pear/pear juice	Neutral	Neutral
Persimmon	Neutral	Neutral
Pineapple	Neutral	Neutral
Pomegranate	Neutral	Beneficial
Prickly pear	Neutral	Beneficial
Quince	Neutral	Neutral
Raisin	Neutral	Neutral
Raspberry	Neutral	Neutral
Sago palm	Neutral	Neutral
Spanish melon	Neutral	Neutral
Starfruit (carambola)	Neutral	Neutral
Strawberry	Neutral	Avoid
Water & lemon	Neutral	Neutral
Watermelon	Neutral	Neutral
Youngberry	Neutral	Neutral

Oils

IN GENERAL, Type Os do best on monounsaturated oils (such as olive oil) and oils rich in omega series fatty acids (such as flax oil). Type O secretors have a bit of an edge in breaking down oils over non-secretors, and probably benefit a bit more from their consumption as well.

BLOOD TYPE O: OILS			
Portion: 1 tblsp			
	African	**Caucasian**	**Asian**
Secretor	3–8	4–8	5–8
Non-Secretor	1–7	3–5	3–6
		Times per week	

Tier One

FOOD	TYPE O SECRETOR	TYPE O NON-SECRETOR
Castor oil	Avoid	Avoid
Coconut oil	Avoid	Neutral
Corn oil	Avoid	Avoid
Cottonseed oil	Avoid	Avoid
Flaxseed (Linseed) oil	Beneficial	Neutral
Olive oil	Beneficial	Beneficial
Peanut oil	Avoid	Avoid
Safflower oil	Avoid	Avoid
Soy oil	Avoid	Avoid
Sunflower oil	Avoid	Avoid
Wheat germ oil	Avoid	Avoid

Tier Two

FOOD	TYPE O SECRETOR	TYPE O NON-SECRETOR
Evening primrose oil	Avoid	Avoid

Neutral: General Nutritional Supplementation

FOOD	TYPE O SECRETOR	TYPE O NON-SECRETOR
Almond oil	Neutral	Beneficial
Black currant seed oil	Neutral	Neutral
Borage seed oil	Neutral	Avoid
Canola oil	Neutral	Avoid
Cod liver oil	Neutral	Avoid
Sesame oil	Neutral	Neutral
Walnut oil	Neutral	Beneficial

Herbs, Spices, and Condiments

MANY SPICES have mild to moderate medicinal properties, often by influencing the levels of bacteria in the lower colon. Many common gums, such as guar gum and carrageenan, should be avoided as they can enhance the effects of lectins found in other foods.

Tier One

FOOD	TYPE O SECRETOR	TYPE O NON-SECRETOR
Algae, blue-green	Avoid	Avoid
Aspartame	Avoid	Avoid
Carrageenan	Avoid	Avoid
Corn syrup	Avoid	Avoid
Cornstarch	Avoid	Avoid
Dextrose	Avoid	Avoid
Dulse	Beneficial	Beneficial
Fructose	Avoid	Avoid
Guar gum	Avoid	Avoid
Guarana	Avoid	Avoid
Ketchup	Avoid	Avoid
Maltodextrin	Avoid	Avoid
MSG	Avoid	Neutral
Pepper (black/white)	Avoid	Avoid
Pickle relish	Avoid	Avoid
Vinegar	Avoid	Avoid

Tier Two

FOOD	TYPE O SECRETOR	TYPE O NON-SECRETOR
Carob	Beneficial	Neutral
Curry	Beneficial	Beneficial
Mace	Avoid	Avoid
Nutmeg	Avoid	Neutral
Parsley	Beneficial	Beneficial
Turmeric	Beneficial	Neutral

Neutral: General Nutritional Supplementation

FOOD	TYPE O SECRETOR	TYPE O NON-SECRETOR
Allspice	Neutral	Neutral
Almond extract	Neutral	Neutral
Anise	Neutral	Neutral
Apple pectin	Neutral	Neutral
Arrowroot	Neutral	Neutral
Barley malt	Neutral	Avoid
Basil	Neutral	Beneficial
Bay leaf	Neutral	Beneficial
Bergamot	Neutral	Neutral
Caraway	Neutral	Neutral
Cardamom	Neutral	Neutral
Chili powder	Neutral	Neutral
Chives	Neutral	Neutral
Chocolate	Neutral	Neutral
Cinnamon	Neutral	Avoid
Clove	Neutral	Neutral
Coriander	Neutral	Neutral
Cream of tartar	Neutral	Neutral
Cumin	Neutral	Neutral
Dill	Neutral	Neutral
Gelatin, plain	Neutral	Neutral
Honey	Neutral	Avoid
Licorice root	Neutral	Beneficial
Maple syrup	Neutral	Avoid
Marjoram	Neutral	Neutral
Mayonnaise	Neutral	Avoid
Mint	Neutral	Neutral
Molasses	Neutral	Neutral
Mustard (prepared, vinegar free)	Neutral	Neutral
Mustard (dry)	Neutral	Neutral
Oregano	Neutral	Beneficial
Paprika	Neutral	Neutral
Pepper (Peppercorn/ red flakes)	Neutral	Neutral
Peppermint	Neutral	Neutral

Rice syrup	Neutral	Avoid
Rosemary	Neutral	Neutral
Saffron	Neutral	Beneficial
Sage	Neutral	Avoid
Salad dressing (OK'd ingredients)	Neutral	Neutral
Savory	Neutral	Neutral
Sea salt	Neutral	Neutral
Soy sauce	Neutral	Avoid
Spearmint	Neutral	Neutral
Stevia	Neutral	Avoid
Sucanat	Neutral	Avoid
Sugar (brown/white)	Neutral	Avoid
Tamari, wheat free	Neutral	Avoid
Tamarind	Neutral	Neutral
Tarragon	Neutral	Beneficial
Thyme	Neutral	Neutral
Vanilla	Neutral	Avoid
Vinegar (apple cider)	Neutral	Avoid
Wintergreen	Neutral	Neutral
Worcestershire sauce	Neutral	Avoid
Yeast (brewer's)	Neutral	Beneficial

Beverages

TYPE O NON-SECRETORS may wish to have a glass of wine occasionally with their meals; they derive substantial benefit to their cardiovascular system from moderate use. Type Os derive some benefit from green tea. It contains polyphenols that block the production of harmful polyamines.

Tier One

FOOD	TYPE O SECRETOR	TYPE O NON-SECRETOR
Coffee (regular/decaf)	Avoid	Avoid
Liquor (distilled)	Avoid	Avoid
Soda (misc./diet/cola)	Avoid	Avoid

Tier Two

FOOD	TYPE O SECRETOR	TYPE O NON-SECRETOR
Beer	Avoid	Avoid
Seltzer water	Beneficial	Beneficial
Tea (black regular/ decaf)	Avoid	Avoid
Tea (green)	Beneficial	Beneficial
Wine (white)	Avoid	Avoid

Neutral: General Nutritional Supplementation

FOOD	TYPE O SECRETOR	TYPE O NON-SECRETOR
Wine (red)	Neutral	Beneficial

Individualized Therapies For Chronic Conditions

As you can see by referring to your Risk Profile, Type O is more susceptible to certain chronic conditions
and diseases than the other blood
types. The following section details
those conditions, the Type O connection, and a wide range of thera-
pies, in addition to the Tier-Two Diet, based on your blood type.

> *See Type O Health Risk Profile, page 122.*

Type O–Specific Digestive Conditions

GERD
Ulcers
Crohn's Disease

GERD

Gastro-esophageal reflux disease (GERD), or chronic heartburn, affects
more than 20 million Americans on a daily basis. Heartburn has nothing
directly to do with the heart. The name is derived from the sympto-
matic burning in the upper abdomen and chest. GERD can be caused
by a number of conditions, including a hiatal hernia. However, the more

common reason so many people are afflicted with chronic heartburn is poor dietary habits. When you don't eat right for your type, you upset the acidic balance, and acid backs up through the sensitive opening that connects your esophagus with your stomach. Type Os, with your naturally elevated acidic state, are much more prone to develop GERD when you don't adhere to your diet.

Prevent and treat GERD with the following therapies:

- Avoid coffee, chocolate, mints, and black tea, all of which can provoke GERD by increasing stomach acid.
- Avoid sugars and sweets, which tend to cause problems for people with GERD.
- Add five to fifteen drops of Gentian (*Gentiana lutea*) to a glass of water and drink it thirty minutes before a meal. By taking this bitter thirty minutes before eating, your digestive secretions will be better prepared to digest your meal. An interesting note is that digestive bitters evolved as a cultural tradition in several European countries.
- Ginger: Several components of ginger protect the cells lining the stomach. I've found that a teaspoon of fresh ginger juice taken several times daily can be a very effective strategy for GERD.
- Don't get too full. Try to leave the table a bit hungry.

Ulcers
Bacteria is a primary factor in the development of ulcers. Until fairly recently, ulcers were believed to be the result of excess stomach acid induced by stress. But in the early 1980s, scientists determined that a common bacterium, *Helicobacter pylori*, was responsible for most cases of ulcers. This bacteria is a bit of an exception to the rule that high stomach acid levels tend to keep the stomach sterile. *H. pylori* can readily live in acidic conditions because of its ability to create a "local pocket" of lowered acidity around itself.[2]

Ulcers are usually accompanied by generalized pain, nausea, vomiting, and a lack of appetite. When ulcers bleed, stools become dark black and tarlike.

Early in the 1950s, it was first discovered that Type Os had about twice the incidences of ulcers of all kinds than the other blood types. These findings have been replicated so many times (over twenty-five studies in the last twenty years alone), with the same consistent result, that the conclusions are virtually unquestionable.[3] Why is this so?

Like other bacteria in the gut, *H. pylori* has a favorite blood type, and it happens to be Type O. Recently, it has been found that this bacterium manufactures a lectin-like molecule, called an adhesion, which facilitates its binding to the cells of the stomach and duodenum wall. This binding is enhanced by cells that bear Type O antigens. Research also shows that Type Os have more inflammation from *H. pylori* than the other blood types. Type O non-secretors have the highest rate of *H. pylori*.

H. pylori infection is about 90 percent curable with antimicrobials and acid-inhibiting medicines, so regular screening for early diagnosis is recommended. There are also natural remedies that can help control *H. pylori*:

BLADDERWRACK, AND OTHER FUCOSE-CONTAINING SEA-WEEDS.   As far back as 1958, scientist George Springer identified several plants that contained substances that were blood group active.[4] One, the common seaweed bladder wrack (*Fucus vesiculosus*), was found to contain substantial amounts of fucose, the sugar that is the Type O antigen. *H. pylori* likes to attach to the Type O antigen, using sugars that mimic this blood type as decoy molecules. Since *H. pylori* like Type O so much, let's give them what they want! In this case, we can flood their "suction cups" with fake-O (bladderwrack fucose in lieu of the real thing) and they will go skating off the stomach lining, unable to attach and cause problems.

The particular fucose sugars found in bladder wrack, called fucoidins, have been shown to also have an anti-inflammatory effect by blocking a series of mediators called complement. Thus they can be even more beneficial in Type O people, who have been shown to have more inflammatory changes to their stomach tissues when infected by *H. pylori*. This is particularly true for non-secretors. Other species of seaweed that are rich in fucoidins include ascophyllum, at about 6 to 8 percent and laminaria at between 5 and 20 percent. Find fresh dried forms and use them instead of the tinctures, which have little or no fucose in them.

BISMUTH.   Bismuth compounds have both anti–*H. pylori* and ulcer-healing properties. Several companies manufacture compounds containing bismuth. An example is the over-the-counter drug Pepto-Bismol. However, if you are sensitive to dyes you may want to find alternatives. Never take bismuth for longer than two weeks.

BERBERINE.   An alkaloid found in the herbs goldenseal (*Hydrastis canadensis*), Coptis (*Coptis chinensis*), Oregon grape, and barberry, berberine has been found to potently inhibit the growth of *H. pylori*.

PROBIOTIC BACTERIA.   Certain strains of friendly Bifidobacteria (*B. bifidus*, *B. breve*, and *B. infantis*) have the ability to make you more resistant to ulcers.

For healing the gastric mucosa (stomach lining) try the following remedies:

- Marshmallow root, taken as a tea or a capsule.
- Slippery elm (particularly non-secretors).
- Sho-saiko-to, a traditional Chinese medicine, suppresses gastric secretion and protects the gastric mucosa, even during times of high stress.
- Thyme leaf, oregano leaf, and rosemary leaf: These common culinary spices are powerful antioxidants and have mild anti-inflammatory activity. Additionally, all of these spices promote improved resistance against bacteria (*like H. pylori*) and other microorganisms (like Candida) that can affect *Type O* digestion.
- Ginger rhizome: contains anti-inflammatory, anti-ulcer, and antioxidant compounds, and promotes gastric motility.

▪ FROM THE BLOOD TYPE OUTCOME REGISTRY ▪

Mark E.
Child
Type O
Improved: Chronic bowel problems

"My son, Michael, is 9½ years old. From the time he was two, he has had difficulty with his bowel movements. There were times he would hold his movement for up to ten days. We went to our doctor, and Michael had to have enemas, suppositories, laxatives, and mineral oil. At the age of nine his condition was worse than ever. In desperation I read your book. Within thirty-six hours of starting the Type O diet, his problem totally disappeared! After a week, we were all ready to splurge on something off our list! We didn't go totally bonkers, but by Monday morning Michael was beginning to show signs of his problem returning. We went back on the program and his condition immediately disappeared again. This program has allowed Michael's self esteem to soar! After seven and a half years and four different doctors, you solved his problem in thirty-six hours."

- Clove fruit: Rich source of eugenol; an anti-inflammatory and anti-ulcer compound.
- *Azardirachta indica* (neem), an indigenous adaptogen from India, can also buffer against stress-induced ulcer formation.

Crohn's Disease

I often treat inflammatory bowel disease, or Crohn's, with the following remedies:

- Get plenty of soluble and insoluble fiber. Perhaps the best source of soluble fiber is the little known *arabinogalactans* (AG) in the Western larch tree. As we've learned, larch arabinogalactan is very useful for immune support as well. In the digestive tract, larch AG has been shown to increase the concentration of short-chain fatty acids, such as butyrate, which are an important energy source for the intestinal cells. Larch also helps to decrease the concentration of ammonia (a toxic byproduct of protein synthesis) in the gut. The kidneys usually excrete ammonia. Larch AG is available under the trade name ARA-6 (North American Pharmacal, Norwalk, CT). An excellent source of insoluble fiber are raw flaxseeds, one tablespoon of which can be added to a glass of water at night, allowing them to swell and soften overnight. The resulting mixture can be taken in the morning.
- Avoid gums, such as carageenan, ghatti, and acacia, which are often used as food stabilizers. Look for foods that are stabilized by other methods.
- Take a probiotic formula containing beneficial bacteria for your blood type.
- Take kelp as a lectin-blocker, especially if you are a non-secretor.
- Avoid lectins bound by amino sugars. The worst for Type O is the wheat germ lectin, which is bound by the sugar n-acetyl glucosamine, while other lectins are bound by the sugars mannose, fucose, n-acetyl galactosamine, and galactose.
- Take measures to reduce your stress levels.
- Use a product called Seacure, a peptide made from whitefish. This product is extremely reliable in normalizing the cells in the Type O gastrointestinal tract. It is available in health food stores.
- Use ghee (clarified butter), which is a good source of butyrate.

Type O–Specific Metabolic Conditions

Syndrome X
Blood-Clotting Disorders

Syndrome X

Syndrome X is a condition created by a combination of obesity, high triglycerides, and insulin resistance, which can lead to diabetes and heart disease. For Type Os, the trigger is carbohydrate intolerance. Many common grain lectins have the effect of inhibiting the breakdown of fats through their effects on insulin. When Type Os adopt low-fat diets rich in metabolically inactivating lectins, they gain weight.

For many years, heart experts have been saying that high triglycerides are not an independent risk for heart disease—only in combination with other factors. However, increasing evidence is pointing to elevated triglycerides as a risk factor on their own, and this partially explains the anomaly of the Type O pathway to heart disease.

Obesity is the gateway to Syndrome X. The entire syndrome can be prevented by attacking the issues that cause weight gain.

In general, Type Os are wise to develop as much active tissue mass as possible, both through diet and exercise, to ensure that you have a supercharged metabolism. For this reason, animal protein is utilized most efficiently, while the lectins in certain grains, breads, legumes, and beans tend to produce a state of insulin resistance resulting in an increase in body fat. The worst offender is the lectins found in wheat germ and whole wheat products. Wheat has the extreme opposite effect of animal protein—so much so that many Type Os report weight loss and gradual decrease in water retention solely by eliminating wheat from their diets. For Type Os who experience difficulty in losing weight, it is often beneficial to rely on sweet potatoes, squash, root vegetables, and pumpkins for your carbohydrates, rather than relying on grains.

Approach your weight loss program as a long-term strategy, and take it slow. The following approach outlines the most crucial elements for successful weight loss. Start with the Type O Diet, Tier Two, and add the following strategies for greater results. I recommend that if you are seriously overweight or have any medical conditions, you should consult with your doctor before you embark on this or any other plan.

1. LEARN YOUR METABOLIC PROFILE. Knowing your muscle mass, percentage of body fat, and basal metabolic rate can be more im-

portant than knowing your weight. These are the indicators of metabolic balance. Your goal is not just to lose pounds, but to build muscle. I suggest that you have a bioelectrical impedence analysis. If that's not feasible, there are some do-it-yourself methods for learning more about your metabolic state. These methods are not scientifically accurate, but they'll provide clues to your general fitness and whether or not you're carrying excess water weight.

Test for Extracellular Water—Edema:
Push your finger firmly down on your shin bone and hold it for five seconds. If you push against muscle or fat, the skin will bounce back up. If there is water between the cells, it will be dis-

---

▪ FROM THE BLOOD TYPE OUTCOME REGISTRY ▪

Lynn N.
Type O
Young female
Improved: Diabetes/weight loss

"I was diagnosed as a type 2 diabetic about a year ago, and controlling my blood glucose level has been a struggle, to say the least. *Eat Right 4 Your Type* is amazing! I had tried vegetarianism for a while, and, until now, never understood why my health failed to improve, nor why I failed to lose a significant amount of weight. Having tried just about everything else, I decided to purchase the book and give Dr. D'Adamo's dietary advice a chance. At first, I must admit, I was skeptical because, 'After all, all humans have the same digestive system, don't they?' Nevertheless, I was intrigued. Now, I'm excited to experience more energy and lower blood glucose levels after following the Type O diet for a mere few weeks. Also, I have eliminated indigestion, heartburn, and flatulence by simply avoiding wheat and corn products. I now eat small amounts of grains such as spelt, kamut, barley, quinoa, buckwheat, rye, and brown rice. Generally, I follow the Type O diet to the letter. However, I have yet to wean myself from coffee. Fortunately, it hasn't been too difficult eschewing typical African-American foods such as ham hocks and cornbread. As an overweight, diabetic African-American woman who is a single parent, full-time college student, apartment manager, and foreign language tutor, it is imperative that I take care of myself. I'm pleased to announce that I'm losing weight and feeling great!"

placed laterally, and the dimple won't fill in immediately. The longer the indentation remains, the more water is present, meaning you're holding excess weight as water.

Measure Your Hip to Waist Ratio:
Excess weight is most unhealthy—and most conducive to metabolic problems—when it is centered in your abdomen, as opposed to your hips and thighs. Here's a quick test to learn about your fat distribution: Stand straight in front of a full-length mirror. Using a tape measure, measure the distance around the smallest part of your waist. Now measure the distance around the largest part of your buttocks. Divide your waist measurement by your hip measurement. A healthy ratio for women is .70 to .75. A healthy ratio for men is .80 to .90.

2. ELIMINATE INSULIN-MIMICKING LECTINS. Most Type Os can lose weight easily and rapidly, simply by eliminating the foods from their diets that promote insulin resistance. Wheat, corn, potatoes, and certain beans contain lectins that have insulin-like effects on the Type O fat cell receptors. When they bind to the receptors, they send a signal to your fat cells to stop burning fat, and to store extra calories as fat. When you eat large amounts of insulin-mimicking lectins that are wrong for your blood type, it has the effect of increasing body fat and decreasing active tissue mass.

Type O Weight Loss Key

INSTEAD OF . . .	EAT . . .
Wheat	Sweet potatoes
Potatoes	Squash
Corn	Root vegetables
Beans	Pumpkin

Type O Contributors to Insulin Resistance and Obesity
- high carbohydrate diet
- deficiency of essential fatty acids, especially Omega 3 oils as found in fish
- history of following low-calorie diets
- skipping meals

- refined sugars and starches
- low-fiber intake
- low intake of vegetables and fruit antioxidant phytochemicals
- use of artificial sugars
- inappropriate lectins in your diet
- lack of exercise or sedentary lifestyle
- stimulants such as coffee, smoking, and alcohol

▪ FROM THE BLOOD TYPE OUTCOME REGISTRY ▪

Alice S.
Type O
Young female
Improved: Weight loss

"I am a large size woman for whom weight loss was basically impossible. I tried the *ER4YT* way of eating for several reasons: weight management, help with digestive difficulties, and help with migraines. After three months, I have lost thirty pounds (basically without instituting a serious exercise program!). My digestive problems have decreased, and I have seen a slight change in the frequency and severity of my migraines. In addition, my doctor noticed that my resting pulse and blood pressure had lowered. I'm very pleased with my results. After the first shock of realizing that everything that I ate and liked to eat was on the avoid list, I have adapted to this way of eating and do not feel deprived or unhappy."

---

3. AVOID STIMULANTS.   Many people use stimulants as a weight loss method, but this approach is counterproductive for Type Os. Often stimulants contain some form of caffeine. There is strong evidence that even moderate amounts of caffeine can activate the Type O sympathetic nervous system, resulting in a higher adrenaline release. This adrenaline release mimics hypoglycemia, even when your blood sugar levels are not actually low.

The primary symptoms of this sympathetic, catecholamine–induced hypoglycemia include sweating, tremor, palpitations, sensation of hunger, restlessness, and anxiety. Other symptoms you might experience are caused by an insufficient supply of glucose to the brain, resulting in blurred vision, weakness, slurred speech, vertigo, and difficulties in concentration.

In addition to the Type O diet, you can maximize your metabolism with supplements of bladder wrack and kelp.

4. REDUCE CARBOHYDRATE CRAVING. If you crave any form of stimulants or carbohydrates, your serotonin levels are low, and your brain is demanding stimulants to raise your serotonin levels. Try taking 5HTP, tyrosine, or glutamine between meals to cut down on your cravings.

For women, I've found that low estrogen levels can produce carbohydrate craving. One or two capsules of the herb maca can help normalize your estrogen levels.

Type O Healthy Heart Supplements— Especially for Non-Secretors

l-carnitine
hawthorn
magnesium
pantethine (active B_5)
CoQ_{10}

Blood-Clotting Disorders

Type O's "thin blood" can become a serious problem when there is a wound or surgical procedure that involves bleeding. Here are some ways to keep your clotting factors in proper balance:

- At least a week prior to surgery, begin a daily protocol of 2,000 milligrams vitamin C, and 30,000 IU vitamin A. These vitamins promote wound healing.
- Before surgery, be sure to have plenty of vitamin K in your system. Vitamin K is essential to blood clotting. Eat lots of greens, especially kale, spinach, and collard greens, and supplement your diet with liquid chlorophyll.
- Avoid using aspirin, which has blood-thinning properties.
- Avoid blood thinners such as garlic and gingko biloba two weeks before surgery.

An additional word of caution: Many Type Os have the misconception that their thin blood protects them from forming dangerous blood clots. This is not necessarily true. For example, phlebitis often starts as an inflammatory condition of the veins, which interferes with blood flow.

Birth Control Note

Type Os should avoid using birth control pills because of the general higher risk of bleeding disorders.

Type O–Specific Immune Conditions

Candida Infection
Thyroid Disease
Inflammatory Conditions

Candida Infection

Candida albicans is a vastly overdiagnosed ailment. In general, I've found Type Os more inclined to Candida hypersensitivity than other blood types, with the greatest susceptibility being for Type O non-secretors.

Several herbal preparations and other substances have been shown to be effective for controlling Candida albicans. However, unless the underlying health of the bowel is taken into consideration, the condition does tend to relapse. That is why your best defense against Candida problems is following the correct diet for your blood type.

- Increase your consumption of olive oil.
- An intriguing lectin found in the root of the stinging nettle plant has been shown to agglutinate Candida albicans, an effect I have verified in my own laboratory. It can be a useful supplement for Type Os suffering from this condition.
- Probiotic bacteria: Virtually all probiotic bacteria have some anti-Candida activity. The presence of substantial quantities of friendly Lactobacilli in your gut is one of the best protections against Candida. The most important species of Lactobacilli for antagonizing Candida are *L. acidophilus*, *L. reuteri*, and *L. casei*.
- Thyme leaf, oregano leaf, and rosemary leaf: These common culinary spices promote improved resistance against bacteria, such as *H. pylori*, and other microorganisms, such as Candida. They can prevent Candida from attaching to your cells, and can even displace Candida that has already attached.

- Kelp (*Laminaria digitata*) or bladder wrack, promotes resistance against Candida and bacterial attachment.

Autoimmune Thyroid Disease

Type Os on high wheat diets have more problems with autoimmune thyroid disease. Both hyperactive (Grave's) and underactive (Hashimoto's) dysfunctions are most common in Type Os.[5] Several Type Os with autoimmune Hashimoto's thyroiditis have successfully controlled their condition with the Blood Type Diet alone, probably the result of lectin avoidance. Grave's disease should always receive appropriate medical supervision.

The thyroid gland has a powerful influence on many parts of the body. Hashimoto's thyroiditis and Grave's disease result from immune system destruction or stimulation of thyroid tissue. Symptoms of low (hypo) or overactive (hyper) thyroid function are nonspecific and can develop slowly or suddenly. These include fatigue, nervousness, cold or heat intolerance, weakness, changes in hair texture or amount of hair, and weight loss or gain. Autoimmune thyroid diseases afflict as many as 4 out of 100 women and are frequently found in families where there are other autoimmune diseases. Experience has shown that the majority are Type O. The diagnosis of specific thyroid disease is readily made with the appropriate laboratory tests.

The symptoms of *hypothyroidism* (low thyroid activity) are controlled with replacement thyroid hormone pills. Side effects and complications from over- or under-replacement of this powerful hormone can occur. Treatment of *hyperthyroidism* (too much thyroid activity) requires long-term anti-thyroid drug therapy or destruction of the thyroid gland with radioactive iodine or surgery. Both of these treatment approaches carry certain risks and long-term side effects.

Hyperactive thyroid tissue is much more sensitive to the agglutinating effects of lectins found in wheat and soybeans than healthy thyroid tissue.[6] Perhaps this explains why several very exciting outcomes on my Web site reported that their thyroid conditions went into spontaneous complete remission by simply following the Blood Type Diet. In every instance the person was Blood Type O, so I am left to speculate that the low lectin diet somehow had the effect of removing a necessary factor in the continued inflammatory or autoimmune response. It could also be that while a normal thyroid doesn't express large amounts of blood type antigens, a sick one can generate enormous amounts. Thyroid tissue that is inflamed generates large amounts of Type A antigen. This would be a major problem if you carried anti-A in your serum, particularly if you are Type O and make four variations of anti-A.

Inflammatory Conditions

Blood Type O is prone to a greater range of inflammatory problems than the other blood types because of the fucose sugar, which acts as its blood type antigen. Fucose sugars serve as adhesion molecules for lectinlike molecules called selectins. This adhesion allows the easy migration of white blood cells from the bloodstream into the areas of inflammation. Type O might also be a bit more predisposed to inflammatory conditions because of lower basal cortisol levels, since cortisol is, in effect, an anti-inflammatory hormone.

▪ FROM THE BLOOD TYPE OUTCOME REGISTRY ▪

Rick D.
Type O
Middle-aged Male
Outcome: Joint and muscle inflammation and pain

"I stopped drinking coffee and my wife has me sort of following my Blood Type Diet. I find a *big* difference in my joints and muscles. I always had pain in my joints. Every day. Now I have a bit in the morning when I get up and once I get going I'm okay. I tested having a coffee about three weeks in to this diet and wow, within an hour I was feeling the difference. I have gout and inflammation of the joints and it flared up every other week or so. Now it rarely happens."

Type Os who consume a lot of grains are highly susceptible to autoimmune disease. The lectins exacerbate the tendency for hyperimmunity, which is characteristic of autoimmune diseases.

All Type Os are at increased risk for inflammatory conditions. Elderly Type Os are prone to osteoarthritis, a chronic deterioration of the bone cartilage. Women are at greater risk than men. Your best defense is the Type O diet. Be particularly careful to avoid wheat and dairy products, which can cause inflammation.

The following supplements can prevent and treat inflammation:

- Jamaican sarsaparilla root, an adaptogen used to calm inflammation, is commonly found in formulas that promote athletic performance.

- Astragalus: This Chinese herb balances the activity of inflammatory and immune processes.
- Thyme leaf, oregano leaf, and rosemary leaf: These common culinary spices are powerful antioxidants and have mild anti-inflammatory activity.
- Ginger rhizome: Contains anti-inflammatory, anti-ulcer, and antioxidant compounds.
- Clove fruit: A rich source of eugenol, an anti-inflammatory and anti-ulcer compound.
- Curcumin (turmeric extract): A chemoprotective, especially for non-secretors.

To learn more about staying healthy and well balanced, log on to the blood type Web site: www.dadamo.com.

Live Right 4
Type A

CONTENTS

The Type A Profile

As a Blood Type A emerging onto the stage of the twenty-first century, the challenges that loom before you are far more complex than your ancestors could have imagined. Many neurochemical factors in the Type A genetic disposition favor a structured, rhythmic, harmonious life, surrounded by a positive, supportive community. The harried pace and increasing sense of isolation experienced by so many in today's society often make these needs difficult to achieve. Type A best exemplifies the powerful interconnectedness of mind and body. This was vital to the shift away from hunting and procurement to building and growing. However, Type A's more internalized relationship to stress, which served your ancestors so well, can be a challenge for the modern Type

continued on page 178

Type A Health Risk Profile

CHARACTERISTICS	MANIFESTATIONS
MIND/BODY Naturally high basal cortisol levels and tendency to overproduce cortisol in response to stress	• Overreaction to stress • Difficulty recovering from stress • Disrupted sleep patterns • Daytime brain fog • Repressed anxiety, hysteria, introversion • Increased blood viscosity • Easy to overtrain with excess exercise • Disruptive to GI friendly bacteria • Suppresses immune function • Promotes muscle loss and fat gain
DIGESTION Oversensitivity to Epidermal Growth Factor	• Protective against ulcers • Creates excess mucus production • Can lead to overgrowth of tissue in esophagus and stomach
Low stomach acid production	• Makes it difficult to digest protein • Blocks action of digestive enzymes • Promotes excess bacterial growth in stomach and upper intestine • Can impair vitamin and mineral absorption
Lack of enzyme, intestinal alkaline phosphatase	• Produces high serum cholesterol, especially LDL • Makes it difficult to break down fat
METABOLISM High levels of blood-clotting factors	• "Thicker" blood—tendency to aggregation • Blood clots more easily
IMMUNITY Low antibody IgA levels	• Creates vulnerability to ear and respiratory infections • Creates susceptibility to GI infections
Low antibody IgE levels	• Promotes asthma and allergies
Tumor markers resemble Type A antigen	• Weakened NK cell activity • Impairs immune system's ability to discriminate between friend and foe

INCREASED RISKS	VARIATIONS
• Obsessive-compulsive disorder (OCD) • Heart disease • Insulin Resistance Syndrome X/type 2 diabetes • Hypothyroidism • Cancer • High stress can further exacerbate virtually all health challenges	ELDERLY: • High cortisol levels are linked to Alzheimer's disease and senile dementia • Disruptions in stress hormones may lead to age-related loss of muscle tissue
• Barrett's esophagus • Esophageal cancer • Respiratory infections • Stomach cancer	CHILDREN: Excess mucus production increases risk of ear infections.
• Stomach cancer • Gallstones • Jaundice	NON-SECRETOR: Slightly higher levels of stomach acid make animal protein more digestible ELDERLY: Decrease in stomach acid levels makes animal protein harder to digest
• Coronary artery disease • Osteoporosis • Colon cancer • Hypercholesterolemia	NON-SECRETOR: Slightly higher levels of intestinal alkaline phosphatase
• Coronary artery disease • Cerebral thrombosis • Problematic in cancer	ELDERLY: • Increased risk of strokes from embolisms • Increased risk of occlusive heart diseases
• Celiac disease • Rheumatic heart disease • Kidney disease	NON-SECRETOR: Higher risk, especially children, who tend to have greater incidence of ear infections
• Most cancers	

A. With the daily piling-on of stressors today, it's harder to efficiently recover once Type A stress hormones are spiked. The consequences of chronic stress are clearly expressed in the Type A profile, with the heightened susceptibility to cardiovascular disease and cancer. Maintaining a balance of stress hormones is perhaps the single most important thing Type As can do for their health.

The key factor in the evolution of Type A can be traced to the struggle for survival long ago, when there was a rapidly dwindling supply of meat. Having exhausted the great game herds of Africa, humans pushed farther out from their ancestral home into Europe and Asia, over time becoming omnivorous to compensate for a limited availability of meat. The adaptations that produced Blood Type A were based on the need to fully utilize nutrients from carbohydrate sources. These biological adaptations can still be observed today in the Type A digestive structure. Low levels of hydrochloric acid in the stomach and high intestinal disaccharide levels permit more efficient digestion of carbohydrates. These are also the very factors that make it difficult to digest and metabolize animal protein and fat.

The sensitive Type A hormonal balance, which includes the ever-present effects of high cortisol levels, makes you more susceptible to diabetes, heart disease, and cancer, but there is good news: Type As can significantly minimize all blood type–related risk factors by simply adhering to the Blood Type A Diet and Prescription.

The Type A Prescription, a proactive mix of lifestyle strategies, hormonal equalizers, exercise therapies, and specialized dietary guidelines, will maximize your health, decrease your natural risk factors, and help you overcome disease. The result: high performance, mental clarity, greater vitality, and increased longevity.

The Type A Prescription

THE TYPE A prescription is a combination of dietary, behavioral, and environmental therapies to help you live right for your type:

- LIFESTYLE STRATEGIES to structure your life for health and longevity
- ADAPTED LIFESTYLE STRATEGIES for children, the elderly, and non-secretors
- EMOTIONAL EQUALIZERS and stress relievers

- SPECIALIZED DIET PLAN: Tier One for maximum health
- TARGETED DIET PLAN: Tier Two to overcome disease
- INDIVIDUALIZED THERAPIES for chronic conditions
- THERAPEUTIC SUPPLEMENT PROGRAM for extra support

Lifestyle Strategies

Keys

🗝 Cultivate creativity and expression in your life.

🗝 Establish a consistent daily schedule.

🗝 Go to bed no later than 11:00 P.M. and sleep for eight hours or more. Don't linger in bed. As soon as you wake up, get moving!

🗝 Take at least two breaks of twenty minutes each during the workday. Treat them as mini-vacations. Use this time for meditation and reflection.

🗝 Don't skip meals.

🗝 Eat more protein at the start of the day, and less at the end.

🗝 Don't eat when you're nervous.

🗝 Schedule smaller, more frequent meals—six instead of three.

🗝 Engage in thirty–forty-five minutes of calming exercise at least three times a week.

🗝 Plan regular screening for heart disease and cancer prevention.

🗝 Always chew your food thoroughly to enhance digestion. Low stomach acid makes digestion more difficult.

The following are guidelines for building a lifestyle plan that will maximize Type A health and longevity.

1. Reset Your Twenty-Four-Hour Clock

Since cortisol, bone growth, immune function, and many other critical biological functions operate on a twenty-four-hour circadian rhythm, you need to be careful to maintain a regular schedule and avoid erratic sleep patterns. You can reset your daily schedule, create exposure to a bright light or sunshine between 6 and 8 A.M., or regulate the light in your sleeping environment. Two supplements have also been used in re-setting rhythms—the well-known melatonin, and a less well-known form of vitamin B_{12} called methylcobalamin.

The gentlest and most effective way to phase-shift the human circadian rhythm is by using a combination of bright light exposure and methylcobalamin. Basically, methylcobalamin helps bright light do its

About the Important Circadian Rhythm

Cortisol is released in a twenty-four-hour schedule, referred to as a circadian rhythm. Extraordinarily, our bodies contain more than one hundred circadian rhythms. Each unique cycle influences an aspect of the body's function, including body temperature, hormone levels, heart rate, blood pressure—even pain threshold. Almost no area of the body is unaffected by circadian rhythms. Scientists can't explain precisely how our brain keeps track of this very complex, multifaceted twenty-four-hour time schedule, but we do know our brains rely on outside influences, such as sunlight and darkness, to remain tracked. Under ideal circumstances, cortisol's release schedule would produce the highest levels between 6 and 8 A.M., with a gradual decline throughout the day. Researchers propose that the circadian secretion of cortisol helps cue many of the body's other cyclical rhythms. While this is still debatable, it's clear that if cortisol levels are elevated while sleeping, the result will be a disruption of some of the body's other twenty-four-hour clocks. For example, an elevated level of cortisol at midnight will disrupt bone regeneration the following day by shifting the relative balance of bone growth metabolism away from making new bone and toward bone turnover. A similar process occurs with skin regeneration. When cortisol levels remain raised at night, skin is unable to regenerate, resulting in premature aging. The immune system will be disrupted as well if cortisol levels remain high during periods of sleep. It's a vicious cycle, because high cortisol causes sleep deprivation, and sleep deprivation causes an increase in cortisol. This isn't a surprise, since sleep deprivation is a huge stress. If you were to force yourself to stay awake during your usual sleep time, the result would be this: At some point you'd become sleepy, because your body temperature would be decreasing and your cortisol levels would be rising rapidly. Now you'd move from just being sleepy to being *very* sleepy. At this point, you'd notice that you felt chilled. As your body temperature plummeted, your blood sugar would begin falling precipitously as well.

If your cortisol levels were spiked too high, you would begin to experience the same patterns during the day, until your energy was depleted, and "brain fog" was a constant state.

job. Methylcobalamin also improves the quality of your sleep and helps you feel refreshed upon waking. Athough methylcobalamin does not impact total levels of cortisol, it can help shift the peak of cortisol secretion, helping place your cortisol clock back on schedule.

Methylcobalamin: 1–3 mg per day taken in the morning

Melatonin: Melatonin is a hormone, and as such it is best used under a health professional's direction. In my experience, it is safe for Type As, and can benefit you in other ways—i.e. alleviating problems with EGF receptor overexpression and immune function. However, using hormones as supplements should only be considered when other, gentler measures have failed.

2. Eat Right for Strength and Balance

In addition to eating right for Type A, pay special attention to these guidelines for keeping stress levels in balance:

- Limit sugar, caffeine, and alcohol. These are short-term "fixes" that ultimately increase stress and slow down your metabolism. One cup of coffee, or one cup every six hours, is usually acceptable for Type As. This amount does not provoke much of a stress response. It mostly effects catecholamines, which are easily eliminated by Type As. If you are a coffee drinker, be careful to limit other caffeine-containing foods. Too much caffeine will generate a cortisol response.

- Don't undereat or skip meals. Use appropriate blood type snacks between meals if you get hungry. Avoid low-calorie diets. Remember, food deprivation is a huge stress. It raises cortisol levels, lowers metabolism, encourages fat storage, and depletes healthy muscle mass.

- Eat a balanced breakfast, with more protein-containing food. For Type As, breakfast should be thought of as the "King of Meals," particularly if you're trying to lose weight. It is the most important meal of the day for balancing your metabolic needs and your stress response. Eat like a king in the morning, like a pauper at night.

- Smaller, more frequent meals will counteract digestive problems caused by low stomach acid. Don't eat when you're nervous or because you're nervous. Your stomach initiates the digestive process with a combination of digestive secretions and the muscular contractions that mix food with them. When you have low levels of digestive secretions, food tends to stay in the stomach longer. In addition, be attentive to food combining. You'll digest and metabolize foods more efficiently if you avoid eating starches and proteins at the same meal. The use of digestive bitters thirty minutes prior to a meal can also help rev up your digestion.

3. Make Exercise Your Safety Valve

Heightened cortisol levels make it harder for Type As to recover from stress. Research has demonstrated that overall cortisol levels can be lowered through a regular program of exercises that provide focus and calming effects. Make these activities a regular—and life saving—part of your lifestyle:

PRACTICE HATHA YOGA.   Hatha yoga has become increasingly popular in Western countries as a method for coping with stress, and in my experience is an excellent form of exercise for Type As.

PRACTICE THE MARTIAL ART, TAI CHI.   Tai Chi, a type of martial art that is basically a form of moving meditation, has also been studied for its antistress effects. Tai Chi clearly drops levels of salivary cortisol, drops blood pressure, and improves mood after a stress-provoking event. Its effects were actually very similar to the antistress effects of taking a walk at 6 km per hour and were superior to just reading as an antidote to stress.

PRACTICE MEDITATION AND DEEP BREATHING.   Meditation has been studied for its effects on stress hormones. It was found that after meditation, serum cortisol levels were significantly reduced. Breathing is a critical component of meditation and yoga. A technique called alternate nostril breathing is a powerful tool in managing your stress levels. Left nostril breathing generates a more relaxing effect or toning down of sympathetic activity. Right nostril breathing might increase sympathetic activity. The switching back and forth, or alternate nostril breathing technique, tends to generate a relative balance between the sympathetic and parasympathetic nervous systems and is a tremendous antistress measure.

While it is fine for Type As to participate in more intense physical activity when you're healthy and in good condition, be aware that these forms of exercise do not act as safety valves for stress in your blood type. I have seen Type As excel at weight lifting and aerobic events, but even then they've had to be very diligent about not overtraining. The warning signs that you're overdoing it include: chronically cold hands, excessive fatigue two hours after exercise, or lightheadedness upon standing. If you are exercising a lot and are experiencing any of these, reduce your training load.

I suggest the following schedule for healthy Type As:

CARDIOVASCULAR ACTIVITY	WEIGHTS	FLEXIBILITY/STRETCHING
25 minutes	20 minutes	30 minutes
2–3 times weekly	2–3 times weekly	3–4 times weekly

ADAPTED LIFESTYLE STRATEGIES	TYPE A CHILDREN

Structure your Type A child's life to include these essential strategies for healthy growth, wellness, and diminished risk for disease.

Young Children
- Reduce exposure to TV; avoid programs or movies that contain violence, horror, danger, or war. This exposure will raise cortisol levels. Emphasize music, books, and art.
- As early as age two or three, a child can join you in a daily deep breathing and stretching exercise session.
- Avoid being in crowds of people—a big stress producer for Type As.
- Cultivate a love of nature and science in children.
- Serve six small meals instead of three big ones.
- Schedule one or two time-out quiet periods each day.
- Set a firm schedule for bedtime, and make sure your child gets between eight and ten hours of sleep a night to maintain the circadian rhythm and avoid cortisol imbalance.
- Play stress-reducing music and use aromatherapy in your child's room.
- There is a tendency for Type As to internalize emotions. Be extra sensitive to signs that your child is upset or troubled. Encourage them to talk it over with you.

Older Children
- Limit exposure to violent movies or TV, encouraging comedies instead. Laughter reduces stress; violence spikes cortisol levels.
- Limit extracurricular school activities to one or two.
- Encourage your child to choose sports activities that don't increase stress levels. Examples: martial arts and dance. Type As are not well suited to repetitive endurance sports.
- Teach problem solving as a way to handle frustration. Type As tend to become easily discouraged.

- Schedule meals at the same time every day.
- Cultivate an appreciation for nature and solitude with activities such as long walks, camping, and bird watching.
- Talk to your child. Encourage him or her to open up to you without fear of judgment or reprisal. Type As have a tendency to internalize their emotions, so there is perhaps a greater need to watch for signs of problems.

ADAPTED LIFESTYLE STRATEGIES | TYPE A SENIORS

Type A's unique profile offers special challenges for seniors—all of which can be effectively addressed with the right strategies. Pay attention to the following:

- Stomach acid production, already low in Type As, decreases even more in about 20 percent of elderly people. It is particularly important to follow the Type A Diet to keep your stomach acid at a level that enables proper digestion. Take a supplement of L-histidine twice daily, drink a weak tea of bitter herbs before a meal, and avoid carbonated beverages.
- Maintaining a circadian rhythm can be difficult for seniors. Overall, elderly people tend to have more problems with interrupted sleep and insomnia. You may need to increase your intake of vitamin B_{12}, or take a melatonin supplement.
- After age sixty, your sense of smell begins to decline, sometimes dramatically. Your sense of smell also plays a role in taste. Both taste and smell serve to activate your digestive juices and announce, "It's time to eat." Often people with a declining sense of taste and smell tend to undereat. Inability to smell strong odors can also be dangerous, as you are less likely to detect food that has spoiled. Undereating is a special problem for Type A seniors. Your delicate immune system also makes you more sensitive to bacterial infections.
- The consequences of stress, especially high cortisol levels, can be systemic. In particular, be aware that increased cortisol levels can lead to bone loss. Daily relaxation and stretching exercises will help prevent osteoporosis. They will also increase your mental acuity. High cortisol levels have been linked to Alzheimer's disease and senile dementia.

Emotional Equalizers

For emotional health and avoidance of Type A–related mind-body imbalances, incorporate the following behaviors into your daily life.

Keys

🔑 Speak up when you feel anxious or overwhelmed. Don't repress or ignore your concerns. Sing!

🔑 Before you add an activity or responsibility, give up one you already have.

🔑 Use natural light therapy in your work space.

🔑 Be decisive. Procrastination raises cortisol levels.

🔑 Schedule a full day of solitude and silence once a month.

🔑 When exercising, stop *before* you reach your limit.

🔑 Break your mental and physical work into segments.

🔑 Supplement your diet with stress-relieving adaptogens (below).

1. Identify Your Tendencies

Research supports the link between high cortisol levels and *"Type C Behavior"* traits. This personality type is thought to be cancer prone, which would be consistent with what is known about Type As; almost all common cancers have a higher reported incidence in Type A than in the other blood types. Some of the common attributes of *"Type C Behavior"* correlate to the expected effects of having higher cortisol levels. For example, people who exhibit this behavior tend to repress their true anxieties while appearing confident and well-adjusted; erect emotional blockades to forming close relationships; often feel unworthy of love; tend to put more into a relationship than they get out of it, often give in to the wishes of others while ignoring their own needs, feel a large amount of self-pity; and worry about small, inconsequential matters. High cortisol levels are associated with shyness and wary behavior in children; "cynically hostile" men; teenage mothers with postpartum depression and anxiety; hyperactive children with internalizing behavior; and children who stutter and have anxiety about communicating.

Many of the conceptions in Japanese pop psychology about the personalities of Type As center on their great ability to handle details and fine points. I find this interesting, in light of the observed connection between Type As and obsessive-compulsive disorder. Perhaps what is "detail orientation" in a healthy Type A may exhibit itself as OCD at the far end of the spectrum.

Evaluate whether you fit any of the personality characteristics that researchers suggest are more typical of your blood type—in particular, a tendency to be introverted, excessively detail-oriented, and even obsessive-compulsive. It is not my intention to label you. Your personality is quite individual, and genetic predispositions only form a small part of the picture. You might consider, though, what this data means to you. In my experience, these prototypical behaviors tend to emerge most strikingly when resistance is low and stress is high.

If you are a Type A who identifies with the characteristics of introversion and the so-called *"Type C Personality"* traits, examine your tendencies to internalize ideas and emotions. Do you feel constrained by your job or your relationship? Do you have someone with whom to share your feelings? Are you sufficiently challenged by your job or hobbies? Do you have the feeling that you adequately express yourself? Do you let your feelings well up inside you before you let anyone else in on the secret?

My own studies show that the introverted, analytical characteristics are especially true of Type A men. Other studies, as noted, have demonstrated that high cortisol is associated with shyness and stuttering in children, and postpartum depression and anxiety in new mothers.

For Type As, mental balance is often achieved when you have ample opportunities to express yourself—be it through art or writing, verbally, or physically. You can also benefit from mood-balancing herbs, such as St. John's wort, or calming herbs, such as chamomile, valerian, and passion flower.

Remember to take breaks when you're involved in work that takes a lot of focus and concentration. As a Type A myself, I've noticed that I am much more productive if I don't work to the point of exhaustion, but rather "bracket" my mental activities with other activities, such as cabinetry. I often switch between mental and physical projects several times a day. The effect is rehabilitating. It allows me to distance myself from each activity, affording greater objectivity and creativity. This strategy also reduces my tendency to neurose over details to the point that a project is ruined. It was Winston Churchill who first wrote of having the ability to "rest" parts of his mind by simply using other parts of his mind. Churchill must have been a Type A! In the midst of World War II, he always managed to find time for his watercolors.

2. Use Adaptogens to Improve Your Stress Response

The term "adaptogen" has been used to categorize plants that improve the nonspecific response to stress. Many of these plants have a bidirectional or normalizing influence on your physiology—if something is too low, they bring it up; too high, they bring it down. The most effective adaptogens for Type A stress control are:

KOREAN OR CHINESE GINSENG (*Panax ginseng*).   Korean and Chinese ginseng are more suited to males. An abundance of research has demonstrated that it can enhance your response to physical or chemical stress, as well as have a beneficial effect on your central nervous, cardiovascular, and endocrine systems.

SIBERIAN GINSENG (*Eleutherococcus senticosus*).   Siberian ginseng is suited to both males and females, and has also been proven to help adapt your body to stressful circumstances.

WITHANIA SOMNIFERA (ASHWAGANDHA).   It has been called Indian ginseng, and is considered to be the preeminent adaptogen from the Ayurvedic medical system. It has similar antistress and anabolic activity to Korean and Chinese ginseng.

OCIMUM SANCTUM OR "HOLY BASIL."   This is a sacred and revered plant in Indian custom and religion. It is loosely categorized as an adaptogen and can promote a better stress response in Type As.

BOERHAAVIA.   Classically thought of as a liver herb, Boerhaavia is also effective as a stress-relieving herb for Type A. It can have a dramatic effect in buffering against elevation of plasma cortisol levels under stressful conditions, in the process preventing a drop in immune system performance. For Type As who have been under prolonged stress to the point where cortisol levels have been exhausted, Boerhaavia's bidirectional adaptogenic activity restores cortisol levels.

TERMINALIA ARJUNA.   This classic heart tonic from the traditional medical system of India is useful to the heart disease–prone Type A. It has the antistress benefit of helping to lower cortisol.

INULA RACEMOSA.   This is another Asian herb with a primary focus on cardiovascular health that mimics the antistress (cortisol-lowering) effect of terminalia.

GINGKO BILOBA.   Thought of usually as an aid to memory, this herb actually has significant antistress (cortisol-buffering) activity and is an excellent and well-balanced herb for Type As.

3. Fight Stress with the Right Supplements
When you are under a great deal of mental, emotional, or physical stress, several supplements are of particular importance for Type As.

VITAMIN C.   Evidence shows that vitamin C, in amounts greater than 500 mg per day, provides a buffer against high cortisol when you are exposed to a lot of stress.

B VITAMINS.   Type As must get extra amounts of B_1, B_5, and B_6 (and ensure you are getting enough B_{12} if your diet is strictly vegetarian) to have an optimal stress response. Vitamins B_1 and B_6 help improve the cortisol function of the adrenal gland and simultaneously normalize the rhythmic activity of the gland. Stress in virtually all forms places extra demands on your B_5 status, increasing overreaction and exhaustion in the face of stress.

ZINC.   About 15 to 25 mg of supplemental zinc can reduce cortisol.

TYROSINE.   Tyrosine is an amino acid that is most appropriate in conditions of acute stress. Strong research shows that taking 3 to 7 grams of tyrosine prior to stressful circumstances substantially reduces the acute effects of stress and fatigue on performance.

PHOSPHATIDYLSERINE.   Phosphatidylserine, found in trace amounts in lecithin, helps regulate the stress-induced activation of the HPA axis. (Note: 400 to 800 mg is needed to achieve results, and this supplement is very expensive.)

PLANT STEROLS AND STEROLINS.   Plant sterols and sterolins are phytochemicals generally described as plant "fats," which are chemically very similar to cholesterol, but appear to have adaptogenic biological activity. In particular, they help to prevent immune system suppression during stress, and normalize cortisol and DHEA levels.

4. Reduce Stress in Your Environment

The following factors are known to increase cortisol levels and mental exhaustion for Type As.[1] Be aware of them and limit your exposure.

- Crowds of people
- Unproductive meetings
- Financial concerns
- Long telephone calls
- Negative emotions
- Anxiety for others
- Cold or hot weather conditions
- Sunbathing
- Lack of sleep
- Coffee (more than 1 cup)
- Smoking
- Dieting (low calories)
- High-carbohydrate breakfast
- Too much sugar and starch
- Violent movies
- Strong chemicals
- Strong smells or perfumes
- Loud noise
- Overwork
- Too much exercise
- Arguments

Other ways to create a harmonious setting:

MUSIC.   Music can be a powerful modulator of stress. Properly used, some music can reduce or buffer your stress response.[2] However, other types of music can actually increase your internal stress response, so music can be a double-edged sword. Studies have shown the following types of music to lower cortisol:
A waltz by J. Strauss
A piece of modern classical by H. W. Henze
"Ambient" music by Brian Eno

AROMATHERAPY.   Calming scents are chamomile and lemon. Use them liberally.

5. Seek Appropriate Treatment for Anxiety.
If you are being treated for an anxiety disorder or suffer from OCD:

- Treatments for OCD often focus on serotonin imbalances and are treated with drugs such as Luvox. Doctors fail to make the cortisol connection and address high levels of cortisol. I believe OCD is cortisol related, not serotonin related. Pursue a course of treatment that focuses on stress reduction.
- OCD patients have been known to have low levels of melatonin. Ask your doctor about taking a melatonin supplement.

6. Take Control
Take charge of the factors you can control. It might be impossible at the present moment to walk away from a stressful job, relationship, or home situation. However, there are things you can do to ease your stress. You can develop new responses to defuse anger or conflict. You can learn to manage your time better. You can just say no to new demands. You can make decisions. This last one is most important. When a matter remains unresolved, it acts as a chronic stressor. Unresolved issues have a similar effect to a virus on your computer's hard drive. They eat up all the available memory and make it impossible to run "programs" like good health and peace of mind. Unmanaged emotions compromise the quality of your life and your health. They limit mental clarity, productivity, and your ability to adapt to stress. Positive, embracing feelings are your best protection against stress—which is why the calming exercises are absolutely critical for Type As.

Type A Two-Tier Diet

The Two-Tier Diet is designed to offer a more individualized program. It has been my experience that some people do very well on the basic Tier One Diet—that is, a moderate degree of adherence to the primary beneficial and avoid foods, with heavy reliance on neutral foods for general nutritional supplementation. Others need a more rigid plan, especially if they suffer from chronic conditions. Adding the Tier Two Diet will increase compliance in order to overcome disease and restore a state of well-being.

> *SECRETOR or NONSECRETOR?*
> *Before you start the diet, take the easy home saliva test to determine your secretor status. See page 358*

Your secretor status can influence your ability to fully digest and metabolize certain foods. For this reason, each food list contains a separate column of rankings for secretors and non-secretors. Although the majority of people are secretors and can safely follow the recommendations in the secretor column, the variations can make a big difference if you are among the approximately 20 percent who are non-secretors.

In rare cases, your A_1, A_2, Rh, and MN status will influence a food ranking. Those distinctions are listed below the appropriate chart.

BENEFICIAL: These foods possess components which enhance the metabolic, immune or structural health of your blood type.

NEUTRAL: These foods usually have no direct benefit or harmful effect, based on your blood type, but many of them supply nutrients needed for a well-balanced diet.

AVOID: These foods contain components that are harmful for your blood type.

The Blood Type Diet Tier System

Tier One: Maximize Health

Make these choices as soon as possible to maximize your health. Using Tier One choices in combination with neutral foods for general nutritional supplementation will suffice for most healthy individuals.

Tier Two: Overcome Disease

Add these choices if you are suffering from a chronic disease or wish to follow the diet at a higher compliance level. If you are adhering to the Tier Two Diet, use caution when you incorporate neutral foods for general nutritional supplementation.

Individualized Dietary Guidelines

If you are a healthy Type A, the Tier One Diet will provide the combination of foods you need for good health. To make the most of it, pay special attention to these guidelines:

Keys

- Avoid excessive use of meat products. Low levels of hydrochloric acid and intestinal alkaline phosphatase make it indigestible for Type A, and can create a range of metabolic problems.
- Limit neutral meats, such as chicken and turkey, to two to three times a week.
- Derive your primary protein from soy products and fresh seafood.
- Include modest amounts of cultured dairy foods in your diet, but avoid fresh milk products, which cause excess mucous production. Cultured dairy products have a probiotic effect; they promote healthy intestinal flora and a stronger immune environment.
- Eat your beans; beans provide an essential high-protein vegetable source for Type A.
- Don't overdo the grains, especially wheat-derived foods. Avoid wheat if you have a weight problem or a tendency to produce mucus.
- Eat lots of beneficial fruits and vegetables.
- Liberally consume nuts and seeds. Higher quantities of this food group have significant cardiovascular advantages for you.
- Drink green tea for extra immune system benefits.
- Consume vitamin A-rich foods such as yellow squash, carrots, spinach, and broccoli to boost intestinal alkaline phosphatase levels.

Type A Dietary Strategies

These strategies are designed to help the healthy Type A avoid the problems that can arise from your specific neurological, digestive, metabolic, and immune makeup.

Increase Your Stomach Acid Levels

Signs of low stomach acid include frequent belching and cracks on the sides of the mouth. These strategies will help counter low stomach acid.

TAKE 500 MILLIGRAMS OF L-HISTIDINE TWICE A DAY. This is an amino acid supplement. It improves gastric acid production, especially if you have allergic symptoms.

USE BITTER HERBS. Herbs such as Gentian (*Gentiana* spp) have long been used by naturopaths to stimulate gastric secretions. They can be taken as a weak tea thirty minutes before a meal.

AVOID CARBONATED BEVERAGES. Stay away from drinks such as mineral water, seltzer, and soda. The carbonation decreases gastrin production, which decreases stomach acidity.

TAKE BETAINE. In the form of betaine hydrochloride, it can increase the acidity of the stomach, and it has some extra benefits. Betaine is also recommended to reduce blood levels of a substance called homocysteine (associated with heart disease). It is used by the body to generate S-adenosylmethionine (SAM-e), a substance that has been receiving media attention as a natural antidepressant and as a healing agent for the liver. In traditional Chinese medicine, anxiety and depression are associated with imbalances of liver energy, or *chi*. Kola nuts contain substantial amounts of betaine, as well as a few other liver protectants, such as d-catechin, l-epicatechin, kolatin, and kolanin. They also contain caffeine, so use them sparingly, and not at all if you have digestive problems.

TAKE DENDROBIUM. This increases acid output and gastrin concentration.

If you suffer from cracks on the lips or sides of the mouth, use a topical licorice gel for temporary relief.

Prevent Lectin Damage/Lower Polyamines

AVOID LECTINS THAT ARE TYPE A RED FLAGS.

kidney beans	*Non-secretors: Avoid wheat and corn*
lima beans	
potatoes	
cabbage	
eggplant	
bananas (secretors only)	
tomatoes	

TIP: Replace tomatoes with a friendlier cocktail. Type As can get their lycopene from the Membrane Fluidizer Cocktail that I have often recommended for Type Bs. Using guava, grapefruit, or watermelon juice as the base, add ½ to 1 tablespoon of high-quality flaxseed oil, and 1 tablespoon of good-quality lecithin. Shake well. The lecithin emulsifies the oil, making a sort of smoothie out of the mixture, which is actually quite palatable. This will increase the absorption of lycopenes from these foods to a level not unlike tomato paste, but without the tomato lectin. Having a few dried apricots as a snack is also a good idea.

Type As can help block the actions of dietary lectins by using polysaccharide sacrificial molecules, such as those found in :

- NAG (N-Acetylglucosamine)
- Fucus vesiculosis—kelp
- Laminaria
- Larch arabinogalactan

Routinely Consume Cultured Foods

The regular consumption of the right cultured foods for your type is one of the critical *Live Right* strategies for Type As. By eating foods teeming with favorable bacteria, you gain significant health advantages, including improved digestive and immune function, better resistance to bacteria, viruses, and other pathogens, improved detoxification, antitumor properties, improved hormonal regulation, better absorption of your nutrients, vitamins, and minerals, and numerous other health effects beneficial to your blood type.

Type As, should routinely eat a range of cultured soy products, including miso, tempeh, and natto. Yogurt and kefir, when made with live culturing organisms, are also powerful foods for Type As and can be eaten two to three times per week. In addition, virtually any bean, pulse, grain, root vegetable, green vegetable, fruit, spice, or beverage can be cultured and used as a great addition to the diet.

Type A Non-Secretor Lectin Blockers:

Chondroitin sulphate (nutriceutical)
Bladder wrack (herbal)
Kelp (herbal)
Glucosamine N-Acetyl (amino acid)
Mannose

The Phony Soy Controversy

Many Type As and Type ABs have expressed concern about soy products after reading warnings that soy products may be protease inhibitors—that is, they inhibit the enzyme secreted by the pancreas that facilitates protein digestion. Let's dispel this myth once and for all. It is true that soy contains a protease inhibitor, named Bowman-Birk Soy Protease Inhibitor (BBI). However, BBI, far from being of harm to Type As and Type ABs, is actually a very good friend. Here's why:

- BBI protease inhibitor from soy has well-recognized anti-carcinogenic properties.
- BBI protease inhibitor from soy is a significant inhibitor of Human Leucocyte Elastase (HLE), an enzyme that dissolves the protein elastin and also degrades and inactivates a number of plasma proteins. Elastase probably plays a physiological function in neutrophil migration, phagocytosis, and tissue remodeling. HLE apparently plays a pathological role in pulmonary emphysema, rheumatoid arthritis, endometriosis, infections, and inflammation.

Thus Type As and Type ABs on soy-based diets can look forward to having lower levels of inflammation, allergy, cancer, and infection—thanks to this "poison" in soy.[3] Another beneficial effect of soy with special importance to Type A is the ability of the phytochemical genestein to block the effects of the enzyme aromatase. Aromatase is an enzyme that produces estrogen and other steroids. Aromatase is located in estrogen-producing cells of the body. Many estrogen-positive cancers are inhibited by blocking this enzyme. Aromatase inhibitors are increasingly the drug of choice for managing metastic breast cancers that have retained estrogen sensitivity. Other aromatase inhibitors include high-lignan flaxseed oil and the flavones Apigenin (found in chamomile) and Chrysin (found in passion flower).

Cultured soy products, including miso, natto, okara, soy sauce, and tempeh, are a treasury of health-promoting compounds for Type A. While not good for all blood types, they are superb antioxidants, improve the absorption rate of iron, decrease the incidence of iron deficiency anemia, and improve the availability of zinc in the diet.

Miso is a cultured paste made from soy beans. It has significant antioxidant activity and enhances the bioavailability of minerals like iron and zinc. Like most cultured soy products, miso has substantially higher quantities of the isoflavones diadzein and genistein, which are thought to play roles in soy's anticancer effect. However, its most beneficial contribution to your health probably lies in its ability to decrease the risk of developing cancer.

Natto is a traditional Japanese food, made by fermenting boiled soy beans with *Bacillus natto*. Like miso, it has substantial health-promoting qualities. Antitumor compounds have been identified in natto, and it contains substantial quantities of isoflavones. Natto enhances iron absorption and zinc bioavailability, and also appears to favorably impact both B and T cell immune performance. Natto also has highly beneficial blood-thinning properties, due to its ability to break down clots. This has special importance for Type A non-secretors, who tend to form clots more easily than Type A secretors.

Okara Koji is okara cultured by *Aspergillus oryzae*, a culturing agent also used to make miso. Okara has substantial quantities of antioxidants, such as gamma-tocopherol, delta-tocopherol, genistin, daizein, genistein, and 3-hydroxyanthranilic acid. It also aids the absorption of iron.

Components of Japanese-style cultured or fermented soy sauce contain antioxidant and anticarcinogenic compounds. Soy sauce also has a beneficial effect on iron absorption.

Tempeh is a cultured soy food indigenous to Indonesia. A potent antioxidant has been isolated from tempeh (3-hydroxyanthranilic acid). Similar to other cultured soy products, tempeh enhances iron availability. Culturing soy beans to make tempeh also favorably impacts the content and formation of fat-soluble vitamins and provitamins, such as beta-carotene and plant sterols. Tempeh is also high in isoflavones. Tempeh can also contain vitamin B_{12}, especially important for Type A vegetarians.

Edamame, boiled soy beans in the pod, are an excellent choice for Type A. I often eat them as a quick snack.

Meat and Poultry

MANY OF THE DISEASES related to a high-animal protein diet are much more common in Type A than in the other blood types. Type A lacks some of the enzymes and stomach acids needed to effectively digest animal protein. Red meat generates polyamines in Type As, and increases cancer risk. Type A non-secretors have been shown to have slightly enhanced abilities to break down animal proteins, but should still derive most of their protein from non-meat sources.

BLOOD TYPE A: MEATS AND POULTRY			
Portion: 4–6 oz. (men); 2–5 oz. (women and children)			
	African	**Caucasian**	**Asian**
Secretor	0–2	0–3	0–3
Non-Secretor	2–5	2–4	2–3
A$_2$	Increase by 1 serving weekly		
MM	Decrease by 1 serving weekly		
	Times per week		

Tier One

FOOD	TYPE A SECRETOR	TYPE A NON-SECRETOR
Bacon/ham/pork	Avoid	Avoid
Beef	Avoid	Avoid
Buffalo	Avoid	Avoid
Duck	Avoid	Neutral
Goat	Avoid	Neutral
Goose	Avoid	Neutral
Heart	Avoid	Avoid
Horse	Avoid	Avoid
Lamb	Avoid	Neutral
Liver (calf)	Avoid	Avoid
Mutton	Avoid	Neutral
Rabbit	Avoid	Neutral
Squirrel	Avoid	Avoid
Turtle	Avoid	Neutral
Veal	Avoid	Avoid
Venison	Avoid	Avoid

Tier Two

FOOD	TYPE A SECRETOR	TYPE A NON-SECRETOR
Partridge	Avoid	Neutral
Pheasant	Avoid	Neutral
Quail	Avoid	Neutral

Neutral: General Nutritional Supplementation

FOOD	TYPE A SECRETOR	TYPE A NON-SECRETOR
Chicken	Neutral	Neutral
Cornish hens	Neutral	Neutral
Grouse	Neutral	Neutral
Guinea hen	Neutral	Neutral
Ostrich	Neutral	Neutral
Squab	Neutral	Neutral
Turkey	Neutral	Beneficial

Fish and Seafood

FISH AND SEAFOOD represent a nutrient-rich source of protein for most Type As. Because of this, fish is probably the best food source to build active tissue mass—especially for Type A non-secretors. Many forms of fish are rich in Omega series fatty acids, which can help lower the risk of cardiovascular disease, in addition to helping control the production of cellular growth factors. In general, many of the seafoods to avoid contain lectins or polyamines. Since Type A non-secretors have much lower levels of blood type A antigen in their digestive tracts, they are less liable to be susceptible to the lectin activities of many types of seafood. Higher levels of stomach acid and enzymes also help non-secretors metabolize deep-ocean fish somewhat better than Type A secretors. The escargot snail *Helix pomatia* is recommended as it possesses a beneficial lectin that strengthens the Type A immune system.

BLOOD TYPE A: FISH AND SEAFOOD			
Portion: 4–6 oz. (men); 2–5 oz. (women and children)			
	African	**Caucasian**	**Asian**
Secretor	1–3	1–3	1–3
Non-Secretor	2–5	2–5	2–4
A₂	Increase by 2 servings weekly		
	Times per week		

Tier One

FOOD	TYPE A SECRETOR	TYPE A NON-SECRETOR
Crab	Avoid	Avoid
Flounder	Avoid	Neutral
Gray Sole	Avoid	Neutral
Grouper	Avoid	Neutral
Haddock	Avoid	Neutral
Hake	Avoid	Neutral
Halibut	Avoid	Neutral
Lobster	Avoid	Avoid
Lox	Avoid	Avoid
Mackerel	Beneficial	Beneficial
Mussels	Avoid	Neutral
Octopus	Avoid	Neutral
Pickerel	Beneficial	Beneficial
Pollack	Beneficial	Beneficial
Red snapper	Beneficial	Beneficial
Salmon	Beneficial	Beneficial
Sardine	Beneficial	Beneficial
Scallop	Avoid	Neutral
Shad	Avoid	Neutral
Shrimp	Avoid	Avoid
Snail (Helix spp, escargot)	Beneficial	Beneficial
Sole	Avoid	Avoid
Tilefish	Avoid	Neutral
Whitefish	Beneficial	Beneficial
Whiting	Beneficial	Beneficial

Tier Two

FOOD	TYPE A SECRETOR	TYPE A NON-SECRETOR
Anchovy	Avoid	Neutral
Barracuda	Avoid	Avoid
Bass (bluegill)	Avoid	Neutral
Bass (striped)	Avoid	Avoid
Beluga	Avoid	Neutral
Bluefish	Avoid	Neutral

Carp	Beneficial	Beneficial
Catfish	Avoid	Avoid
Caviar	Avoid	Neutral
Clam	Avoid	Avoid
Cod	Beneficial	Beneficial
Conch	Avoid	Avoid
Crab (horseshoe)	Avoid	Avoid
Eel/Japanese eel	Avoid	Avoid
Frog	Avoid	Neutral
Harvest fish	Avoid	Beneficial
Herring/kippers (fresh)	Avoid	Neutral
Herring/kippers (pickled)	Avoid	Avoid
Mollusks	Avoid	Avoid
Monkfish	Beneficial	Beneficial
Opaleye fish	Avoid	Neutral
Oyster	Avoid	Avoid
Perch (silver)	Beneficial	Beneficial
Perch (yellow)	Beneficial	Beneficial
Scup	Avoid	Neutral
Squid	Avoid	Avoid
Trout (rainbow)	Beneficial	Beneficial
Trout (sea)	Beneficial	Beneficial

Neutral: General Nutritional Supplementation

FOOD	TYPE A SECRETOR	TYPE A NON-SECRETOR
Abalone	Neutral	Neutral
Bass (sea)	Neutral	Neutral
Bullhead	Neutral	Neutral
Butterfish	Neutral	Neutral
Croaker	Neutral	Neutral
Cusk	Neutral	Beneficial
Drum	Neutral	Beneficial
Halfmoon fish	Neutral	Beneficial
Mahimahi	Neutral	Neutral
Mullet	Neutral	Beneficial
Muskellunge	Neutral	Beneficial

Orange roughy	Neutral	Neutral
Parrot fish	Neutral	Neutral
Perch (ocean)	Neutral	Neutral
Perch (white)	Neutral	Beneficial
Pike	Neutral	Neutral
Pompano	Neutral	Beneficial
Porgy	Neutral	Neutral
Rosefish	Neutral	Beneficial
Sailfish	Neutral	Beneficial
Scrod	Neutral	Neutral
Shark	Neutral	Neutral
Smelt	Neutral	Neutral
Sturgeon	Neutral	Neutral
Sucker	Neutral	Beneficial
Sunfish	Neutral	Neutral
Swordfish	Neutral	Beneficial
Tilapia	Neutral	Neutral
Trout (brook)	Neutral	Beneficial
Tuna	Neutral	Neutral
Weakfish	Neutral	Neutral
Yellowtail	Neutral	Neutral

Dairy and Eggs

DAIRY PRODUCTS can be used in small quantities by Type A secretors, and to a lesser degree by Type A non-secretors. Be especially cautious if you suffer from recurrent sinus infections or colds, since dairy products can be mucus forming for Type As. Eggs in small quantities can serve as a complementary protein source, especially for Type A non-secretors, who tend to metabolize them more efficiently.

BLOOD TYPE A: EGGS			
Portion: 1 egg			
	African	**Caucasian**	**Asian**
Secretor	1–3	1–3	1–3
Non-Secretor	2–3	2–5	2–4
		Times per week	

BLOOD TYPE A: MILK AND YOGURT

Portion: 4–6 oz. (men); 2–5 oz. (women and children)

	African	Caucasian	Asian
Secretor	0–1	1–3	0–3
Non-Secretor	0–1	1–2	0–2
		Times per week	

BLOOD TYPE A: CHEESE

Portion: 3 oz. (men); 2 oz. (women and children)

	African	Caucasian	Asian
Secretor	0–2	1–3	0–2
Non-Secretor	0	0–1	0–1
A$_2$	Decrease milk and yogurt by 2 servings weekly		
MM	Increase eggs by 2 weekly; decrease milk, cheese, and yogurt by 2 servings weekly		
	Times per week		

Tier One

FOOD	TYPE A SECRETOR	TYPE A NON-SECRETOR
American cheese	Avoid	Avoid
Blue cheese	Avoid	Avoid
Brie	Avoid	Avoid
Butter	Avoid	Avoid
Buttermilk	Avoid	Avoid
Camembert	Avoid	Avoid
Casein	Avoid	Avoid
Cheddar cheese	Avoid	Avoid
Colby cheese	Avoid	Avoid
Cream cheese	Avoid	Avoid
Edam cheese	Avoid	Avoid
Emmenthal cheese	Avoid	Avoid
Gouda	Avoid	Avoid
Gruyère	Avoid	Avoid
Half & half	Avoid	Avoid
Ice cream	Avoid	Avoid
Jarlsberg cheese	Avoid	Avoid
Milk (cow-skim or 2%)	Avoid	Avoid
Milk (cow-whole)	Avoid	Avoid

Monterey Jack cheese	Avoid	Avoid
Muenster cheese	Avoid	Avoid
Neufchatel cheese	Avoid	Avoid
Parmesan cheese	Avoid	Avoid
Provolone cheese	Avoid	Avoid
Swiss cheese	Avoid	Avoid

Tier Two

FOOD	TYPE A SECRETOR	TYPE A NON-SECRETOR
Cottage cheese	Avoid	Neutral
Sherbet	Avoid	Avoid
String cheese	Avoid	Avoid
Whey	Avoid	Neutral

Neutral: General Nutritional Supplementation

FOOD	TYPE A SECRETOR	TYPE A NON-SECRETOR
Duck egg	Neutral	Neutral
Egg (chicken)	Neutral	Neutral
Egg white (chicken)	Neutral	Neutral
Egg yolk (chicken)	Neutral	Neutral
Farmer cheese	Neutral	Neutral
Feta cheese	Neutral	Neutral
Ghee (clarified butter)	Neutral	Neutral
Goat cheese	Neutral	Neutral
Goose egg	Neutral	Neutral
Kefir	Neutral	Neutral
Milk (goat)	Neutral	Avoid
Mozzarella cheese	Neutral	Neutral
Paneer	Neutral	Neutral
Quail egg	Neutral	Neutral
Ricotta cheese	Neutral	Neutral
Salmon roe	Neutral	Neutral
Sour cream (low/non-fat)	Neutral	Avoid
Yogurt	Neutral	Neutral

Beans and Legumes

TYPE AS THRIVE on vegetable proteins found in many beans and legumes, although some beans contain problem lectins. In general, this category, along with appropriate choices of seafood, is more than sufficient to build active tissue mass for Type As. Soy beans are to be emphasized; they are a good source of essential amino acids, they contain a lectin that may help protect against several cancers, and they can help inhibit the growth of blood vessels to cancer cells—a particular Type A susceptibility. Fava beans also contain beneficial cancer-fighting lectins, which may help protect against several cancers of the digestive tract.

BLOOD TYPE A: BEANS AND LEGUMES			
Portion: 1 cup			
	African	**Caucasian**	**Asian**
Secretor	5–7	5–7	5–7
Non-Secretor	3–5	3–5	3–5
MM	Increase by 2 servings weekly		
	Times per week		

Variants: MM—Broad beans, tamarind, tofu, and all soy products are Beneficial.

Tier One

FOOD	TYPE A SECRETOR	TYPE A NON-SECRETOR
Adzuki bean	Beneficial	Neutral
Black bean	Beneficial	Neutral
Black-eyed pea	Beneficial	Neutral
Copper bean	Avoid	Neutral
Fava bean	Beneficial	Neutral
Garbanzo bean	Avoid	Avoid
Kidney bean	Avoid	Neutral
Lentil (domestic)	Beneficial	Beneficial
Lentil (green)	Beneficial	Beneficial
Lentil (red)	Beneficial	Beneficial
Lima bean	Avoid	Avoid
Miso	Beneficial	Beneficial

Navy bean	Avoid	Neutral
Pinto bean	Beneficial	Beneficial
Red bean	Avoid	Avoid
Soy bean	Beneficial	Neutral
Soy flakes	Beneficial	Neutral
Soy granules	Beneficial	Neutral
Tempeh (fermented soy)	Beneficial	Neutral
Tofu	Beneficial	Neutral

Tier Two

FOOD	TYPE A SECRETOR	TYPE A NON-SECRETOR
Green bean	Beneficial	Beneficial
Soy cheese	Beneficial	Neutral
Soy milk	Beneficial	Neutral
Tamarind bean	Avoid	Avoid

Neutral: General Nutritional Supplementation

FOOD	TYPE A SECRETOR	TYPE A NON-SECRETOR
Broad bean	Neutral	Neutral
Cannellini bean	Neutral	Neutral
Jicama	Neutral	Neutral
Mung bean (sprouts)	Neutral	Neutral
Northern bean	Neutral	Neutral
Snap bean	Neutral	Neutral
White bean	Neutral	Neutral

Nuts and Seeds

NUTS AND SEEDS can serve as an important secondary source of protein for Type As. In addition, several nuts, such as walnuts, can help lower polyamine concentrations by inhibiting the enzyme ornithine decarboxylase. Flaxseeds are particularly rich in lignins, which can help lower the number of receptors for the epidermal growth factor, needed for the growth of many common cancers. Peanuts also appear to benefit

Type As. Peanut lectin can inhibit early changes in breast cancer tissues, by blocking the estrogen-producing enzyme aromatase.

BLOOD TYPE A: NUTS AND SEEDS			
Portion: Seeds (handful) Nut Butters (1–2 tbsp)			
	African	Caucasian	Asian
Secretor	4–7	4–7	4–7
Non-Secretor	5–7	5–7	5–7
MM	Increase by 2 servings weekly		
	Times per week		

Tier One

FOOD	TYPE A SECRETOR	TYPE A NON-SECRETOR
Flaxseed	Beneficial	Beneficial
Walnut (black)	Beneficial	Beneficial
Walnut (English)	Beneficial	Beneficial
Peanut	Beneficial	Beneficial
Peanut butter	Beneficial	Beneficial

Tier Two

FOOD	TYPE A SECRETOR	TYPE A NON-SECRETOR
Brazil nut	Avoid	Avoid
Cashew/cashew butter	Avoid	Avoid
Pistachio	Avoid	Avoid

Neutral: General Nutritional Supplementation

FOOD	TYPE A SECRETOR	TYPE A NON-SECRETOR
Almond	Neutral	Neutral
Almond butter	Neutral	Neutral
Almond cheese	Neutral	Neutral
Almond milk	Neutral	Neutral
Beechnut	Neutral	Neutral
Butternut	Neutral	Neutral
Chestnut	Neutral	Neutral

Filbert (hazelnut)	Neutral	Neutral
Hickory	Neutral	Neutral
Litchi	Neutral	Neutral
Macadamia	Neutral	Neutral
Pecan/pecan butter	Neutral	Neutral
Pine nut (pignola)	Neutral	Neutral
Poppy seed	Neutral	Neutral
Safflower seed	Neutral	Avoid
Sesame butter/tahini	Neutral	Neutral
Sesame seed	Neutral	Neutral
Sunflower butter	Neutral	Avoid
Sunflower seed	Neutral	Avoid

Grains and Starches

IN CONTRAST TO animal proteins, where Type A non-secretors have a bit of an edge, because of their insulin sensitivities, Type A non-secretors should be careful of their consumption of complex carbohydrates—a concern not generally applicable to Type A secretors. In particular, non-secretors should watch their consumption of wheat and corn, whose lectins can exert an insulinlike effect, lowering active tissue mass and increasing total body fat. Type A secretors should also be wary of overconsuming whole wheat products; in great enough amounts, the agglutinin in whole wheat can aggravate inflammatory conditions and lower active tissue mass. This lectin can often be milled out of the grain, or destroyed by sprouting. Amaranth, an ancient grain, should be included in the basic Type A diet; it contains a lectin that may be beneficial in preventing colon cancer.

BLOOD TYPE A: GRAINS AND STARCHES			
Portion: 1 cup dry (grains or pastas)			
	African	**Caucasian**	**Asian**
Secretor	7–10	7–9	7–10
Non-Secretor	5–7	5–7	5–7
A₂	Decrease by 1 serving weekly		
Rh–	Decrease by 1 serving weekly		
	Times per week		

Tier One

FOOD	TYPE A SECRETOR	TYPE A NON-SECRETOR
Amaranth	Beneficial	Beneficial
Buckwheat/kasha	Beneficial	Neutral
Essene bread (manna bread)	Beneficial	Neutral
Oat flour	Beneficial	Neutral
Rice cake/flour	Beneficial	Neutral
Rye flour	Beneficial	Neutral
Soba noodles (100% buckwheat)	Beneficial	Neutral
Soy flour bread	Beneficial	Neutral
Wheat bread (sprouted commercial)	Beneficial	Neutral

Tier Two

FOOD	TYPE A SECRETOR	TYPE A NON-SECRETOR
Artichoke pasta (pure)	Beneficial	Beneficial
Teff	Avoid	Neutral
Wheat (bran)	Avoid	Avoid
Wheat (germ)	Avoid	Avoid
Wheat (whole wheat products)	Neutral	Avoid

Neutral: General Nutritional Supplementation

FOOD	TYPE A SECRETOR	TYPE A NON-SECRETOR
Barley	Neutral	Neutral
Corn (white/ yellow/blue)	Neutral	Avoid
Cornmeal	Neutral	Avoid
Couscous (cracked wheat)	Neutral	Avoid
Ezekiel bread (commercial)	Neutral	Neutral

Gluten flour	Neutral	Avoid
Gluten free bread	Neutral	Neutral
Kamut	Neutral	Neutral
Millet	Neutral	Neutral
Oat/oat bran/ oatmeal	Neutral	Neutral
Popcorn	Neutral	Avoid
Quinoa	Neutral	Neutral
Rice (cream of)	Neutral	Neutral
Rice bran	Neutral	Neutral
Rice (all forms)	Neutral	Neutral
Rice milk	Neutral	Neutral
Rice (wild)	Neutral	Neutral
Rye/100% rye bread	Neutral	Neutral
Sorghum	Neutral	Neutral
Spelt	Neutral	Neutral
Spelt flour/ products	Neutral	Neutral
Tapioca	Neutral	Neutral
Wheat (gluten flour products)	Neutral	Avoid
Wheat (refined unbleached)	Neutral	Avoid
Wheat (semolina flour products)	Neutral	Avoid
Wheat (white flour products)	Neutral	Avoid

Vegetables

VEGETABLES CAN BE Type A's first line against chronic disease. They provide a rich source of antioxidants and fiber, in addition to helping to lower the production of polyamines in the digestive tract. Onions are highly beneficial for Type As: They contain significant amounts of the antioxidant quercetin. Many vegetables are rich in potassium, which helps lower extra water weight. Although not technically a vegetable, the common domestic mushroom contains cancer-fighting lectins. Artichoke is quite beneficial to the liver and gallbladder, weak spots for

Type As. Parsnips contain polysaccharides, which are a great stimulant to the immune system.

Tomatoes contain a lectin that reacts with the saliva and digestive juices of Type A secretors. It apparently does not react with Type A non-secretors. Yams are typically high in the amino acid phenylalanine, which inactivates the fat-busting enzyme intestinal alkaline phosphatase (already quite low in Type As) and should be minimized or avoided completely.

BLOOD TYPE A: VEGETABLES			
Portion: 1 cup cooked or dry			
	African	**Caucasian**	**Asian**
Secretor	Unlimited	Unlimited	Unlimited
Non-Secretor	Unlimited	Unlimited	Unlimited
MM	Try to use mostly Tier One Beneficials		
	Times per week		

Variants: A$_2$—Red pepper is Neutral. MM—Onions, bok choy, domestic mushrooms, chicory, and tomatoes are Beneficial.

Tier One

FOOD	TYPE A SECRETOR	TYPE A NON-SECRETOR
Acacia (arabic gum)	Avoid	Avoid
Artichoke (domestic/globe /Jerusalem)	Beneficial	Beneficial
Beet greens	Beneficial	Beneficial
Broccoli	Beneficial	Beneficial
Carrot/carrot juice	Beneficial	Neutral
Celery/celery juice	Beneficial	Neutral
Chicory	Beneficial	Beneficial
Collard greens	Beneficial	Beneficial
Dandelion	Beneficial	Beneficial
Fennel	Beneficial	Neutral
Garlic	Beneficial	Neutral
Ginger	Beneficial	Beneficial
Horseradish	Beneficial	Neutral
Kale	Beneficial	Beneficial

Kohlrabi	Beneficial	Beneficial
Leek	Beneficial	Beneficial
Lettuce (romaine)	Beneficial	Neutral
Mushroom (silver-dollar)	Beneficial	Avoid
Okra	Beneficial	Beneficial
Onion (green)	Beneficial	Beneficial
Parsnip	Beneficial	Beneficial
Potato (white/red/ blue/yellow)	Avoid	Avoid
Pumpkin	Beneficial	Beneficial
Rappini	Beneficial	Neutral
Spinach/spinach juice	Beneficial	Beneficial
Swiss chard	Beneficial	Beneficial
Turnip	Beneficial	Beneficial
Yucca	Avoid	Avoid

Tier Two

FOOD	TYPE A SECRETOR	TYPE A NON-SECRETOR
Alfalfa sprouts	Beneficial	Neutral
Aloe/aloe tea/aloe juice	Beneficial	Neutral
Cabbage (Chinese/ red/white)	Avoid	Avoid
Caper	Avoid	Avoid
Chili pepper	Avoid	Neutral
Eggplant	Avoid	Neutral
Escarole	Beneficial	Beneficial
Juniper	Avoid	Avoid
Mushroom (maitake)	Beneficial	Neutral
Mushroom (shiitake)	Avoid	Neutral
Olive (black)	Avoid	Avoid
Olive (Greek/ Spanish)	Avoid	Avoid
Onion (red/ Spanish/yellow)	Beneficial	Beneficial

Pepper (green/ yellow/jalapeno)	Avoid	Neutral
Pepper (red/ cayenne)	Avoid	Neutral
Pickle (in vinegar)	Avoid	Avoid
Potato (sweet)	Avoid	Neutral
Rhubarb	Avoid	Avoid
Sauerkraut	Avoid	Avoid
Tomato/tomato juice	Avoid	Neutral
Yam	Avoid	Avoid

Neutral: General Nutritional Supplementation

FOOD	TYPE A SECRETOR	TYPE A NON-SECRETOR
Agar	Neutral	Avoid
Arugula	Neutral	Neutral
Asparagus	Neutral	Neutral
Asparagus pea	Neutral	Neutral
Bamboo shoot	Neutral	Neutral
Beet	Neutral	Neutral
Beet/beet greens juice	Neutral	Neutral
Bok choy	Neutral	Neutral
Brussel sprout	Neutral	Neutral
Cabbage juice	Neutral	Avoid
Cauliflower	Neutral	Neutral
Celeriac	Neutral	Neutral
Chervil	Neutral	Neutral
Cilantro	Neutral	Beneficial
Cucumber/ cucumber juice	Neutral	Neutral
Daikon radish	Neutral	Neutral
Endive	Neutral	Neutral
Fiddlehead fern	Neutral	Neutral
Kelp	Neutral	Neutral
Lettuce (bibb/ Boston/iceberg/ mesclun)	Neutral	Neutral
Mushroom (abalone)	Neutral	Neutral

Mushroom (oyster/ enoki/portobello)	Neutral	Neutral
Mushroom (straw)	Neutral	Neutral
Mustard greens	Neutral	Neutral
Olive (green)	Neutral	Avoid
Oyster plant	Neutral	Neutral
Pea (green/pod/ snow)	Neutral	Neutral
Pickle (in brine)	Neutral	Avoid
Pimento	Neutral	Neutral
Poi	Neutral	Neutral
Radicchio	Neutral	Neutral
Radish	Neutral	Neutral
Radish sprouts	Neutral	Neutral
Rutabaga	Neutral	Neutral
Scallion	Neutral	Neutral
Seaweed	Neutral	Neutral
Senna	Neutral	Avoid
Shallots	Neutral	Neutral
Squash (summer/ winter)	Neutral	Neutral
String bean	Neutral	Neutral
Taro	Neutral	Neutral
Water chestnut	Neutral	Neutral
Watercress	Neutral	Neutral
Zucchini	Neutral	Neutral

Fruits and Fruit Juices

FRUITS ARE RICH in antioxidants, and many, such as blueberries, elderberries, cherries, and blackberries contain pigments that inhibit weight gain. Thus a diet rich in proper fruits and vegetables can help weight loss by tempering the effects of insulin. Also, fruits can help shift the balance of water in the body from high extracellular concentrations to high intracellular concentrations. Many fruits, such as pineapple, are rich in enzymes that can help reduce inflammation and encourage proper water balance. Other fruits, such as red grapefruit or guava, can supply the antioxidant lycopene, in lieu of tomatoes.

Type A non-secretors should limit their consumption of high glucose fruits, such as grapes and figs, if they are sensitive to sugar.

BLOOD TYPE A: FRUITS			
Portion: 1 cup or 1 piece			
	African	**Caucasian**	**Asian**
Secretor	2–4	3–4	3–4
Non-Secretor	2–3	2–3	2–3
Rh–	Decrease by 1 serving weekly		
MM	Try to use mostly Tier One Beneficials		
	Times per week		

Tier One

FOOD	TYPE A SECRETOR	TYPE A NON-SECRETOR
Banana	Avoid	Neutral
Blackberry/blackberry juice	Beneficial	Beneficial
Blueberry	Beneficial	Beneficial
Cherry (bing, sweet, white, etc)	Beneficial	Beneficial
Cherry juice (black)	Beneficial	Beneficial
Cranberry	Beneficial	Beneficial
Fig (fresh, dried)	Beneficial	Beneficial
Grapefruit/grapefruit juice	Beneficial	Beneficial
Honeydew	Avoid	Avoid
Lemon/lemon juice	Beneficial	Beneficial
Orange/orange juice	Avoid	Avoid
Pineapple/pineapple juice	Beneficial	Beneficial
Plantain	Avoid	Neutral
Plum (dark/green/red)	Beneficial	Beneficial
Prune/prune juice	Beneficial	Beneficial
Water & lemon	Beneficial	Beneficial

Tier Two

FOOD	TYPE A SECRETOR	TYPE A NON-SECRETOR
Apricot/apricot juice	Beneficial	Beneficial
Boysenberry	Beneficial	Beneficial
Coconut/coconut milk	Avoid	Neutral
Lime/lime juice	Beneficial	Neutral
Mango/mango juice	Avoid	Neutral

| Papaya/papaya juice | Avoid | Avoid |
| Tangerine/ tangerine juice | Avoid | Neutral |

Neutral: General Nutritional Supplementation

FOOD	TYPE A SECRETOR	TYPE A NON-SECRETOR
Apple	Neutral	Neutral
Apple cider/apple juice	Neutral	Neutral
Asian pear	Neutral	Neutral
Avocado	Neutral	Neutral
Breadfruit	Neutral	Neutral
Canang melon	Neutral	Neutral
Cantaloupe	Neutral	Avoid
Casaba melon	Neutral	Avoid
Christmas melon	Neutral	Neutral
Cranberry juice	Neutral	Beneficial
Crenshaw melon	Neutral	Neutral
Currants (black/red)	Neutral	Neutral
Date	Neutral	Neutral
Dewberry	Neutral	Neutral
Elderberry (dark blue/purple)	Neutral	Beneficial
Gooseberry	Neutral	Neutral
Grape (black/concord/ green/red/juice)	Neutral	Neutral
Guava/guava juice	Neutral	Neutral
Kiwi	Neutral	Neutral
Kumquat	Neutral	Neutral
Loganberry	Neutral	Neutral
Mulberry	Neutral	Neutral
Musk melon	Neutral	Neutral
Nectarine/nectarine juice	Neutral	Neutral
Peach	Neutral	Neutral
Pear/pear juice	Neutral	Neutral
Persian melon	Neutral	Neutral
Persimmon	Neutral	Neutral
Pomegranate	Neutral	Neutral
Prickly pear	Neutral	Neutral

Quince	Neutral	Neutral
Raisin	Neutral	Neutral
Raspberry	Neutral	Neutral
Sago palm	Neutral	Neutral
Spanish melon	Neutral	Neutral
Starfruit (carambola)	Neutral	Neutral
Strawberry	Neutral	Neutral
Watermelon	Neutral	Beneficial
Youngberry	Neutral	Neutral

Oils

IN GENERAL, TYPE As do best on monounsaturated oils (such as olive oil) and oils rich in omega series fatty acids (such as flax oil). Type A secretors have a bit of an edge in breaking down oils over non-secretors, and probably benefit a bit more from their consumption as well.

BLOOD TYPE A: OILS			
Portion: 1 tbsp			
	African	Caucasian	Asian
Secretor	5–8	5–8	5–8
Non-Secretor	3–7	3–7	3–6
A₂	Increase by 1 serving weekly		
	Times per week		

Tier One

FOOD	TYPE A SECRETOR	TYPE A NON-SECRETOR
Flaxseed (linseed) oil	Beneficial	Beneficial
Olive oil	Beneficial	Beneficial
Walnut oil	Beneficial	Beneficial

Tier Two

FOOD	TYPE A SECRETOR	TYPE A NON-SECRETOR
Black currant seed oil	Beneficial	Beneficial
Castor oil	Avoid	Avoid
Coconut oil	Avoid	Avoid

Corn oil	Avoid	Avoid
Cottonseed oil	Avoid	Avoid
Peanut oil	Avoid	Neutral

Neutral: General Nutritional Supplementation

FOOD	TYPE A SECRETOR	TYPE A NON-SECRETOR
Almond oil	Neutral	Neutral
Borage seed oil	Neutral	Neutral
Canola oil	Neutral	Neutral
Cod liver oil	Neutral	Beneficial
Evening primrose oil	Neutral	Neutral
Safflower oil	Neutral	Avoid
Sesame oil	Neutral	Beneficial
Soy oil	Neutral	Neutral
Sunflower oil	Neutral	Neutral
Wheat Germ oil	Neutral	Neutral

Herbs, Spices and Condiments

MANY SPICES HAVE mild to moderate medicinal properties, often by influencing the levels of bacteria in the lower colon. Many common gums, such as guar gum, should be avoided as they can enhance the effects of lectins found in other foods. Molasses is a beneficial sweetener for Type As: it can provide some additional dietary iron. Turmeric (curry powder) contains a powerful phytochemical called curcumin, which helps lower levels of intestinal toxins. Brewer's yeast is a beneficial food for Type A non-secretors, enhancing glucose metabolism and helping insure a healthy flora balance in the intestinal tract.

Tier One

FOOD	TYPE A SECRETOR	TYPE A NON-SECRETOR
Aspartame	Avoid	Avoid
Barley malt	Beneficial	Neutral
Carrageenan	Avoid	Avoid

Gelatin plain	Avoid	Avoid
Guar gum	Avoid	Avoid
Ketchup	Avoid	Avoid
Mayonnaise	Avoid	Avoid
Molasses	Beneficial	Neutral
Molasses (blackstrap)	Beneficial	Neutral
MSG	Avoid	Avoid
Parsley	Beneficial	Neutral
Soy sauce	Beneficial	Neutral
Tamari	Beneficial	Neutral
Turmeric	Beneficial	Neutral
Vinegar (all)	Avoid	Avoid
Worcestershire sauce	Avoid	Avoid

Tier Two

FOOD	TYPE A SECRETOR	TYPE A NON-SECRETOR
Chili powder	Avoid	Neutral
Mustard (prepared, vinegar free)	Beneficial	Beneficial
Pepper (black/white)	Avoid	Avoid
Pepper (pepper-corn/red flakes)	Avoid	Avoid
Pickle relish	Avoid	Avoid
Sucanat	Avoid	Avoid
Wintergreen	Avoid	Neutral

Neutral: General Nutritional Supplementation

FOOD	TYPE A SECRETOR	TYPE A NON-SECRETOR
Allspice	Neutral	Neutral
Almond extract	Neutral	Neutral
Anise	Neutral	Neutral
Apple pectin	Neutral	Neutral
Arrowroot	Neutral	Neutral
Basil	Neutral	Neutral
Bay leaf	Neutral	Neutral
Bergamot	Neutral	Neutral
Caraway	Neutral	Neutral

Cardamom	Neutral	Neutral
Carob	Neutral	Neutral
Chives	Neutral	Neutral
Chocolate	Neutral	Neutral
Cinnamon	Neutral	Neutral
Clove	Neutral	Neutral
Coriander	Neutral	Neutral
Corn syrup	Neutral	Avoid
Cornstarch	Neutral	Avoid
Cream of tartar	Neutral	Neutral
Cumin	Neutral	Neutral
Curry	Neutral	Neutral
Dextrose	Neutral	Avoid
Dill	Neutral	Neutral
Dulse	Neutral	Neutral
Fructose	Neutral	Neutral
Guarana	Neutral	Neutral
Honey	Neutral	Neutral
Licorice root	Neutral	Neutral
Mace	Neutral	Neutral
Maltodextrin	Neutral	Avoid
Maple syrup	Neutral	Neutral
Marjoram	Neutral	Neutral
Mustard (prepared, with vinegar)	Neutral	Neutral
Mustard (dry)	Neutral	Neutral
Nutmeg	Neutral	Neutral
Oregano	Neutral	Neutral
Paprika	Neutral	Neutral
Peppermint	Neutral	Neutral
Rice syrup	Neutral	Avoid
Rosemary	Neutral	Neutral
Saffron	Neutral	Neutral
Sage	Neutral	Neutral
Salad dressing (OK'd Ingredients)	Neutral	Neutral
Savory	Neutral	Neutral
Sea salt	Neutral	Neutral
Spearmint	Neutral	Neutral
Stevia	Neutral	Neutral
Sugar (brown/white)	Neutral	Avoid

Tamarind	Neutral	Neutral
Tarragon	Neutral	Neutral
Thyme	Neutral	Neutral
Vanilla	Neutral	Neutral
Yeast (baker's)	Neutral	Beneficial
Yeast (brewer's)	Neutral	Beneficial

Beverages

TYPE A NON-SECRETORS may wish to have a glass of wine occasionally with their meals; they derive substantial benefit to their cardiovascular system from moderate use. Green tea should be part of every Type A's health plan. Type As who are not caffeine sensitive might consider having one cup of coffee daily; it contains many enzymes also found in soy that can help their immune systems function more effectively.

Tier One

FOOD	TYPE A SECRETOR	TYPE A NON-SECRETOR
Liquor (distilled)	Avoid	Avoid
Seltzer water	Avoid	Neutral
Soda (club)	Avoid	Neutral
Soda (misc./diet/ cola)	Avoid	Avoid
Tea (black regular)	Avoid	Neutral
Tea (green)	Beneficial	Beneficial
Wine (red)	Beneficial	Beneficial

Tier Two

FOOD	TYPE A SECRETOR	TYPE A NON-SECRETOR
Beer	Avoid	Neutral
Coffee (regular/decaf)	Beneficial	Beneficial

Neutral: General Nutritional Supplementation

FOOD	TYPE A SECRETOR	TYPE A NON-SECRETOR
Wine (white)	Neutral	Beneficial

Individualized Therapies
for Chronic Conditions

As you can see by referring to your Risk Profile, Type A is more susceptible to certain chronic conditions and diseases than the other blood types. The following section details those conditions, the Type A connection, and a wide range of therapies, in addition to the Tier Two Diet, based on your blood type.

See Type A Health Risk Profile, page 176.

Type A–Specific Digestive Conditions

Barrett's Esophagus
Gallbladder and Liver Disease

Barrett's Esophagus

Barrett's esophagus is a precancerous condition that evolves from chronic GERD. Although GERD itself is most prevalent in Type Os, when Type As develop the condition, they are at much greater risk. Up to 20 percent of those with chronic GERD will go on to develop Barrett's esophagus—and up to 10 percent of those will have an increased risk of developing esophageal or stomach cancer. Both cancers are strongly associated with Type As. Furthermore, patients who develop esophageal cancer subsequent to Barrett's typically have a poor prognosis because the cancer is often discovered at an advanced stage. In the cases of Barrett's esophagus that reported outcomes on my Website, 76 percent were Type A. All reported improvement in swallowing and a lessening of heartburn and stomach pain upon adopting the Type A diet and the following additional strategies:

- Avoid coffee, chocolate, mints, and black tea, all of which can provoke GERD. Normally, coffee is beneficial for Type As, as it increases stomach acid. However, if you suffer from GERD, avoid it.
- Cultivate a taste for green tea. Numerous studies have shown that green tea (*Camellia sinensis*) blocks the chemically induced precancerous changes in the esophagus, stomach, and numerous other sites. The active component of green tea is a class of chemicals called green tea polyphenols. Though the complete mechanism of action for these polyphenols is not fully understood, several theories sug-

Type A Diet Tip—Green Tea:

Although it is the most widely drunk beverage in the world, green tea can taste a little thin or watery to palates jaded by espresso and cappuccino. One way that I enjoy green tea is in the Japanese manner, called *Gen Mai Cha,* which blends green tea with toasted brown rice. The brown rice gives the tea a warm, full-bodied flavor that is very satisfying. These blends are usually available in health food stores and gourmet shops. Try to get the best quality green tea you can; look for what is called "first flush" (first clippings off the plant) as it has the highest percentage of polyphenols. Another trick to enjoying green tea is to not overbrew it. When making standard black tea, many people will steep it for minutes at a time. Do this with green tea and you will wind up with a very bitter brew! Steep green tea for only thirty-five to forty-five seconds, and you'll have unleashed the subtleties of its flavor and aroma without having leached out all the tannins and astringents.

gest that they inhibit a tumor-promoting enzyme called ornithine decarboxylase, enhance antioxidants such as glutathione peroxidase, and also have anti-inflammatory activities. These properties of tea polyphenols make them effective chemopreventive agents against stomach and esophageal cancer. Drink at least three cups a day.

- Avoid sugars and sweets, which tend to cause problems for people with GERD.
- Add five to fifteen drops of Gentian (*Gentiana lutea*) to a glass of water and drink it thirty minutes before a meal. Research shows that Type As take a lengthy forty-five minutes to produce peak gastrin levels, compared to fifteen minutes for Type Os. Gentian, a bitter, has been shown to increase gastrin. By taking this bitter thirty minutes before eating, your digestive secretions will be better prepared to digest your meal. An interesting note is that digestive bitters evolved as a cultural tradition in several European countries. This is one tradition that many Type As would benefit from by adding to their dietary regimen.
- Ginger: Several components of ginger protect the cells lining the stomach. I've found that a teaspoon of fresh ginger juice taken several times daily can be a very effective strategy for GERD.
- Fenugreek: A digestive aid.

**Parenting Tip:
Conquering Chronic Ear Infections**

Ear infections (*otitis media*) are a childhood medical problem accounting for almost 50 percent of all pediatric visits. It has been estimated that about two-thirds of the infants in the United States will
have an ear infection prior to age two. While any blood type can
have an ear infection (or recurrent ear infections), Type A children
(or even children with Type A mothers) have about a 50 percent
higher rate of infections and once having an infection are 26 times
more likely to have a repeat infection.[4] Certain strains of bacteria
most likely to cause ear infections have very strong preferences for
the Type A antigen. The conventional treatment using antibiotics is
ineffective and ultimately more damaging than doing nothing. A
better course of action includes these blood type strategies:

- Type A mothers-to-be should take measures to ensure
  maximum health prior to giving birth.
- New mothers should consider breast feeding for a minimum
  of four months as it provides protection. Bottle feeding is
  associated with a higher rate of ear infections. If you do bottle
  feed, never lay a baby on his or her back during feeding. This
  increases the likelihood of regurgitation into the middle ear.
- Avoid foods with a strong association to ear infection,
  including cow's milk, wheat, egg whites, peanuts, soy, corn,
  tomatoes, chicken, and apples. Also, when you introduce solid
  foods to your infant, begin with fruits and vegetables from the
  beneficial lists that are easily digestible. Delay the introduction
  of grains, legumes, nuts, and seeds until the infant's digestive
  tract has developed stronger barrier mechanisms (at least 3
  months but preferably 6–9 months).

Gallbladder and Liver Disease

The gallbladder is a small sac that sits just beneath the liver. It serves as
a sort of storage room for bile. It is the job of the gallbladder to concentrate bile and then release it when food is passing through the small intestine. Sometimes components of bile—especially cholesterol and
bilirubin—come out of solution and form crystals in the gallbladder, much
as sugar crystallizes when we make rock candy. These pieces of hard matter are called gallstones. Research shows that gallstones are much more
frequent in Type As, as are other liver-related problems. Jaundice in all
forms was first linked to Type A over seventy-five years ago. Continuing
studies have indicated that cirrhosis in general has a much higher occur-

> **▪ FROM THE BLOOD TYPE OUTCOME REGISTRY ▪**
>
> *Tom M.*
> *Type A*
> *Middle-aged male*
> *Improved: Barrett's esophagus*
>
> "It has been difficult to strictly follow the Type A diet (old habits are hard to break). The greatest benefit has been from the near elimination of red meat from my diet. I have noticed an improvement in the way I feel overall. I am not overweight and am in generally good health with the exception that I suffer from Barrett's esophagus. I have been able to cut my daily dose of Zantac in half."

rence in Type As—a fact that I have observed clinically.[5] There is some evidence that bile duct cirrhosis is produced by free-radical damage, perhaps secondary to the liver detoxifying foreign compounds. If true, this would be another good reason for Type As to consume abundant amounts of antioxidant rich fruits and vegetables and drink green tea.

The best thing you can do to protect your liver and gallbladder is to keep your weight under control. Other suggestions:

- Avoid oral contraceptives, which have been linked to gallstones.
- Dandelion root is a great herb for Type As. It is safe and gentle and will help to improve overall liver function.
- Potent, bitter substances, such as artichoke leaf extract, stimulate digestive enzymes and support liver and gallbladder health by promoting bile flow and enhancing cholesterol metabolism.
- Bupleurum is a traditional Chinese herb and has been shown to increase the excretion of bile acids and cholesterol, reducing levels in the blood.
- Curcumin, a chemical component of the Ayurvedic spice turmeric, appears to discourage the formation of gallstones.
- Lecithin is a rich source of phospholipids such as choline, which help to regulate bile stability and enhance its secretion. Increasing the amount of lecithin in the bile decreases the tendency for cholesterol to crystallize into a gallstone. Since the composition of lecithin in bile is responsive to dietary manipulations, a tablespoon or two a day of soy lecithin can be a good gallstone preventive.
- Eat tuna, a rich source of phosphatides.

If Your Type A Child Is Autistic: The Solution Might Be in the Liver

There has been some interest recently in the use of secretin, a hormone that stimulates the liver to produce bile, and triggers pancreatic activity, as a therapy in autism. Autism impacts the normal development of the brain in the areas of social interaction and communication skills.

Children and adults with autism typically have difficulties in verbal and nonverbal communication, social interactions, and leisure or play activities. The disorder makes it hard for them to communicate with others and relate to the outside world. In some cases, aggressive and/or self-injurious behavior may be present. Persons with autism may exhibit repeated body movements (hand flapping, rocking), unusual responses to people, or attachments to objects and resistance to changes in routines. Although autism is thought by some to be limited to males, one in five autistic children is female. One study on secretin and autism reported a study of three children with autism and gastrontestinal problems. The study indicated that after secretin infusion, gastrointestinal function improved, and the children became more sociable and communicative. Although there is not yet a published study, an informal accounting shows a marked prevalence of Type As among autistic children. Recently, there has been positive feedback on the efficacy of the Blood Type Diet in some Type A children with autism. Since the Type A Diet limits several dietary lectins thought to interfere with secretin, it is not too far-fetched to consider that improvement in these children may have actually resulted from enhancement of their own secretin metabolism. As a young mother wrote of her three-year-old Type A daughter, Anna: "Due to using your book, we have cured our three-year-old of autism and have finally found a cure for the constipation she has had since birth.

- Season with coriander. Coriander seeds (*Coriandrum sativum*) have been shown to enhance the synthesis of bile acid by the liver and increase the degradation of cholesterol to fecal bile acids and neutral sterols, which also lowers cholesterol. Coriander seeds also increase HDL cholesterol.
- Take milk thistle (*Silybum marianum*), an antioxidant, with the additional benefit of reaching very high levels in the liver and bile ducts. If you have liver or gallbladder problems—or a family history of them—add a milk thistle supplement to your protocol. (NOTE: Do not use for malignancies other than liver disease.)

Osteoporosis Alert:
Type A Post-Menopausal Women

Post-menopausal women naturally have a higher risk of bone loss, leading to osteoporosis, as a result of estrogen depletion. Type A women have an increased risk because of low levels of intestinal alkaline phosphatase. Repeated studies have shown that this enzyme positively impacts calcium metabolism. Furthermore, higher stomach acid predicts better calcium absorption. Although conventional wisdom in the nutrition community holds that high protein diets accelerate bone loss, the scientific literature shows that the opposite is true. This presents a special challenge for Type A women—especially if you are not using some form of estrogen replacement. It is very important for you to check your secretor status. Type A nonsecretors have extremely low levels of intestinal alkaline phosphatase, which is involved in calcium delivery. To promote healthy bones:

1. Eat canned salmon and sardines with the bones.
2. Regularly consume low-fat yogurt, soy milk, and goat milk.
3. Include lots of broccoli and spinach in your diet.
4. Take daily dose of supplemental calcium citrate—300 to 600 mg.
5. Follow the Type A exercise regimen and do as much walking as you can.
6. In the last year, I've been using a sea-derived calcium on my clinic patients which appears to possess extraordinary absorption properties. Called "AquaMin," this calcium is derived from several species of Irish sea kelp and appears to be efficiently utilized by all the blood groups.

Type A–Specific Metabolic Conditions

Obesity/Low Metabolism
High Cholesterol
Heart Disease
Excessive Blood Clotting

Obesity/Low Metabolism

In many ways, Type A is the exact opposite of Type O when it comes to metabolism. While animal protein speeds up the Type O metabolic rate and makes it more efficient, it has a very different effect on Type A. Many meat-eating Type As report feeling fatigued and lacking energy, especially when they engage in aerobic exercise and restrict complex carbohydrates. Another common Type A problem with excess meat consumption is fluid retention, the result of the inability to properly digest high-protein foods. While Type Os burn their meat as fuel, Type As tend to make a toxic mess out of it.

Type As who struggle with low metabolism and weight gain have another challenge—the effects of high cortisol. For you, being in a condition of stress equals weight gain. That's because stress hormones promote insulin resistance and hormonal imbalance. They also catabolize (burn) muscle tissue instead of fat. Obesity itself leads to cortisol resistance; it becomes a dangerously vicious circle for Type As. High cortisol is also associated with leptin, a hormone related to the obesity gene, which increases your appetite.[6]

In addition to controlling stress, here are some other suggestions for Type As who need to lose weight:

1. LEARN YOUR METABOLIC PROFILE. Knowing your muscle mass, percentage of body fat, and basal metabolic rate can be more important than knowing your weight. These are the indicators of metabolic balance. Your goal is not just to lose pounds, but to build muscle. I suggest that you have a bioelectrical impedence analysis. If that's not feasible, there are some do-it-yourself methods for learning more about your metabolic state. These methods are not scientifically precise, but they'll provide a general idea of your fitness level—and whether or not you're holding excess water weight.

Test for Extracellular Water—Edema: Push your finger firmly down on your shin bone and hold it for five seconds. If you push against muscle or fat, the skin will bounce back up. If there is water between the cells, it will be displaced laterally, and the dimple won't fill in immediately. The longer the indentation remains, the more water is present—meaning you're carrying excess weight as water.

Measure Your Hip to Waist Ratio: Excess weight is most unhealthy—and most conducive to metabolic problems—when it is centered in your abdomen, as opposed to your hips and thighs. Here's a quick test to learn about your fat distribution: Stand straight in front of a full-length mirror. Using a tape measure, measure the distance around the smallest part of your waist. Now measure the distance around the largest part of your buttocks. Divide your waist measurement by your hip measurement.

▪ FROM THE BLOOD TYPE OUTCOME REGISTRY ▪

Sarah P.
Type A
Young female
Improved: Weight loss

"I successfully followed the principles for Blood Type A for approximately four months and experienced tremendous health benefits. My mucus was gone (amazing), I lost ten pounds in three months, and felt right with my body for the first time in years. However, when I went through a period of fatigue nine months after starting the diet, I decided that based on the recent hoopla, I should eat a high-protein diet a la Dr. Atkins, The Zone, Protein Power, etc. I gobbled meat, cheese, heavy creams, and high-fat nuts with some lettuce in between. After a week, I'd gained five pounds, felt sullied from all that meat, and confused. All of these plans claim that the pounds just fall off, but for me it was the opposite. Must be all those O types creating the rave (as they tend to!) I came out of the fog and realized that the Type A diet was perfect for me—job burn-out and lack of career direction were the major contributors to my fatigue. I'm back on Type A foods, and I toast my soy milk latte to Dr. D'Adamo."

A healthy ratio for women is .70 to .75. A healthy ratio for men is .80 to .90.

2. PAY ATTENTION TO WHEN YOU EAT.   Often, how much you eat is less important than when you eat it. Eat the same amount of calories early in the day and most people lose weight, eat them at night and most people gain weight. Skipping breakfast or eating only a small amount of food for breakfast will have detrimental effects on your slow Type A metabolism. Cortisol and thyroid hormones will both be impacted. The same applies to skipping lunch. If you are serious about losing weight, a critical strategy is to eat a well-balanced breakfast, a well-balanced lunch, and an adequate dinner—early in the evening. Resist the late night munchies.

3. SUPPLEMENT YOUR DIET WITH METABOLISM BOOSTERS.
   - CoQ10: 60 mg twice daily. Coenzyme Q10 is critical for energy metabolism and heart health. Supplementation has been shown to reduce blood pressure, blood sugar levels, and triglycerides, while improving HDL cholesterol. Since CoQ10 is an antioxi-

dant, it also reduces the oxidant stress often seen in obesity and increases body levels of antioxidant vitamins.

- l-Carnitine: 1–2 g l-Carnitine is needed to move fats into your mitochondria (the "energy packet" within the cell), where they can then be used as a source of energy. Evidence demonstrates that l-Carnitine reduces insulin resistance.
- Biotin is a vitamin needed in fat metabolism. Evidence shows that at the correct dose, biotin can lower blood sugar, improve tolerance to sugar, and decrease insulin resistance.
- Lipoic Acid: 100–600 mg per day can help promote improved sugar handling capabilities. Lipoic acid is also a critical nutrient in energy metabolism and is an acclaimed and powerful antioxidant.
- Magnesium: 200–300 mg a day. Overweight individuals, especially with extremely poor sugar-handling capabilities, are often deficient in this mineral.
- Zinc: 25 mg. Zinc is needed for growth hormone function, thyroid function, and a balanced stress response.
- L-glutamine: 200–500 mg, twice daily.

High Cholesterol
A number of studies show that Type As and Type ABs are more likely to be at risk of heart disease and death by virtue of elevated cholesterol. Type As need to recognize that they are not metabolically equipped to deal with dietary fat, and consumption of a high-fat diet will probably result in high cholesterol levels. The key is diet. However, here are some supplements that will help keep cholesterol levels in check:

PANTETHINE.   Pantethine is the active form of vitamin B_5, or pantothenic acid. However, pantothenic acid is not the equivalent of pantethine. You'll need to find out if your health food store or pharmacy stocks pantethine. It is made by several reputable companies and shouldn't be too difficult to locate. Numerous studies attest to the ability of pantethine to lower cholesterol anywhere from 18–24 percent. Pantethine also lowers concentrations of the lipoprotein particles that are responsible for the plaque that develops into "hardening of the arteries." Pantethine, in 600 mg per day doses for six to nine months, was shown to lower triglycerides 37.7 percent in diabetic subjects—greater than the other drugs tested. Perimenopausal women are at a much greater risk of heart disease. One Italian study showed that after sixteen weeks of treatment, pantethine produced significant reductions of total cholesterol, LDL-cholesterol, and LDL-C/HDL-C ratio.[7] Pantethine is safe (huge doses have been given to animals with no ill effects), and well-tolerated by Type As. A great side-effect for Type As is that pantethine also promotes an improved ability to adapt to stress without exhausting your adrenal resources.

SOY.   A number of studies have shown that the consumption of soy products can reduce cholesterol levels. The effectiveness is greatest in people with very high levels (over 355 mg/dL), which can be reduced by as much as 20 percent. In the 260 to 333 mg/dL category, the possible reduction is less than 10 percent. About 50 grams of soy protein a day are needed for the maximum effect. To put this into perspective, consider that one cup of soy milk contains 4 to 10 grams, 4 ounces of tofu contains 8 to 13 grams, and a 3 ounce soy burger has 18 grams.

FIBER.   Fiber comes in two varieties—soluble and insoluble. Of the two, it is soluble fiber that is believed to reduce blood cholesterol, by binding to bile acids in the intestine. Since bile acids are made from cholesterol, their removal from the digestive tract forces more to be synthesized from cholesterol, resulting in a lowering of blood cholesterol. Unfortunately, you have to eat a lot of soluble fiber to have any significant effect on your cholesterol: anywhere from 60 to 100 grams daily. Additionally, as the amount of soluble fiber in your diet increases, the levels of good cholesterol (HDL) go down as well. Having a high-fiber diet is good medicine; going to the extremes advocated to accomplish cholesterol lowering seems irrational to me; we're just mopping the floor and neglecting to turn off the faucet. Psyllium powder is perhaps the best source of soluble fiber; a teaspoon three times daily can lower cholesterol as much as 15 percent.

MAGNESIUM.   Many people with high cholesterol and triglycerides are magnesium deficient, so you may need a supplement. A typ-

---

• FROM THE BLOOD TYPE OUTCOME REGISTRY •

Barry F.
Type A
Middle-aged male
Improved: Cardiovascular

"Lab tests indicate dramatic decrease in blood cholesterol and triglycerides, lost twenty-plus pounds, digestion working much better, energy more stable throughout the day, clearer thinking. Everything got better on the plan. I practice acupuncture and herbal medicine and regularly recommend this to my patients."

ical dose for Type A is 250–500 mg daily. Green leafy vegetables are a good food source.

FISH OIL, FLAXSEED OIL.   There is some evidence that fish oil supplementation increases HDL cholesterol and lowers homocysteine levels, a newly recognized cardiac risk factor. Flaxseed oil and walnuts are also good sources of the omega-3 acid alpha linolenic acid.

PROBIOTIC BACTERIA AND CULTURED FOODS.   Friendly bacteria have a modest abilty to lower cholesterol levels.

PYROXIDAL (VITAMIN B$_6$)   Aids protein metabolism and helps regulate water balance.

Heart Disease

In addition to eating right for your blood type, keeping your stress levels in check, and lowering your cholesterol, here are some supplements that promote heart health:

HAWTHORN.   Traditional naturopathic wisdom holds that hawthorn has solventlike effects on the arteries. It is currently used to treat angina, hypertension, arrhythmias, and congestive heart failure.

COENZYME Q10.   This has positive effects on the heart, as well as protecting against periodontal disease, where low-grade infections can have additional damaging effects on the arteries. Supplemental CoQ10 alters the natural history of cardiovascular illnesses and has the potential for prevention of cardiovascular disease through the inhibition of LDL cholesterol oxidation and by the maintenance of optimal cellular function throughout the ravages of time and internal and external stresses.

ANTIOXIDANTS.   Recent evidence suggests that one of the important mechanisms predisposing people to the development of atherosclerosis is oxidation of the cholesterol-rich, low-density lipoprotein particle. Low-density lipoprotein oxidation can be prevented by naturally occurring antioxidants such as vitamin C, vitamin E, and beta-

---

Type A and Menopause

If you are in perimenopause or menopause, talk to your physician about using the fraction "estriol" (2 to 4 mg) to relieve symptoms and protect yourself from bone loss and cardiovascular problems that come with estrogen depletion. Estriol is safer for you than the conventional ERT, Premarin. Dong quai and primrose oil are generally safe for Type As. The herb black cohosh can help relieve hot flashes.

carotene. Antioxidants are best derived from the diet or from food-derived supplements.

BEWARE OF EXTRA IRON.   If you suffer from anemia—a Type A tendency—take care with extra iron supplements. A survey of over 1,900 Finnish men between the ages of forty-two and sixty revealed a 4 percent increase in heart attack risk with each 1 percent increase in serum ferritin. Ferritin is the protein the body uses to store iron. Apparently, high iron levels catalyze the formation of free radicals, which damage the artery wall.

Herbal Aids:

Terminalia arjuna: This classic heart tonic from the traditional medical system of India is useful to the heart disease–prone Type A. It has the additional benefit of helping to lower cortisol.

Inula racemosa: another Asian herb with a primary focus on cardiovascular health, which mimics this antistress (cortisol lowering effect) of terminalia.

Excessive Blood Clotting

Type A is associated with higher levels of the clotting chemicals factor VIII and von Willebrand's disease. Both of these clotting conditions are associated with increased risk of heart attack.

LEMON AND WATER.   Although not documented in the literature, one of my teachers, John Bastyr, used to say that the juice of three to four lemons has almost the clot-inhibiting action of Coumadin. This is a good tonic for Type As first thing in the morning, as it has the added benefit of reducing mucus production, a particular Type A problem.

STRESS REDUCTION.   There is good evidence that Type As react to stress by increasing the viscosity (thickness) of their blood. Practicing good relaxation techniques, yoga or tai chi, can be valuable adjuncts to a healthy heart protocol.

GINGKO BILOBA/ASPIRIN.   Gingko inhibits the platelet-activating factor, which may help minimize excessive clot formation. Aspirin appears to lower the rate of coronary artery disease, in part by its inhibitory effects on factor VIII. Low-dose aspirin may also help lower your risks of colon cancer, another disease with a known preference for Type A. I wouldn't advise taking both gingko and low-dose aspirin; they tend to amplify the effects of each.

Other A-friendly substances with abilities to reduce platelet aggregation include ginger, garlic, and bromelain.

Type A–Specific Immune Conditions

Cancer

(In particular, Breast, Stomach, Colon, Prostate)

Cancer

Without question, the best way to protect yourself from cancer is to follow the Type A Diet and reduce your stress levels. Over the years, I've developed a number of supplementary strategies. However, I want to emphasize that none of the suggestions in this section are meant to replace the recommendations of your surgeons and oncologists. My experience is that the best approach to take with an adversary like cancer is to place as many independent and mutually supportive strategies at your disposal as possible. My patients are routinely utilizing the best that conventional medicine has to offer. I advise you to do the same. The strategies we will discuss are accessory strategies, which attack cancer from an angle currently ignored or not emphasized within conventional medicine. Some of these angles are actually being explored, and I suspect they will eventually be incorporated into the mainstream. Until that time, view these strategies as additional fences placed around a bad neighbor's yard.

If you are suffering from a cancerous condition, I do not encourage you to use these strategies alone. My experience is that the most successful outcomes are the result of using the best of conventional medicine, supplemented with the best of natural medicine.

1. TAKE YOUR PROBIOTICS. Cultured foods provide a treasure trove of activity antagonistic to cancer. See page 193 for specific details.

2. USE LECTINS TO FIGHT CANCER. Lectins are not always bad for you. Substantial research has demonstrated that certain lectins agglutinate malignant cells. These lectins happen to be A-like in composition. As a rule, malignant cells are agglutinated by very low concentrations of a particular lectin and normal cells are not agglutinated unless the concentration is many times higher. The higher proportion of malignant cells agglutinated results from the sizable increase in surface receptors on the malignant cells, which results from their incredibly high reproduction rate.

Peanut lectin has been shown to inhibit the growth of several breast cancer cell lines, in addition to allowing for the destruction of breast cancer cells.[8] Amaranth lectin, fava bean lectin, and the lectin in the common edible mushroom are all of potential benefit in fighting colon cancer.

Perhaps it is the preponderance of soy products used in macrobiotic cooking (and the concurrent high intake of soybean lectin) that has resulted in the many positive responses to cancer ascribed to this form of diet. Soybeans are typically thought of as anticarcinogenic, by virtue of their estrogen-like components. The lectins in soy, which can comprise up to 5 percent of the dry weight, can entangle cancer cells—especially in the colon and breast.

3. IMPROVE YOUR NATURAL KILLER CELL ACTIVITY.   To boost your NK activity—crucial for fighting cancer—follow these guidelines:

- Increase your intake of green vegetables.
- Increase your intake of soybean products.
- Increase your intake of omega-3 fatty acids.
- Decrease your intake of polyunsaturated vegetable fats.
- Keep dietary fat intake between 20 and 25 percent of calories (22 percent is probably about ideal).
- Maintain proper body weight.
- Exercise. If you are trying to improve the activity of your NK cells, exercise will help, but don't go overboard. Stick with the Type A exercise prescriptions.
- Get plenty of fresh air and sunlight
- Use modest amounts of alcohol (males especially).
- Moderate your work hours.
- Don't smoke.
- Decrease stress. Stress in virtually any way, shape, or form will

Helix Pomatia: The Antimetastatic Lectin

The lectin contained in *Helix pomatia* (snail) has been widely researched for its anticancer properties. In particular, it has demonstrated the ability to unmask A-like cancerous and precancerous cells, so the Type A antibodies will recognize them as enemy and launch an attack.[9] It does this by attaching to the A marker found on cancer cells called LLC, which acts as an internal passport, allowing the "bad guys" to cross the road blocks (lymph nodes) and into the systemic circulation.

I routinely suggest the inclusion of *Helix pomatia* as a dietary supplement for women with breast cancer. I have also witnessed some remarkable and quick alterations in lymphatic swelling in several of my lymphoma patients consuming this food (and its lectin) routinely.

negatively effect NK cell function. In studies of women with stage I and II breast cancer, higher NK activity was predicted by the perception of factors such as positive emotional support from a spouse or intimate other, an empathetic doctor, and the ability to find means of outside support. Generally, tests assessing a woman's overall stress level upon being diagnosed with breast cancer strongly correlated to NK cell activity. In these women, a high degree of stress predicted a lower ability of NK cells to destroy cancer cells. High stress also significantly predicted a poorer response to interventions aimed at improving NK cell activity.[10]

4. MODIFY EGF. Epidermal Growth Factor (EGF) is a polypeptide hormone that aids the growth and repair of our protective epithelial tissue. EGF is widely distributed in the body, with high concentrations detectable in saliva, the prostate gland, and the duodenum of the small intestine. The receptor for EGF (EGF-R) is specific for a carbohydrate that is closely related to the Type A antigen.

The connection between EGF-R and the A antigen becomes clear when you study the data.[11] EGF-R plays an important role in a variety of human cancers that show a higher incidence for Type A. Of all the dietary factors that you can control, the type and quantity of fat you consume might have the largest impact on EGF. The essential polyunsaturated fatty acid, linoleic acid, is an important promoter of cancer progression. You have several options:

- Reduce the amount of this fat in your diet.
- Take a melatonin supplement before bedtime. Melatonin inhibits the uptake of plasma linoleic acid.
- Inhibit the activity of 5-lipoxygenase, a compound that is related to cancer cell growth. Tamoxifen is a 5-lipoxygenase inhibitor. So is olive oil. Other medicinal plants that perform this function:
  - ginger (has at least eight 5-lipoxygenase inhibitory compounds)
  - turmeric
  - stinging nettles
  - saw palmetto
  - boswellia
  - rosemary
- The antioxidants quercetin and luteolin appear to inhibit the stimulatory effects of EGF, probably by inhibiting its activity on the EGF receptor.
- Wheat germ lectin activates the EGF receptor as efficiently as

EGF itself, making the use of wheat lectin products inadvisable for cancer patients. Mannan-binding protein and other mannose-specific lectins appear to inhibit the activation of the EGF receptor. As such, these are excellent foods for Type As.

Foods with mannose-binding lectins include:

- onion (*Allium cepa*)
- garlic (*Allium sativum*)
- corn (*Zea mays*)
- leek (*Allium porrum*)
- aloe (*Aloe arborescens*)
- saffron (*Crocus sativus*)

To a lesser degree (mannose-glucose specific):

- fava beans (*Vicia fabia*)
- peas (*Pisum sativum*)
- sweet pea (*Lathyrus odoratus*)
- lentils (*Lens culinaris*)

5. ASK YOUR DOCTOR ABOUT THE TYPHOID VACCINE. George F. Springer, M.D., spent over twenty years harnessing the potential of the immune system to combat cancer. Originally a pioneer in work with blood type antigens, Springer dedicated his life and his unique expertise to breast cancer after his wife died from this disease. His work eventually led him to the development of what is known as "Springer's vaccine." His reported five- and ten-year survival rates for stage II, III, and IV breast cancer with this novel T (Thomson-Friedenreich) and Tn antigen therapy are nothing short of amazing when compared against standard treatments.

Springer's work capitalized on the difference between healthy and cancerous cells to create a vaccine that specifically stimulated the immune system to fight cells with these stumps (T and Tn antigens).

His vaccine consisted of three parts:

- chemically degraded Type O blood cells (providing T and Tn antigens)
- the Salmonella typhii vaccine or typhoid vaccine (which contains T and Tn antigens)
- calcium phosphate (he believed the T and Tn antigens could stick to this)

Springer gave the vaccine to breast cancer patients subcutaneously (under the skin), initially at six week intervals, eventually extending the gap to twelve weeks. For people receiving chemotherapy, he waited three to four weeks after cessation of the last round of chemotherapy prior to beginning his treatment. In the case of radiation, he waited one to three months after the last dose of radiation prior to initiating treatment. He recommended that his patients receive this vaccine "ad infinitum."

Springer passed away in the spring of 1998, and the vaccine he used with such great results is, as far as we know, currently unavailable. The *S. typhii* vaccine, a component of his vaccine, is readily available. Three variations of this vaccine are available on the market; however, one of the injectable forms (preferably the typhoid vaccine manufactured by Wyeth-Ayerst) should be used if attempting to boost T and Tn antibodies. The oral form should not be used.

As a public health measure, the typhoid vaccine is easy to get. Dosing schedule is usually two injections, one month apart. A booster is usually recommended every three years. The vaccine should never be given during pregnancy or during an active infection. It should not be given until at least one month after the last dose of chemotherapy, or one to three months after the last dose of radiation.

This vaccine is generally very well tolerated; however, occasionally some flu-like symptoms will occur and persist for one to two days following the vaccination. Localized redness, swelling, and discomfort can occur at the injection site, especially for those with an active cancer, and may last one to two days.

While this vaccine cannot be expected to produce the outcomes Springer achieved, it is one of the only options I know of that might promote increased amounts of T and Tn antibodies. As such, it offers a potential to work in an area that is ignored in most cancer protocols. At its worst, it will offer you a degree of protection against typhoid. This vaccine is safe for all blood types. Re-vaccinate every six years.

Springer's work was truly ahead of its time. Perhaps someday it will be widely embraced and used. Until that day, we are left with the typhoid vaccine, and a legacy giving us a new insight into immunity, cancer, and the architecture of a breast cancer cell.

> *To learn more about staying healthy and well balanced, log on to the blood type Web site: www.dadamo.com.*

Live Right 4
Type B

CONTENTS

The Type B Profile

AS A TYPE B, you carry the genetic potential for great malleability and the ability to thrive in changeable conditions. Unlike your blood type predecessors, Type O and Type A, who have staked their claims to opposite ends of every spectrum, your position is fluid rather than stationary, with the ability to move in either direction along the continuum. It's easy to see how this flexibility served the interests of early Type Bs, who needed to balance the twin forces of the animal and vegetable kingdoms. At the same time, it can be extremely challenging to balance two poles, and Type Bs tend to be highly sensitive to the effects of slipping out of balance.

The primary challenges that can get in the way of optimum health for Type B include a tendency to produce higher than normal cortisol

continued on page 240

Type B Health Risk Profile

CHARACTERISTICS	MANIFESTATIONS
MIND/BODY Naturally high basal cortisol levels and tendency to overproduce cortisol in response to stress	• Overreaction to stress • Difficulty recovering from stress • Disrupted sleep patterns • Daytime brain fog • Disruptive to GI friendly bacteria • Suppresses immune function
Tend to clear nitric oxide rapidly, through the B gene allele's influence on enzymatic production of NO	*When out of balance:* • Overly emotional reaction to stressful situations • Lethargy, lack of motivation • Broad systemic effects
DIGESTION Moderate to high levels of the enzyme intestinal alkaline phosphatase	• Promotes easy breakdown of fats • Offers added protection against coronary artery disease • Strengthens bones
METABOLISM Strong influence of lectins on metabolic balance	• Lectins slow metabolism • Lectins create insulin resistance
IMMUNITY Many bacteria have B-like antigens	• B antigens don't mount attacks against infections that resemble their own
Susceptibility to slow-growing viral infections	• Dysfunctional immune reactions

INCREASED RISKS	VARIATIONS
• Depression • Insulin resistance • Hypothyroidism • High stress can further exacerbate virtually all health challenges	ELDERLY • High cortisol levels are linked to Alzheimer's disease and senile dementia • Disruptions in stress hormones may lead to age-related loss of muscle tissue CHILDREN • High cortisol levels may be a factor in autism
When out of balance: • Chronic viral infections • Chronic Fatigue Syndrome, MS, Lou Gehrig's disease • Excessively high or low blood pressure	
Low risk factors for diabetes and heart disease when metabolism is in a balanced state	SECRETORS: • Affect of lectins more pronounced
• Hypoglycemia • Obesity • "Leaky gut"	ELDERLY: • Lack of libido
• Influenza (severe) • E. coli (severe when contracted) • Gastroenteritis • Urinary tract infections • Staph infections • Sinus infections	CHILDREN. Risk of neonatal strep infection, especially if mother is Type B ANCESTRY: Asians have special risk of TB NON-SECRETORS: • Have the highest rate of VTIs of all
• Autoimmune disease • Type 1 diabetes	ANCESTRY: Type B African Americans have special risk of type 1 diabetes and auto-immune disease

levels in situations of stress; sensitivity to the B-specific lectins in select foods, resulting in inflammation, and greater risk for developing Syndrome X; susceptibility to slow-growing, lingering viruses—such as those responsible for multiple sclerosis, CFS, and lupus; and a vulnerability to autoimmune diseases. In addition, idiosyncratic ethnic and racial variations require mixed strategies.

If I were to generalize, I would say that a healthy Type B, living right for his or her type, tends to have fewer risk factors for disease and tends to be more physically fit and mentally balanced than any of the other blood types. Type Bs tend to have a greater ability to adapt to altitude and statistically are the tallest of the blood types. The Type B prescription is a combination of dietary, behavioral, and environmental therapies to help you live right for your type.

The Type B Prescription

THE TYPE B prescription is a combination of dietary, behavioral, and environmental therapies to help you live right for your type:

- LIFESTYLE STRATEGIES to structure your life for health and longevity
- ADAPTED LIFESTYLE STRATEGIES for children, the elderly, and non-secretors
- EMOTIONAL EQUALIZERS and stress relievers
- SPECIALIZED DIET PLAN: Tier One for maximum health.
- TARGETED DIET PLAN: Tier Two to overcome disease
- INDIVIDUALIZED THERAPIES for chronic conditions
- THERAPEUTIC SUPPLEMENT PROGRAM for extra support

Lifestyle Strategies

Keys

🔑 Visualization is a powerful technique for Type Bs. If you can visualize it, you can achieve it.

🔑 Find healthy ways to express your nonconformist side.

🔑 Spend at least twenty minutes a day in some creative task that requires your complete attention.

🔑 Go to bed no later than 11:00 P.M. and sleep for eight hours or more.

🔑 Use visualization to relax during breaks.

🔑 Engage in a community, neighborhood, or other group activity that gives you a meaningful connection to a group. Type Bs are natural born networkers.

✎ Be spontaneous.

Structure your life for Type B health and longevity by making these adjustments to your lifestyle:

1. Eat Right for Strength and Balance

Type B shares some of Type A's tendency to high cortisol levels. So, in addition to eating right for Type B, pay special attention to these guidelines for keeping cortisol levels in balance:

- Reduce carbohydrate cravings by eating six small meals a day instead of three larger meals.
- When you feel tired, eat some protein.
- Don't undereat or skip meals, especially if you're expending a lot of energy in exercise. Food deprivation is a huge stress.
- Plan ahead to have foods on hand for a quick energy snack. This is especially important if you're on the go during the day. It's very difficult to find food on the road that isn't high in sugar, wheat, or corn.

2. Obey Your Circadian Rhythm

One of the best ways I have found for Type Bs to deal with stress is through scheduling. This makes a lot of sense, since one of the keys to cortisol regulation is maintaining a regular twenty-four-hour circadian rhythm. You can reset your daily schedule, or create exposure to a bright, full spectrum light or sunshine between 6 and 8 A.M., or you can regulate the light in your sleeping environment. Two supplements have also been found effective in resetting rhythms; the well-known melatonin, and a less well-known form of vitamin B_{12} called methylcobalamin.

The gentlest and most effective way to phase-shift the human circadian rhythm is by using a combination of bright light exposure and methylcobalamin. Basically, methylcobalamin helps bright light do its job. Methylcobalamin also improves the quality of your sleep and helps you feel refreshed upon waking. Athough methylcobalamin does not impact total levels of cortisol, it can help shift the peak of cortisol secretion, helping place your cortisol clock back on schedule.

Methylcobalamin: 1 to 3 mg per day taken in the morning

Melatonin: Melatonin is a hormone, and as such it is best used under the direction of a health professional

3. Choose Physical Exercise That Challenges Your Mind As Well As Your Body

Type Bs need to balance meditative activities with more intense physical exercise. You seem to do best with activities that are not too aerobically intense, have an element of mental challenge, and involve other people. Excellent forms of exercise for Type Bs include tennis, martial arts, cycling, hiking, and golf.

For an overall exercise program that combines strength and cardiovascular work with stress reduction, I recommend the following schedule.

CARDIOVASCULAR ACTIVITY	WEIGHTS	FLEXIBILITY/STRETCHING
25 minutes	20 minutes	30 minutes
4–5 times weekly	2–3 times weekly	2–3 times weekly

ADAPTED LIFESTYLE STRATEGIES	TYPE B CHILDREN

Structure your Type B child's life to include these essential strategies for healthy growth, wellness, and diminished risk for disease.

Young Children

- Create a non-restrictive environment. For example, allow your child to select his or her own clothes, even if the colors clash or you don't like the styles.
- Be flexible about rules, where possible—for example, bed times and meal times.
- Find small ways to appeal to your Type B child's nonconformist tendencies—for example, serving a sandwich for breakfast or eggs for dinner.
- Find ways to appeal to your child's organized side—such as check-off lists, an alarm clock, and color-coded clothing bins.
- As early as age two or three, a child can join you in daily deep breathing, stretching, and meditation.
- Encourage creativity and fantasy games.
- Cultivate appreciation of other cultures.
- Limit sugars and artificial sweeteners, which are believed to be a factor in attention deficit disorder.

Older Children

- Be open about your child's need to flaunt social customs in harmless ways—haircut, clothing, pierced ears—while encouraging activist tendencies in a positive direction.
- Encourage daily visualization exercises.
- Encourage your child to choose sports activities that challenge him or her mentally, as well as physically. Or balance intense physical exercise with intense mental activities, such as chess.
- Teach problem-solving as a way to manage stress. Help your child understand that there are "good" and "bad" stresses.

ADAPTED LIFESTYLE STRATEGIES	TYPE B SENIORS

- Type Bs have a tendency to suffer memory loss and decreased mental acuity as they age. "Exercise" your mind by doing tasks that require concentration, such as crossword puzzles.
- A daily regimen of stretching, yoga, and meditation will lower cortisol levels and increase your mental acuity. High cortisol levels have been linked to Alzheimer's disease and senile dementia.
- Be especially careful with hygeine and safe food preparation. Type Bs are particularly vulnerable to bacterial infections. If your sense of smell has declined, and you have trouble judging freshness by smell, try to have a younger friend or relative accompany you grocery shopping.
- Maintaining a circadian rhythm—important for control of cortisol levels—can be difficult for seniors. Overall, elderly people tend to have more problems with interrupted sleep and insomnia. You may need to increase your intake of vitamin B_{12}, or take a melatonin supplement.
- Reserve time for relaxation, meditation, or visualization.

Emotional Equalizers

The complex circuits of mind and body expressed in Type B continue to amaze me. When you are in "balance," which is the way you are meant to be, you are able to block stress, anxiety, and depression, using your powerful gift for relaxation and visualization. I have always noted these qualities in my Type B patients, and at last genetic and biochemical research is providing some clues, with newly revealed links to nitric oxide, and a clearer understanding of your unique use of stress hormones. When you are functioning optimally, nitric oxide clears quickly—meaning that the communication between your bodily systems is more efficient.

The collective research that has been done on the Blood Type B personality seems to confirm these neurochemical attributes. When you are in a state of balance, you can be flexible, creative, sensitive, and mentally agile, with a strong intuitive sense. Out of balance, you suffer from the effects of high cortisol and a susceptibility to viral infections, chronic fatigue, mental fogginess, and autoimmune diseases. Your focus in achieving mind-body integrity needs to be on lowering your cortisol levels and increasing your mental acuity.

1. Identify Your Tendencies

Research indicates that Type Bs tend to exhibit so-called *"Type B Behavior"* patterns. People who exhibit these patterns tend to be easy going. They're able to take upsets in stride, keep their priorities in perspective, and understand their limitations. They are less driven than other blood types and make sure to find time to relax.

Type Bs seem to have a remarkable capacity for reducing stress by practicing visualization and relaxation techniques. In my practice, I never attempt to treat a Type B who has high blood pressure using medications until I first suggest that the patient try using relaxation and visualization. More often than not, simple visualization techniques work as well, or better, at controlling system-wide biological imbalances in Type Bs than drugs or other interventions. Perhaps Type Bs' ability to use these tools so much more effectively than the other blood types is related to their special ability to efficiently modulate the effects of nitric oxide communication between their body systems. For example: a Type B who needs to control his or her blood pressure can use visualization to achieve nerve balance, which then sends a message to the blood vessels via nitric oxide to be less spastic.

When Type Bs fail to maintain this essential chemical balance, they suffer the effects of their naturally high cortisol levels without reprieve. In a state of maladaptation, Type Bs become extremely tired, depressed and lacking in motivation. Perhaps this is the reason they are sometimes defined as "lazy" in Japanese pop psychology. Many of my patients who suffer from chronic fatigue syndrome are Type Bs.

Type Bs are more emotionally complex than the other blood types— perhaps reflecting the balance between Type O and Type A. They tend to be unconventional thinkers, uncomfortable with rigid rules.

Evaluate whether or not you fit any of the personality characteristics that researchers suggest are more typical of your blood type—in particular, a tendency to be drawn toward the unconventional, to be uncomfortable with rigid rules, and to be impatient with linear thinking. Ask yourself whether you have a tendency to get easily frustrated, and become lethargic and unmotivated when things are more difficult than you expect. It is not my intention to label you. Your personality is quite individual, and genetic predispositions only form a small part of the picture. You might consider, though, what this data means to you. In my experience, these prototypical behaviors tend to emerge most strikingly when resistance is low and stress is high.

2. Use Meditation and Visualization

Type Bs have a remarkable ability to reduce stress through meditation and visualization. Of all the meditation techniques, TM, or transcendental meditation, has been the most thoroughly studied for its antistress effects. Evidence indicates that cortisol decreases during meditation—especially for long-term practitioners—and remains somewhat lower after meditation.

Breathing is a critical component of meditation. Not surprisingly, a technique called "alternate nostril breathing" is a powerful tool in managing your physiology. Left nostril breathing generates a more relaxing effect, or toning down, of sympathetic activity. Right nostril breathing generates an increase in parasympathetic activity. The alternate nostril breathing technique generates a relative balance between the sympathetic and parasympathetic nervous systems and is a tremendous antistress measure.

PRACTICE THE MARTIAL ART, TAI CHI.   Tai Chi is ideal for Type Bs, as it requires focus and concentration. A form of moving meditation, Tai Chi has also been studied for its antistress effects. Tai Chi clearly drops levels of salivary cortisol, lowers blood pressure, and improves mood after a stress-provoking event.

COMBINE MUSIC WITH GUIDED IMAGERY.   The combination of music with guided imagery has been studied for its effects on stress and mood in healthy adults. Type Bs are known to benefit from visualization, and this is an ideal technique for you. Stress-releasing music that has been shown to be effective includes a waltz by J. Strauss, a piece of modern classical by H. W. Henze, and the album "Discreet Music" by Brian Eno.

3. Use Adaptogens to Improve Your Stress Response

The term "adaptogen" has been used to categorize plants that improve the nonspecific response to stress. Many of these plants actually have a bidirectional or normalizing influence on your physiology—if something is too low, they act to bring it up; too high, they bring it down. These balancing effects make adaptogens ideal for Type Bs.

PANAX GINSENG (KOREAN GINSENG).   Ginseng appears to make the HPA axis more sensitive or responsive, perhaps thereby allowing your body to make more cortisol when it is required but allowing a quicker normalization of cortisol once the stress is removed. These activities lie at the very core of the definition of adaptogen, which implies a capability for a bidirectional or normalizing effect on physiological function. While Panax ginseng is safe for all blood types, it has historically been reserved for men. It has been my experience that some women do not respond as well to this herb as to Siberian ginseng. Also, with Panax, *more* is not always better. Go for quality rather than quantity.

ELEUTHEROCOCCUS SENTICOSUS (SIBERIAN GINSENG). Eleutherococcus is more well known by its common name, Siberian ginseng (and is occasionally seen in health food or vitamin stores as Ci Wu Jia). Although it is called ginseng, technically speaking it not a ginseng at all. Russian researchers in the 1940s and 1950s did a great deal of research on plants that function as adaptogens. Eleutherococcus was arguably the plant that consistently produced the best adaptogenic effects in their research. The research found that ingestion of extracts from this plant increased the ability to accommodate to adverse physical conditions, improved mental performance, and enhanced the quality of work under stressful conditions. This plant appears to have a normalizing effect on the stress response, allowing better performance in the face of more stressful conditions. Siberian ginseng is one of the more effective herbs at improving low blood pressure.

WITHANIA SOMNIFERA (ASHWAGANDHA).   This has been called Indian ginseng, and is considered to be the preeminent adaptogen from the Ayurvedic medical system. It has shown similar antistress and anabolic activity to Panax ginseng. Withania counteracts many of the biological changes accompanying extreme stress, including changes in blood sugar, adrenal weight, and cortisol levels. It slightly improves thyroid problems caused by stress.

BACOPA MONNIERA LEAF EXTRACT (25 percent bacosides). This provides antioxidant support for the brain and nervous system. It also helps support consistent mood and mental clarity for Type Bs.

"HOLY BASIL" (*O. SANCTUM*) LEAF EXTRACT (2 percent ursolic acid). This lowers cortisol and reduces stress-related breakdown in physiological function. It also enhances physical and emotional endurance and lowers elevated blood sugar by improving glucose metabolism.

LICORICE ROOT. Licorice root (not DGL) strengthens the adrenals and promotes endocrine health in Type Bs and promotes antiviral immune system function. Always take licorice supplements along with a potassium supplement. I strongly recommend working with the supervision of a skilled herbalist or physician.

TRIBULUS TERRESTRIS. This is an adaptogenic herb that promotes a balanced response to stress.

4. Fight Stress with the Right Supplements

The Type B diet provides a rich variety of all the necessary vitamins and minerals. However, when you are under a great deal of physiological or mental/emotional stress, several supplements might be useful:

VITAMIN C. Evidence shows that vitamin C, in amounts greater than the RDA, is needed to optimally support the adrenal glands function and buffer against high cortisol when you are exposed to a lot of stress. Beware. Almost all vitamin C supplements are made from genetically engineered corn. Check the ingredients.

B VITAMINS. Vitamins B_1 and B_6 are important to help improve cortisol function of the adrenal gland and simultaneously normalize the rhythmic activity of the gland. A vitamin B_5 deficiency severely compromises the function of the adrenal cortex (responsible for cortisol production). Stress in virtually all forms tends to place extra demands on your B_5 status. Vitamin B_5 will both allow your adrenal cortex to respond more appropriately to stress without getting exhausted and buffer against a tendency to create excessively high amounts of cortisol.

ZINC. 15 to 25 mg or so of zinc acts to substantially reduce cortisol.

TYROSINE. Tyrosine is an amino acid that is most appropriate in conditions of acute stress. Strong research shows that taking tyrosine in doses of between three and seven grams prior to circumstances characterized by psychosocial and physical stress substantially reduces the acute effects of stress and fatigue on performance.

PHOSPHATIDYLSERINE. Phosphatidylserine, found in trace amounts in lecithin, is a useful supplement to help regulate the stress-induced activation of the HPA axis and prevent large increases in cortisol levels. (NOTE: 400 to 800 mg is needed to achieve results, and this supplement is very expensive.)

PLANT STEROLS AND STEROLINS. Plant sterols and sterolins are phytochemicals generally described as plant "fats," which are chemically very similar to cholesterol, but appear to have "adaptogenic" biological activity. They help prevent immune system suppression during stress, and help to normalize cortisol and DHEA levels.

ARGININE.   This amino acid is one of the building blocks of nitric oxide synthesis.

CITRULLINE.   This amino acid is involved in the energy cycle and nitric oxide synthesis. A good source is watermelon.

SPECIAL STRATEGIES	THE TYPE B CHILD AND ADD

Although there are no clear studies of blood type and attention deficit disorder, I've observed many Type B children over the years who have extreme difficulties with concentration and memory retention, often in combination with a history of chronic infections (viruses, ear infections, etc.). This makes sense when you consider that when Type Bs are ill (or out of balance) one of the first things to suffer is mental acuity. I have had great success with Type B children suffering the symptoms of ADD. These techniques require time and patience for Mom and Dad, but the results are worth it. It's certainly more effective at getting to the root of the problem than drugs such as Ritalin.

1. The Type B diet is the centerpiece of the strategy. You'll find that it will help prevent the chronic infections that often accompany ADD. Be especially firm about avoiding foods that have high lectin activity for Type Bs. Cut out all chicken, corn, and peanuts. Try replacing wheat with spelt or other wheat-free grains and see if it has an effect.
2. Emphasize a regular bedtime schedule to help normalize the circadian rhythm. Make sure your child gets at least eight to ten hours of sleep a night.
3. Encourage activities that require concentration and quiet. Set aside time every day—even if it is only twenty minutes—to sit with your child and work on a puzzle, build a model, draw, or play chess.
4. Discourage sports that are overly intense and competitive, in favor of moderate physical exercise, such as bike riding, hiking, swimming, and martial arts such as Tae Kwon Do.
5. Cut back on sugar, which can promote insulin resistance. Some research has shown a connection between excess sugar consumption and ADD.

Type B Two-Tier Diet

The Two-Tier Diet is designed to offer a more individualized program. It has been my experience that some people do very well on the basic Tier One Diet—that is, a moderate degree of adherence to the primary beneficial and avoid foods, with heavy reliance on neutral foods for general nutritional supplementation. Others need a more rigid plan, especially if they suffer from chronic conditions. Adding the Tier Two Diet will increase the compliance to help overcome disease and restore a state of well-being.

Your secretor status can influence your ability to fully digest and metabolize certain foods. For this reason, each food list contains a separate column of rankings for secretors and non-secretors. Although the majority of people are secretors and can safely follow the recommendations in the secretor column, the variations can make a big difference if you are among the approximately 20 percent who are non-secretors.

> SECRETOR or NONSECRETOR?
> Before you start the diet, take the easy home saliva test to determine your secretor status. See page 358.

In rare cases, your Rh and MN will influence a food ranking. Those distinctions are listed below the appropriate chart.

The Blood Type Diet Tier System

Tier One: Maximize Health

Make these choices as soon as possible to maximize your health. Using Tier One choices in combination with neutral foods for general nutritional supplementation will suffice for most healthy individuals.

BENEFICIAL: These foods possess components that enhance the metabolic, immune, or structural health of your blood type.

NEUTRAL: These foods usually have no direct benefit or harmful effect, based on your blood type. But many of them supply nutrients needed for a well-balanced diet.

AVOID: These foods contain components that are harmful for your blood type.

Tier Two: Overcome Disease

Add these choices if you are suffering from a chronic disease or wish to follow the diet at a higher compliance level. If you are adhering to the Tier Two Diet, use caution when you incorporate neutral foods for general nutritional supplementation.

Individualized Dietary Guidelines

If you are a healthy Type B, the Tier One Diet will provide the combination of foods you need for good health. To make the most of it, pay special attention to these guidelines:

Keys

🍴 Eat small to moderate portions of high-quality, lean, organic meat several times a week for strength, energy, and efficient metabolism. Meat should be prepared medium to rare for the best health

---

Special Tips for Type Bs Making a Change from Vegetarian Diets

Many new subscribers to the Type B Diet have been longtime vegetarians. A high percentage of people of Asian ancestry (Japan, China, Mongolia, and India) are Type B, and these cultures emphasize grains and fish. Soy is preferred to dairy—especially that derived from cows. These cultural intolerances are not classic food intolerances. However, you will need to proceed more slowly in adapting to the Type B Diet. Here are some guidelines:

1. If you are not used to eating dairy products, introduce them gradually, after you have been on the Type B Diet for several weeks. Begin with cultured dairy products, such as yogurt and kefir, which are more easily tolerated than fresh dairy products.
2. The protein in your diet should emphasize a combination of seafood and dairy, with very limited amounts of beneficial meat. Until you have adapted to the diet, stay away from some of the Type B neutral meats, such as beef, veal, liver, and pheasant.
3. Take a digestive enzyme with your main meal until you adapt to eating meat and dairy. Bromelain, an enzyme found in pineapple, is available in supplemental form. In addition, take ginger, peppermint, or parsley—all good stomach tonics.

effects. If you charbroil, or cook meat well-done, use a marinade composed of beneficial ingredients, such as cherry juice, lemon juice, spices, and herbs.

🔊 Include regular portions of richly oiled cold-water fish. Fish oils can boost your metabolism.

Type B Dietary Strategies

These strategies are designed to help the healthy Type B avoid the problems that can arise from your specific neurological, digestive, metabolic, and immune makeup. On the whole, Type Bs are blessed with hardy and flexible digestive systems, capable of efficiently digesting either animal proteins or carbohydrates. You aren't plagued with the inherited problems of either Type O (high stomach acid) or Type A (low stomach acid) that give them so much trouble digesting certain foods. You also share the benefit of high levels of intestinal alkaline phosphatase with Type O, which protect you from some of the harmful effects of high-protein and high-fat diets.

The key to digestive health for Type Bs is to avoid intestinal toxicity and high indicans. Your susceptibility to infections and your sensitivity to the lectins in your "avoid" foods provide a clear signal: Stay on your diet and your digestive system will respond positively.

Prevent Lectin Damage

AVOID FOODS THAT ARE TYPE B RED FLAGS. The worst are:

chicken
corn
buckwheat
lentils
peanuts
sesame seeds
tomatoes

TIP: Replace tomatoes with the Membrane Fluidizer Cocktail—a great way to get your lycopene. Using guava, red grapefruit, or watermelon juice as the base, add ½ to 1 tablespoon of high-quality flaxseed oil and 1 tablespoon of good quality lecithin. Shake well. The lecithin emulsifies the oil, making a sort of smoothie out of the mixture, which is actually quite palatable. This will increase the absorption of lycopenes from these foods to a level not unlike tomato paste, but without the tomato lectin. Having a few dried apricots as a snack is also a good idea.

Type Bs can help block the actions of dietary lectins by using polysaccharide sacrificial molecules, such as those found in:

- NAG (N-Acetylglucosamine)
- Fucus vesiculosis—kelp
- Laminaria
- Larch arabinogalactan

SPECIAL STRATEGIES	AFRICAN AMERICAN TYPE BS WITH DAIRY INTOLERANCES

It has consistently been my experience that Type Bs of African ancestry encounter some problems on the Type B Diet. In particular, many African Americans are lactose intolerant. Type B African Americans also appear to have more chronic health problems than other Type Bs and are known to produce more anti–blood type antibodies than other Type Bs. I suspect the basis might be anthropological, since the gene for Type B didn't exist in the African ancestral homeland. It is possible that Africans were only exposed to it much later, through migration and intermingling. It is certainly possible that the adaptations made in Type Bs never fully "took" with Type Bs of African descent, leaving them with some idiosyncrasies that remain to this day.

Since dairy foods are so beneficial for Type Bs, their absence in the typical African-American diet may contribute to some of the additional health problems you face. If you are a Type B of African ancestry who is lactose intolerant, you'll need to introduce dairy foods very gradually. Use a lactase enzyme preparation, which will make it possible for you to eat dairy, and start with cultured dairy foods, such as yogurt, before you move to fresh milk products. Simultaneously, make the other adjustments in your diet—emphasizing as many beneficial foods as possible and avoiding the foods that are difficult for Type Bs to digest. I've found that lactose intolerant Type Bs find it easier to incorporate dairy after they have made the other changes to their diets.

Meat and Poultry

TYPE B IS ABLE to efficiently metabolize animal protein, but there are limitations that require careful dietary navigation. Chicken, one of the most popular of food choices, disagrees with Type B, because of the lectin contained in the organ and muscle meat. Turkey does not contain this lectin and can be eaten as an excellent alternative to chicken. The leaner cuts of lamb and mutton should be a part of the Type B diet. They help build muscle and active tissue mass, increasing Type B's metabolic rate. Type B non-secretors have protein requirements similar to Type O and should increase their weekly intake of meat and poultry.

BLOOD TYPE B: MEATS AND POULTRY			
Portion: 4–6 oz. (men); 2–5 oz. (women and children)			
	African	**Caucasian**	**Asian**
Secretor	3–6	2–6	2–5
Non-Secretor	4–7	4–7	4–7
Rh–	Increase by 1 serving weekly		
	Times per week		

Tier One

FOOD	TYPE B SECRETOR	TYPE B NON-SECRETOR
Chicken	Avoid	Avoid
Cornish hens	Avoid	Avoid
Duck	Avoid	Avoid
Goat	Beneficial	Beneficial
Lamb	Beneficial	Beneficial
Mutton	Beneficial	Beneficial
Partridge	Avoid	Avoid
Quail	Avoid	Avoid
Squirrel	Avoid	Avoid

Tier Two

FOOD	TYPE B SECRETOR	TYPE B NON-SECRETOR
Bacon/ham/pork	Avoid	Avoid
Goose	Avoid	Avoid
Grouse	Avoid	Avoid

Guinea hen	Avoid	Avoid
Heart	Avoid	Neutral
Horse	Avoid	Neutral
Rabbit	Beneficial	Beneficial
Squab	Avoid	Neutral
Turtle	Avoid	Avoid
Venison	Beneficial	Beneficial

Neutral: General Nutritional Supplementation

FOOD	TYPE B SECRETOR	TYPE B NON-SECRETOR
Beef	Neutral	Neutral
Buffalo	Neutral	Neutral
Liver (calf)	Neutral	Beneficial
Ostrich	Neutral	Neutral
Pheasant	Neutral	Neutral
Turkey	Neutral	Neutral
Veal	Neutral	Neutral

Fish and Seafood

FISH AND SEAFOOD are an excellent source of protein for Type B. Fish is a treasure trove of dense nutrients, able to build active tissue mass in Type B. This holds particularly true for Type B non-secretors. The highly beneficial forms of fish are rich in omega series fatty acids, which can help increase immune function, in addition to controlling the production of cellular growth factors. Seafood can also be a good source of docosahexaenoic acid (DHA), a nutrient needed for proper nerve, tissue, and growth function—critical for Type B children. Many of the avoid seafoods have lectins or polyamines that are not healthy for Type B. Don't use frozen fish, as the content of polyamines in it is much higher than in freshly caught fish.

BLOOD TYPE B: FISH AND SEAFOOD			
Portion: 4–6 oz. (men); 2–5 oz. (women and children)			
	African	Caucasian	Asian
Secretor	4–5	3–5	3–5
Non-Secretor	4–5	4–5	4–5
		Times per week	

Tier One

FOOD	TYPE B SECRETOR	TYPE B NON-SECRETOR
Anchovy	Avoid	Avoid
Bass (bluegill)	Avoid	Avoid
Bass (sea)	Avoid	Avoid
Bass (striped)	Avoid	Avoid
Beluga	Avoid	Avoid
Clam	Avoid	Avoid
Conch	Avoid	Avoid
Crab	Avoid	Avoid
Croaker	Beneficial	Beneficial
Eel/Japanese eel	Avoid	Avoid
Frog	Avoid	Avoid
Lobster	Avoid	Avoid
Mollusks	Avoid	Avoid
Monkfish	Beneficial	Beneficial
Mussels	Avoid	Avoid
Octopus	Avoid	Avoid
Oyster	Avoid	Avoid
Perch (ocean)	Beneficial	Beneficial
Pickerel	Beneficial	Beneficial
Pollack	Avoid	Avoid
Sardine	Beneficial	Beneficial
Shrimp	Avoid	Avoid

Tier Two

FOOD	TYPE B SECRETOR	TYPE B NON-SECRETOR
Barracuda	Avoid	Neutral
Butterfish	Avoid	Neutral
Caviar	Beneficial	Neutral
Cod	Beneficial	Beneficial
Crab (horseshoe)	Avoid	Avoid
Flounder	Beneficial	Neutral
Grouper	Beneficial	Beneficial
Haddock	Beneficial	Beneficial
Hake	Beneficial	Beneficial
Halibut	Beneficial	Neutral
Harvest fish	Beneficial	Beneficial
Mackerel	Beneficial	Beneficial

Mahimahi	Beneficial	Beneficial
Pike	Beneficial	Neutral
Porgy	Beneficial	Beneficial
Salmon	Beneficial	Neutral
Shad	Beneficial	Beneficial
Snail (*Helix pomatia/ escargot*)	Avoid	Neutral
Sole	Beneficial	Neutral
Sturgeon	Beneficial	Beneficial
Yellowtail	Avoid	Neutral

Neutral: General Nutritional Supplementation

FOOD	TYPE B SECRETOR	TYPE B NON-SECRETOR
Abalone	Neutral	Neutral
Bluefish	Neutral	Neutral
Bullhead	Neutral	Neutral
Carp	Neutral	Beneficial
Catfish	Neutral	Neutral
Chub	Neutral	Neutral
Cusk	Neutral	Neutral
Drum	Neutral	Neutral
Gray sole	Neutral	Neutral
Halfmoon fish	Neutral	Neutral
Herring/kippers (fresh)	Neutral	Neutral
Herring/kippers (pickled)	Neutral	Neutral
Lox	Neutral	Neutral
Mullet	Neutral	Neutral
Muskellunge	Neutral	Neutral
Opaleye fish	Neutral	Neutral
Orange roughy	Neutral	Neutral
Parrot fish	Neutral	Neutral
Perch (silver)	Neutral	Neutral
Perch (white)	Neutral	Neutral
Perch (yellow)	Neutral	Neutral
Pompano	Neutral	Neutral
Red snapper	Neutral	Neutral
Rosefish	Neutral	Neutral
Sailfish	Neutral	Neutral
Scallop	Neutral	Avoid

Scrod	Neutral	Neutral
Scup	Neutral	Neutral
Shark	Neutral	Neutral
Smelt	Neutral	Neutral
Squid	Neutral	Neutral
Sucker	Neutral	Neutral
Sunfish	Neutral	Neutral
Swordfish	Neutral	Neutral
Tilapia	Neutral	Neutral
Tilefish	Neutral	Neutral
Tuna	Neutral	Neutral
Weakfish	Neutral	Neutral
Whitefish	Neutral	Neutral
Whiting	Neutral	Neutral

Dairy and Eggs

DAIRY PRODUCTS can be eaten by almost all Type B secretors, and to a lesser degree by Type B non-secretors. Unlike Type O and Type A, Type B can employ dairy to build active tissue mass, helping to increase metabolism. However, it should be cautioned that some Type Bs are lacking the lactase enzyme, which causes problems with digestion of dairy. Also, Type B non-secretors should be wary of eating too much cheese. They are more immunologically sensitive to many of the microbial strains in many aged cheeses. This is more common to Type Bs of African ancestry, but the sensitivity can also be found in Caucasian and Asian populations. This caution holds particularly true if you suffer from recurrent sinus infections or colds, as dairy products are often mucus producers. Eggs are a good source of DHA for Type B and can be an integral part of your protein requirement, helping to build active tissue mass. The phosphatides serine and choline are very helpful for the Type B nervous and immune system. Try to find dairy products that are both hormone free and organic.

BLOOD TYPE B: EGGS			
Portion: 1 egg			
	African	**Caucasian**	**Asian**
Secretor	3–4	3–4	3–4
Non-Secretor	5–6	5–6	5–6
		Times per week	

BLOOD TYPE B: MILK AND YOGURT

Portion: 4–6 oz. (men); 2–5 oz. (women and children)

	African	Caucasian	Asian
Secretor	3–5	3–4	3–4
Non-Secretor	1–3	2–4	1–3
	Times per week		

BLOOD TYPE B: CHEESE

Portion: 3 oz. (men); 2 oz. (women and children)

	African	Caucasian	Asian
Secretor	3–4	3–5	3–4
Non-Secretor	1–4	1–4	1–4
MM	Decrease milk, cheese, and yogurt by 2 servings weekly		
	Times per week		

Tier One

FOOD	TYPE B SECRETOR	TYPE B NON-SECRETOR
Duck egg	Avoid	Avoid
Farmer cheese	Beneficial	Beneficial
Goat cheese	Beneficial	Beneficial
Goose egg	Avoid	Avoid
Ice cream	Avoid	Avoid
Kefir	Beneficial	Beneficial
Milk (goat)	Beneficial	Beneficial
Mozzarella cheese	Beneficial	Beneficial
Paneer	Beneficial	Beneficial
Quail egg	Avoid	Avoid
Ricotta cheese	Beneficial	Beneficial
Salmon roe	Avoid	Avoid

Tier Two

FOOD	TYPE B SECRETOR	TYPE B NON-SECRETOR
American cheese	Avoid	Avoid
Blue cheese	Avoid	Avoid
Cottage cheese	Beneficial	Neutral
Feta cheese	Beneficial	Beneficial

Milk (cow-skim or 2%)	Beneficial	Neutral
Milk (cow-whole)	Beneficial	Neutral
String cheese	Avoid	Avoid
Yogurt	Beneficial	Beneficial

Neutral: General Nutritional Supplementation

FOOD	TYPE B SECRETOR	TYPE B NON-SECRETOR
Brie	Neutral	Neutral
Butter	Neutral	Neutral
Buttermilk	Neutral	Neutral
Camembert	Neutral	Avoid
Casein	Neutral	Neutral
Cheddar cheese	Neutral	Avoid
Colby cheese	Neutral	Neutral
Cream cheese	Neutral	Neutral
Edam cheese	Neutral	Neutral
Egg (chicken)	Neutral	Neutral
Egg white (chicken)	Neutral	Neutral
Egg yolk (chicken)	Neutral	Neutral
Emmenthal cheese	Neutral	Avoid
Ghee (clarified butter)	Neutral	Beneficial
Gouda	Neutral	Neutral
Gruyère	Neutral	Neutral
Half & half	Neutral	Neutral
Jarlsberg cheese	Neutral	Avoid
Monterey jack cheese	Neutral	Avoid
Munster cheese	Neutral	Avoid
Neufchatel cheese	Neutral	Neutral
Parmesan cheese	Neutral	Avoid
Provolone cheese	Neutral	Avoid
Quark cheese	Neutral	Neutral
Sherbet	Neutral	Neutral
Sour cream (low/ non-fat)	Neutral	Neutral
Swiss cheese	Neutral	Avoid
Whey	Neutral	Beneficial

Beans and Legumes

TYPE B CAN DO WELL on proteins found in many beans and legumes, although this food category does contain more than a few beans with problematic lectins. Beans and legumes, along with good seafood choices, are more than sufficient to build active tissue mass. Soy products should be de-emphasized, as they are rich in a class of enzymes that can interact negatively with the B antigen. Several beans, such as mung beans, contain Type B agglutinating lectins and should be avoided. Type B non-secretors should try to get most of their protein from the primary sources, such as fish and dairy.

BLOOD TYPE B: BEANS AND LEGUMES			
Portion: 1 cup, dry			
	African	**Caucasian**	**Asian**
Secretor	5–7	5–7	5–7
Non-Secretor	3–5	3–5	3–5
			Times per week

Tier One

FOOD	TYPE B SECRETOR	TYPE B NON-SECRETOR
Adzuki bean	Avoid	Avoid
Black bean	Avoid	Avoid
Black-eyed pea	Avoid	Avoid
Garbanzo bean	Avoid	Avoid
Kidney bean	Beneficial	Neutral
Lentil (domestic)	Avoid	Avoid
Lentil (green)	Avoid	Avoid
Lentil (red)	Avoid	Avoid
Mung bean (sprouts)	Avoid	Avoid
Navy bean	Beneficial	Neutral
Pinto bean	Avoid	Avoid
Soy flakes	Avoid	Avoid
Soy granules	Avoid	Avoid
Soy, tempeh	Avoid	Avoid
Soy, tofu	Avoid	Avoid

Tier Two

FOOD	TYPE B SECRETOR	TYPE B NON-SECRETOR
Lima bean	Beneficial	Neutral
Soy cheese	Avoid	Avoid
Soy milk	Avoid	Neutral
Soy, miso	Avoid	Avoid

Neutral: General Nutritional Supplementation

FOOD	TYPE B SECRETOR	TYPE B NON-SECRETOR
Broad bean	Neutral	Neutral
Cannellini bean	Neutral	Neutral
Copper bean	Neutral	Neutral
Fava bean	Neutral	Neutral
Green bean	Neutral	Neutral
Jicama	Neutral	Neutral
Northern bean	Neutral	Neutral
Red bean	Neutral	Neutral
Snap bean	Neutral	Neutral
Soy bean	Neutral	Avoid
Tamarind bean	Neutral	Neutral
White bean	Neutral	Neutral

Nuts and Seeds

NUTS AND SEEDS can be an important secondary source of protein for Type B. Black walnuts can help lower polyamine concentrations by inhibiting the enzyme ornithine decarboxylase. As with other aspects of the Type B diet plan, there are some idiosyncratic elements to the choice of seeds and nuts: Several, such as sunflower and sesame, have B agglutinating lectins and should be avoided.

BLOOD TYPE B: NUTS AND SEEDS			
Portion: Seeds (handful) Nut Butters (1–2 tbsp)			
	African	Caucasian	Asian
Secretor	4–7	4–7	4–7
Non-Secretor	5–7	5–7	5–7
	Times per week		

Tier One

FOOD	TYPE B SECRETOR	TYPE B NON-SECRETOR
Cashew/cashew butter	Avoid	Avoid
Peanut	Avoid	Avoid
Peanut butter	Avoid	Avoid
Pine nut (pignola)	Avoid	Avoid
Pistachio	Avoid	Avoid
Poppy seed	Avoid	Avoid
Pumpkin seed	Avoid	Neutral
Safflower seed	Avoid	Avoid
Sesame butter/tahini	Avoid	Avoid
Sesame seed	Avoid	Avoid
Sunflower butter	Avoid	Avoid
Sunflower seed	Avoid	Avoid
Walnut (black)	Beneficial	Beneficial

Tier Two

FOOD	TYPE B SECRETOR	TYPE B NON-SECRETOR
Filbert (hazelnut)	Avoid	Avoid

Neutral: General Nutritional Supplementation

FOOD	TYPE B SECRETOR	TYPE B NON-SECRETOR
Almond	Neutral	Neutral
Almond butter	Neutral	Neutral
Almond cheese	Neutral	Neutral
Almond milk	Neutral	Neutral
Beechnut	Neutral	Neutral
Brazil nut	Neutral	Neutral
Butternut	Neutral	Neutral
Chestnut	Neutral	Neutral
Flaxseed	Neutral	Neutral
Hickory	Neutral	Neutral
Litchi	Neutral	Neutral
Macadamia	Neutral	Neutral
Pecan/pecan butter	Neutral	Neutral
Walnut (English)	Neutral	Beneficial

Grains and Starches

GRAINS PRESENT a series of problems for Type B—particularly Type B non-secretors. They should be even more careful of their consumption of complex carbohydrates because of their insulin sensitivities. Type Bs should also avoid rye and buckwheat, as these foods contain lectins capable of exerting an insulinlike effect on their bodies, lowering active tissue mass and increasing body fat. Type B secretors should not eat whole wheat products. The agglutinin in whole wheat can aggravate inflammatory conditions and lower active tissue mass. This lectin can often be milled out of the grain or destroyed by sprouting.

BLOOD TYPE B: GRAINS AND STARCHES			
Portion: 1 cup dry (grains or pastas)			
	African	**Caucasian**	**Asian**
Secretor	5–7	5–9	5–9
Non-Secretor	3–5	3–5	3–5
Rh–	Decrease by 1 serving weekly		
	Times per week		

Tier One

FOOD	TYPE B SECRETOR	TYPE B NON-SECRETOR
Buckwheat/kasha	Avoid	Avoid
Corn (white/yellow/blue)	Avoid	Avoid
Cornmeal	Avoid	Avoid
Essene bread (manna bread)	Beneficial	Beneficial
Kamut	Avoid	Avoid
Millet	Beneficial	Beneficial
Popcorn	Avoid	Avoid
Rice (puffed)/rice bran	Beneficial	Beneficial
Rice milk	Beneficial	Beneficial
Rice cake/flour	Beneficial	Beneficial
Rye flour	Avoid	Avoid
Rye/100% rye bread	Avoid	Avoid
Soba noodles (100% buckwheat)	Avoid	Avoid
Sorghum	Avoid	Neutral

Tier Two

FOOD	TYPE B SECRETOR	TYPE B NON-SECRETOR
Amaranth	Avoid	Neutral
Artichoke pasta (pure)	Avoid	Neutral
Couscous (cracked wheat)	Avoid	Avoid
Gluten flour	Avoid	Avoid
Oat flour	Beneficial	Neutral
Oat/oat bran/oatmeal	Beneficial	Neutral
Rice (wild)	Avoid	Neutral
Spelt	Beneficial	Neutral
Tapioca	Avoid	Neutral
Teff	Avoid	Avoid
Wheat (bran)	Avoid	Avoid
Wheat (germ)	Avoid	Avoid
Wheat (gluten flour products)	Avoid	Avoid
Wheat (whole wheat products)	Avoid	Avoid

Neutral: General Nutritional Supplementation

FOOD	TYPE B SECRETOR	TYPE B NON-SECRETOR
Barley	Neutral	Neutral
Ezekiel bread (commercial)	Neutral	Neutral
Gluten-free bread	Neutral	Neutral
Malt	Neutral	Neutral
Quinoa	Neutral	Neutral
Rice (cream of)	Neutral	Neutral
Rice (white/brown/ basmati) bread	Neutral	Neutral
Soy flour bread	Neutral	Avoid
Spelt flour/products	Neutral	Neutral
Wheat (refined unbleached)	Neutral	Avoid
Wheat (semolina flour products)	Neutral	Avoid
Wheat (white flour products)	Neutral	Avoid

Wheat bread (sprouted commercial—not Ezekiel)	Neutral	Neutral

Vegetables

VEGETABLES PROVIDE A RICH source of antioxidants and fiber, and also help to lower the production of polyamines in the digestive tract. Onions are also a powerful friend to Type B. They contain significant amounts of the antioxidant quercetin, a powerful antimutagen. All of the neutral or beneficial vegetables are of great benefit to the Type B trying to lose weight. Artichoke is quite beneficial to the liver and gallbladder, weak spots for Type B. Parsnips are rich in polysaccharides, which are a great stimulant to the immune system. Tomatoes contain a lectin that re acts with the saliva and digestive juices of Type B secretors. Tomatoes do not react with Type B non-secretors.

BLOOD TYPE B: VEGETABLES			
Portion: 1 cup, cooked or raw			
	African	**Caucasian**	**Asian**
Secretor Beneficials	Unlimited	Unlimited	Unlimited
Secretor Neutrals	2–5	2–5	2–5
Non-Secretor Neutrals	2–3	2–3	2–3
Non-Secretor Beneficials	Unlimited	Unlimited	Unlimited
MM	Try to use mostly Tier One Beneficials		
	Times per day		

Tier One

FOOD	TYPE B SECRETOR	TYPE B NON-SECRETOR
Acacia (Arabic gum)	Avoid	Avoid
Aloe/aloe tea/aloe juice	Avoid	Avoid
Beet	Beneficial	Beneficial
Beet greens/beet greens juice	Beneficial	Beneficial
Broccoli	Beneficial	Beneficial
Brussel sprouts	Beneficial	Beneficial
Carrot	Beneficial	Beneficial

Collard greens	Beneficial	Beneficial
Ginger	Beneficial	Beneficial
Kale	Beneficial	Beneficial
Mushroom (shiitake)	Beneficial	Beneficial
Mustard greens	Beneficial	Beneficial
Olives (black)	Avoid	Avoid
Olives (Greek/Spanish)	Avoid	Avoid
Parsnip	Beneficial	Beneficial
Potato (sweet)	Beneficial	Beneficial
Radish	Avoid	Avoid
Radish sprouts	Avoid	Avoid
Rhubarb	Avoid	Avoid
Tomato/tomato juice	Avoid	Neutral

Tier Two

FOOD	TYPE B SECRETOR	TYPE B NON-SECRETOR
Artichoke (domestic/ globe/Jerusalem)	Avoid	Neutral
Cabbage (Chinese/red/ white)	Beneficial	Neutral
Cabbage juice	Beneficial	Neutral
Cauliflower	Beneficial	Beneficial
Eggplant	Beneficial	Neutral
Juniper	Avoid	Avoid
Olive (green)	Avoid	Avoid
Pepper (green/yellow/ jalapeno)	Beneficial	Neutral
Pepper (red/cayenne)	Beneficial	Neutral
Pumpkin	Avoid	Neutral
Yam	Beneficial	Beneficial

Neutral: General Nutritional Supplementation

FOOD	TYPE B SECRETOR	TYPE B NON-SECRETOR
Agar	Neutral	Avoid
Alfalfa sprouts	Neutral	Neutral
Arugula	Neutral	Neutral
Asparagus	Neutral	Neutral
Asparagus pea	Neutral	Neutral

Bamboo shoot	Neutral	Neutral
Bok choy	Neutral	Neutral
Caper	Neutral	Neutral
Carrot juice	Neutral	Neutral
Celeriac	Neutral	Neutral
Celery/celery juice	Neutral	Neutral
Chervil	Neutral	Neutral
Chicory	Neutral	Neutral
Chili pepper	Neutral	Neutral
Cilantro	Neutral	Neutral
Cucumber/cucumber juice	Neutral	Neutral
Daikon radish	Neutral	Neutral
Dandelion	Neutral	Neutral
Endive	Neutral	Neutral
Escarole	Neutral	Neutral
Fennel	Neutral	Neutral
Fiddlehead fern	Neutral	Neutral
Garlic	Neutral	Beneficial
Horseradish	Neutral	Neutral
Kelp	Neutral	Neutral
Kohlrabi	Neutral	Neutral
Leek	Neutral	Neutral
Lettuce (bibb/Boston/ iceberg/mesclun)	Neutral	Neutral
Lettuce (romaine)	Neutral	Neutral
Mushroom (abalone)	Neutral	Neutral
Mushroom (silver dollar)	Neutral	Neutral
Mushroom (maitake)	Neutral	Neutral
Mushroom (oyster/ enoki/portobello)	Neutral	Neutral
Mushroom (straw)	Neutral	Neutral
okra	Neutral	Beneficial
Onion (green)	Neutral	Beneficial
Onion (red/Spanish/ yellow	Neutral	Beneficial
Oyster plant	Neutral	Neutral
Pea (green/pod/snow)	Neutral	Neutral
Pickle (in brine)	Neutral	Neutral
Pickle (in vinegar)	Neutral	Neutral
Pimento	Neutral	Neutral

Poi	Neutral	Neutral
Potato (white/red/blue/ yellow)	Neutral	Avoid
Radicchio	Neutral	Neutral
Rappini	Neutral	Neutral
Rutabaga	Neutral	Neutral
Sauerkraut	Neutral	Neutral
Scallion	Neutral	Neutral
Seaweed	Neutral	Neutral
Senna	Neutral	Neutral
Shallots	Neutral	Neutral
Spinach/spinach juice	Neutral	Neutral
Squash (summer/winter)	Neutral	Neutral
String bean	Neutral	Neutral
Swiss chard	Neutral	Neutral
Taro	Neutral	Neutral
Turnip	Neutral	Neutral
Water chestnut	Neutral	Neutral
Watercress	Neutral	Neutral
Yucca	Neutral	Neutral
Zucchini	Neutral	Neutral

Fruits and Fruit Juices

A DIET RICH in proper fruits and vegetables can help weight loss by tempering the effects of insulin. Also, fruits can help shift the balance of water in the body from high extracellular concentrations to high intracellular concentrations. Pineapples are rich in enzymes that help reduce inflammation and encourage proper water balance. Other fruits, such as red grapefruit and watermelon, can supply lycopene, the same antioxidant found in otherwise problematic tomatoes. Be aware that the B antigen can often result in unique interactions. Avocados, persimmons, and pomegranates contain lectins capable of agglutinating Type B cells. The Type B non-secretor benefits from a broader variety of fruits than does the Type B secretor. However, Type B non-secretors might want to limit the amount of high glucose fruits they consume, like grapes, figs, and dates, if they find themselves overly sensitive to sugar or with a mid-abdominal "paunch."

BLOOD TYPE B: FRUITS			
Portion: 1 cup or 1 piece			
	African	**Caucasian**	**Asian**
Secretor	2–4	3–5	3–5
Non-Secretor	2–3	2–3	2–3
		Times per week	

Tier One

FOOD	TYPE B SECRETOR	TYPE B NON-SECRETOR
Avocado	Avoid	Avoid
Cranberry/cranberry juice	Beneficial	Beneficial
Persimmon	Avoid	Avoid
Pineapple/pineapple juice	Beneficial	Beneficial
Plum (dark/green/red)	Beneficial	Beneficial
Pomegranate	Avoid	Avoid
Watermelon	Beneficial	Beneficial

Tier Two

FOOD	TYPE B SECRETOR	TYPE B NON-SECRETOR
Banana	Beneficial	Neutral
Coconut milk	Avoid	Avoid
Grape (all types)	Beneficial	Beneficial
Papaya/papaya juice	Beneficial	Beneficial
Prickly pear	Avoid	Avoid
Starfruit (carambola)	Avoid	Avoid

Neutral: General Nutritional Supplementation

FOOD	TYPE B SECRETOR	TYPE B NON-SECRETOR
Apple	Neutral	Neutral
Apple cider/apple juice	Neutral	Neutral
Apricot/apricot juice	Neutral	Neutral
Asian pear	Neutral	Neutral
Blackberry/blackberry juice	Neutral	Beneficial
Blueberry	Neutral	Beneficial

Boysenberry	Neutral	Beneficial
Breadfruit	Neutral	Neutral
Canang melon	Neutral	Neutral
Cantaloupe	Neutral	Avoid
Casaba melon	Neutral	Neutral
Cherry (all)	Neutral	Beneficial
Christmas melon	Neutral	Neutral
Crenshaw melon	Neutral	Neutral
Currants (black/red)	Neutral	Beneficial
Date	Neutral	Neutral
Dewberry	Neutral	Neutral
Elderberry (dark blue/ purple)	Neutral	Beneficial
Fig (fresh/dried)	Neutral	Beneficial
Gooseberry	Neutral	Neutral
Grapefruit/grapefruit juice	Neutral	Neutral
Guava/guava juice	Neutral	Beneficial
Honeydew	Neutral	Avoid
Kiwi	Neutral	Neutral
Kumquat	Neutral	Neutral
Lemon/lemon juice	Neutral	Neutral
Lime/lime juice	Neutral	Neutral
Loganberry	Neutral	Neutral
Mango/mango juice	Neutral	Neutral
Mulberry	Neutral	Neutral
Musk melon	Neutral	Neutral
Nectarine/nectarine juice	Neutral	Neutral
Orange/orange juice	Neutral	Neutral
Peach	Neutral	Neutral
Pear/pear juice	Neutral	Neutral
Persian melon	Neutral	Neutral
Plantain	Neutral	Neutral
Prune/prune juice	Neutral	Neutral
Quince	Neutral	Neutral
Raisin	Neutral	Neutral
Raspberry	Neutral	Beneficial
Sago palm	Neutral	Neutral
Spanish melon	Neutral	Neutral
Strawberry	Neutral	Neutral
Tangerine/tangerine juice	Neutral	Neutral

Water & lemon	Neutral	Neutral
Youngberry	Neutral	Neutral

Oils

TYPE B DOES BEST on monounsaturated oils, such as olive oil, and oils rich in omega series fatty acids, such as flaxseed oil. Walnut oil and black currant seed oil are highly beneficial for Type B secretors, who have a bit of an edge in breaking down oil over non-secretors. Make it a point to avoid sesame, sunflower, and corn oils, which contain lectins damaging to the Type B digestion.

BLOOD TYPE B: OILS			
Portion: 1 tbsp			
	African	**Caucasian**	**Asian**
Secretor	5–8	5–8	5–8
Non-Secretor	3–5	3–7	3–6
		Times per week	

Tier One

FOOD	TYPE B SECRETOR	TYPE B NON-SECRETOR
Borage seed oil	Avoid	Avoid
Castor oil	Avoid	Avoid
Coconut oil	Avoid	Avoid
Corn oil	Avoid	Avoid
Cottonseed oil	Avoid	Avoid
Olive oil	Beneficial	Beneficial
Peanut oil	Avoid	Avoid
Safflower oil	Avoid	Avoid
Sesame oil	Avoid	Avoid
Soy oil	Avoid	Avoid
Sunflower oil	Avoid	Avoid

Tier Two

FOOD	TYPE B SECRETOR	TYPE B NON-SECRETOR
Canola oil	Avoid	Avoid

Neutral: General Nutritional Supplementation

FOOD	TYPE B SECRETOR	TYPE B NON-SECRETOR
Almond oil	Neutral	Neutral
Black currant seed oil	Neutral	Beneficial
Cod liver oil	Neutral	Neutral
Evening primrose oil	Neutral	Neutral
Flaxseed (linseed) oil	Neutral	Beneficial
Walnut oil	Neutral	Beneficial
Wheat germ oil	Neutral	Neutral

Herbs, Spices and Condiments

MANY SPICES HAVE mild to moderate medicinal properties. Some exert an influence on the levels of bacteria in the lower colon. Many common gums, such as guar gum, should be avoided. Gums can enhance the effects of lectins found in other foods. Molasses is a beneficial sweetener for Type B and can provide some additional dietary iron. Turmeric, one of the spices in curry powder, contains a powerful phytochemical called curcumin, which helps lower levels of intestinal toxins. Brewer's yeast is a beneficial food for Type B non-secretors. It enhances glucose metabolism and helps insure a healthy flora balance in the intestinal tract. Type B responds best to warming herbs, such as ginger, horseradish, and cayenne pepper.

Tier One

FOOD	TYPE B SECRETOR	TYPE B NON-SECRETOR
Almond extract	Avoid	Avoid
Aspartame	Avoid	Avoid
Carrageenan	Avoid	Avoid
Corn syrup	Avoid	Avoid
Cornstarch	Avoid	Avoid
Curry	Beneficial	Beneficial
Guar gum	Avoid	Avoid
Ketchup	Avoid	Avoid
Licorice root	Beneficial	Beneficial
Molasses (blackstrap)	Beneficial	Beneficial

MSG	Avoid	Avoid
Parsley	Beneficial	Beneficial
Pepper (black/white)	Avoid	Avoid

Tier Two

FOOD	TYPE B SECRETOR	TYPE B NON-SECRETOR
Allspice	Avoid	Avoid
Barley malt	Avoid	Avoid
Cinnamon	Avoid	Avoid
Dextrose	Avoid	Avoid
Gelatin plain	Avoid	Avoid
Guarana	Avoid	Avoid
Maltodextrin	Avoid	Avoid
Soy sauce	Avoid	Avoid
Stevia	Avoid	Neutral
Sucanat	Avoid	Avoid

Neutral: General Nutritional Supplementation

FOOD	TYPE B SECRETOR	TYPE B NON-SECRETOR
Anise	Neutral	Neutral
Apple pectin	Neutral	Neutral
Arrowroot	Neutral	Neutral
Basil	Neutral	Neutral
Bay leaf	Neutral	Neutral
Bergamot	Neutral	Neutral
Caraway	Neutral	Neutral
Cardamon	Neutral	Neutral
Carob	Neutral	Neutral
Chili powder	Neutral	Neutral
Chives	Neutral	Neutral
Chocolate	Neutral	Neutral
Clove	Neutral	Neutral
Coriander	Neutral	Neutral
Cream of tartar	Neutral	Neutral
Cumin	Neutral	Neutral
Dill	Neutral	Neutral
Dulse	Neutral	Neutral

Fructose	Neutral	Avoid
Honey	Neutral	Neutral
Mace	Neutral	Neutral
Maple syrup	Neutral	Neutral
Marjoram	Neutral	Neutral
Mayonnaise	Neutral	Neutral
Mint	Neutral	Neutral
Molasses	Neutral	Neutral
Mustard (prepared, vinegar free)	Neutral	Neutral
Mustard (prepared, with vinegar)	Neutral	Neutral
Mustard (dry)	Neutral	Neutral
Nutmeg	Neutral	Neutral
Oregano	Neutral	Beneficial
Paprika	Neutral	Neutral
Pepper (peppercorn/ red pepper flakes)	Neutral	Neutral
Peppermint	Neutral	Neutral
Pickle relish	Neutral	Avoid
Rice syrup	Neutral	Neutral
Rosemary	Neutral	Neutral
Saffron	Neutral	Neutral
Sage	Neutral	Neutral
Salad dressing	Neutral	Neutral
Savory	Neutral	Neutral
Sea salt	Neutral	Neutral
Spearmint	Neutral	Neutral
Sugar (brown/white)	Neutral	Avoid
Tamari	Neutral	Neutral
Tamarind	Neutral	Neutral
Tarragon	Neutral	Neutral
Thyme	Neutral	Neutral
Turmeric	Neutral	Neutral
Vanilla	Neutral	Neutral
Vinegar (apple cider)	Neutral	Neutral

Beverages

TYPE B NON-SECRETORS may wish to have a glass of wine occasionally with their meals. There are substantial benefits to their cardiovascular system from moderate use. Green tea should be part of every Type B health plan, as it contains polyphenols that block the production of harmful polyamines.

Tier One

FOOD	TYPE B SECRETOR	TYPE B NON-SECRETOR
Tea (green)	Beneficial	Beneficial

Tier Two

FOOD	TYPE B SECRETOR	TYPE B NON-SECRETOR
Liquor (distilled)	Avoid	Neutral
Seltzer water	Avoid	Neutral
Soda (club)	Avoid	Neutral
Soda (misc./diet/cola)	Avoid	Avoid

Neutral: General Nutritional Supplementation

FOOD	TYPE B SECRETOR	TYPE B NON-SECRETOR
Beer	Neutral	Neutral
Coffee (regular/decaf)	Neutral	Avoid
Tea (black regular/decaf)	Neutral	Avoid
Wine (red)	Neutral	Beneficial
Wine (white)	Neutral	Beneficial

Individualized Therapies for Chronic Conditions

As you can see by referring to your Risk Profile, Type B is more susceptible to certain chronic conditions and diseases than the other blood types. The following section details those conditions, the Type B connection, and a wide range of therapies, in addition to the Tier Two Diet, based on your blood type.

See Type B Health Risk Profile, page 238.

Type B–Specific Metabolic Conditions

Syndrome X

Syndrome X

The metabolic balance of Type Bs is dramatically influenced by the rather idiosyncratic effects of lectins in certain foods. Lectins in chicken, corn, buckwheat, lentils, peanuts, and sesame seeds cause insulin resistance and induce polyamine formation, resulting in weight gain, fluid retention, and hypoglycemia.

Type Bs who want to lose weight should absolutely avoid corn, followed by wheat.

Type Bs are similar to Type Os in their reaction to wheat. The lectin found in wheat adds to the problems caused by the other metabolism-slowing foods. When food is not efficiently digested and burned as fuel for the body, it gets stored as fat. In itself, wheat lectin doesn't attack Type Bs as severely as it does Type Os. However, when you add wheat to the mix of corn, lentils, buckwheat, and peanuts, the end result is just as damaging. Type Bs who want to lose weight should definitely avoid whole wheat. Many rye products can be just as damaging as wheat for Type Bs, and they should be watched as well.

When these lectin-containing foods are eliminated from your diet, it has been my experience that Type Bs are very successful in controlling their weight. You don't have any natural physiological barriers to weight loss, such as the thyroid problems that can hamper Type Os, although you can have problems with excess cortisol if you don't take time for periodic stress reduction. Digestively, you're quite balanced. All you need to do to lose weight is to stay on your diet.

Some people are surprised that Type Bs aren't more likely to have problems with weight control, since dairy foods are encouraged on your diet. Of course, if you overeat high calorie foods, you're going to gain weight. The moderate consumption of dairy foods, particularly cultured foods like kefir or yogurt, aids your digestion, promotes healthy bowel flora, and increases active tissue mass. Whole-food, hormone-free dairy can be good for you.

When you stray from the Type B prescriptions, you are susceptible to the various metabolic conditions associated with Syndrome X—in particular, obesity, insulin resistance, and elevated triglyceride levels. If you're a Type B non-secretor, your risk rises substantially.

A classic sign of insulin resistance in Type Bs is the apple-shaped figure, which is characterized by a broad girth at the mid-section. Fat cells located in the abdomen release fat into the blood more easily than fat cells found elsewhere. For example, pear-shaped individuals, with fat located in the hips and thighs, do not have the same health risks. The release of fat from the abdomen begins within three to four hours after a meal is consumed, compared to many more hours for other fat cells. This easy release shows up as higher triglycerides and free fatty acid levels. Free fatty acids themselves cause insulin resistance and elevated triglycerides usually coincide with low HDL, or "good" cholesterol. Overproduction of insulin as a result of insulin resistance syndrome has also been shown to increase the "very bad" cholesterol, VLDL.

If you tend toward the apple shape and have excess abdominal fat, you need to lose weight in order to prevent a progression to more serious conditions.

Type Bs can successfully lose weight by making some adjustments to the Type B Diet. I've also found that Type Bs do particularly well when they keep a diet journal.

Approach your weight loss program as a long-term strategy and take it slow. The following approach outlines the most crucial elements for successful weight loss. Each one of them plays a role. If you are seriously overweight or have any medical conditions, I suggest that you consult with your doctor before you embark on this or any other plan.

1. LEARN YOUR METABOLIC PROFILE.   Knowing your muscle mass, percentage of body fat, and basal metabolic rate can be more important than knowing your weight. These are the indicators of metabolic balance. Your goal is not just to lose pounds, but to build muscle. I suggest that you have a bioelectrical impedence analysis. If that's not feasible, there are some do-it-yourself methods for learning more about your metabolic state. These methods are not scientifically accurate, but they'll provide clues.

> *Test for Extracellular Water—Edema:* Push your finger firmly down on your shin bone and hold it for five seconds. If you push against muscle or fat, the skin will bounce back up. If there is water between the cells, it will be displaced laterally, and the dimple won't fill in immediately. The longer the indentation remains, the more water is present, meaning the more weight you are carrying in water.

> *Measure Your Hip to Waist Ratio:* Excess weight is most unhealthy—and most conducive to metabolic problems— when it is

centered in your abdomen, as opposed to your hips and thighs. Here's a quick test to learn about your fat distribution: Stand straight in front of a full-length mirror. Using a tape measure, measure the distance around the smallest part of your waist. Now measure the distance around the largest part of your buttocks. Divide your waist measurement by your hip measurement. A healthy ratio for women is .70 to .75. A healthy ratio for men is .80 to .90.

2. CUT OUT THE WORST OFFENDERS. To accelerate weight loss, make the following adjustments to your Type B diet:

- Eliminate corn and corn products.
- Eliminate wheat. Although Type Bs don't have as much trouble with wheat gluten as Type Os, you should definitely avoid it if you want to lose weight. Otherwise, use it sparingly.
- The lectins in several foods inhibit absorption and metabolic efficiency for Type Bs. I have observed many Type Bs who have no

---

▪ FROM THE BLOOD TYPE OUTCOME REGISTRY ▪

Michelle W.
Middle-Aged Female
Type B
Outcome: Weight loss—Improved

"I went on the diet January 1, 1998, and I am still on it. I follow it strictly, and for the first three or four months, I actually consumed more calories than before. I did this to test the diet. I knew if I cut my calories I would lose weight. What I wanted to know was if this diet was really different. I didn't want the exclusion of some foods to reflect a lower calorie intake. I ate sugar, and only those things on my list. I started at 270 pounds, and the only health problems I had were 1. I had half my thyroid removed due to cancer over twenty years ago; and 2. a flare up of water retention. In the past, I had always handled water retention by consuming water, lemon juice, and cucumbers. But for about two months prior to my going on the diet, nothing that I tried worked. Your diet reduced the water retention immediately by 80 percent. I have had great weight loss. As of today, I have lost seventy-nine pounds and have eleven more to go. I have tried to deviate from the *ER4YT* diet twice. Once to eat pork rinds, and once to eat chicken. The pork rinds I ate in large quantities and had problems digesting them. The one meal of El Pollo Loco Chicken caused a five pound weight gain."

trouble losing weight once they eliminate these foods: chicken, lentils, peanuts, sesame seeds, and buckwheat.

- Select low and non-fat dairy products, and soft cheeses over hard. They contain less fat and fewer calories.
- Eat seafood several times a week.

3. MONITOR SYMPTOMS OF SLUGGISH METABOLISM.   Be alert to signs that your metabolism isn't operating efficiently. These include:

fatigue
dry skin
cold hands and feet
loss of sexual interest
constipation and water retention
lightheadedness on standing

4. MANAGE YOUR STRESS.   Stress can interfere with your ability to lose weight. Stress hormones promote insulin resistance and hormonal imbalance. They also catabolize (burn) muscle tissue instead of fat. For recommendations, see *Lifestyle Strategies* and *Emotional Equalizers*.

5. SUPPLEMENT YOUR DIET WITH METABOLISM BOOSTERS.

- Magnesium: 200–300 mg day; 300–500 mg when you're highly stressed or fatigued. Type Bs risk having deficiencies in magne-

---

▪ FROM THE BLOOD TYPE OUTCOME REGISTRY ▪

Richard S.
Type B
Middle-aged male
Improved: Weight loss

"At the age of fifty-three I found it difficult to fight off the 'one pound a year syndrome' for people over thirty-five. I exercised regularly and attempted to knock off the ten pounds. My mood has changed considerably, this might be related to my giving up grain alcohol. I have lost eight to nine lbs in a month with few cravings. While I found the Atkins diet somewhat effective, it didn't give me enough stamina for my exercise routine. My wife thinks your diet is crazy, but she is quite supportive because of my mood change and weight loss."

sium—in part, because you assimilate calcium so efficiently. Coincidentally, overweight individuals, especially those with extremely poor sugar handling capabilities, are often deficient in this mineral.

- CoQ10: 60 mg twice daily. Coenzyme Q10 is critical for energy metabolism and heart health. Supplementation has been shown to reduce blood pressure, fasting and two-hour plasma insulin, glucose, and triglycerides, while improving HDL cholesterol. Since CoQ10 is an antioxidant, it helps reduce the oxidant stress often seen in obesity and increases the efficiency of antioxidant vitamins like A, C, E, and beta-carotene.

- L-Carnitine: 500 mg. L-carnitine is needed to move fats into your mitochondria (energy metabolizing cells), where they can then be used as a source of energy. Evidence demonstrates that L-carnitine reduces insulin resistance.

- Biotin: 2–8 mg. Biotin is a vitamin needed in fat metabolism. Evidence shows that at the correct dose, biotin can lower blood sugar, improve tolerance to sugar, and decrease insulin resistance.

- Chromium or chromium-rich yeast: Chromium is another trace mineral associated with sugar regulation. At appropriate levels it is needed to regulate fasting blood sugar levels and improve receptor sensitivity to insulin.

- Zinc: 25 mg. Zinc is needed for growth hormone function, thyroid function, and a balanced stress response.

- Lipoic Acid: 100–600 mg per day can help promote improved sugar-handling capabilities. Lipoic acid is also a critical nutrient in energy metabolism and is an acclaimed and powerful antioxidant.

- Pyridoxal (vitamin B_6) enhances protein metabolism and helps build active tissue mass.

6. WATCH YOUR HABITS.   Alcohol consumption can exacerbate insulin resistance by contributing metabolically to hyperglycemia. Although beer is normally neutral for Type Bs, avoid it if you're trying to lose weight. There may be health benefits to red wine, which is extremely high in phytochemicals, but it does contain extra calories as sugar. If you drink a glass of wine, have it with a meal to offset blood sugar swings.

Don't smoke. If you smoke because you fear the weight gain that might come with quitting, consider this: Chronic cigarette smokers are insulin resistant and hyperinsulinaemic, compared with non-smokers.

Type B–Specific Immune Conditions

Bacterial Infections
Viral/Nervous System Disorders
Autoimmune Disease

Immunity is the Achilles' heel of the unbalanced Type B. While your blood type seems to offer some protection against cancer, you are highly susceptible to bacterial infections, slow growing viral diseases of the nervous system, and certain autoimmune diseases.

Bacterial Infections

Many bacterial infections attack Type Bs with special force. There's a reason. The most common bacteria-producing infections are B-like in nature, and you don't produce antibodies against them.

KIDNEY AND URINARY TRACT INFECTIONS.   Like many infectious diseases, your blood type can influence your susceptibility to and response against the common bacteria responsible for urinary tract infections (UTIs). As a general rule, Type B is most plagued by chronic or recurrent UTIs. Your secretor status also plays a role. Non-secretors are much more likely to contract severe and repeated UTIs. If you're a Type B non-secretor, this is a case of a true synergism.[1] You're bound to be more affected.

'The reason non-secretors have a higher risk is due to several factors—the inability to prevent adherence of unwanted bacteria, the presence of more binding sites for their attachment, and the tendency to have a more difficult time in eliminating bacterial colonization. Evidence indicates that women and children with renal scarring subsequent to recurrent UTIs are more likely to be non-secretors. As many as 55 to 60 percent of non-secretors have been found to develop renal scars, even with the regular use of antibiotic treatment for UTIs. This tendency to scarring does not seem to be dictated as much by the aggressiveness of the bacterial infection, but by the more aggressive inflammatory response created by non-secretors against the bacterial infection.

Many different bacterial organisms can cause UTIs. However, the most common for Type Bs are:

Klebsiella pneumoniae
Proteus sp.
Pseudomonas sp.

To guard against UTIs:

- Cranberries and blueberries both have anti-adhesion activity, so act to prevent bacteria from adhering to the cells in your bladder and urinary tract.
- *Uva ursi* is an excellent herb for combatting urinary tract infections.
- Buchu is another excellent B-friendly bladder herb.
- Consume plenty of cultured dairy foods, which contribute to a balanced urinary tract.

INFLUENZA.   Type Bs have the weakest defense of all the blood types against the most common influenza viruses *(A H1N1 and A H3N2)*. I highly recommend that you take regular doses of elderberry extract—1 teaspoon three to four times daily during the flu season. Elderberry has been used by herbalists for centuries, and it has been shown to inhibit replication of all strains of influenza virus. Elderberry works by producing a greater immune response and by inhibiting neuroaminidase. This is an enzyme whose actions *should* be inhibited, as it enhances the ability of microorganisms to invade and destroy tissue. Neuroaminidase also helps lectins behave more disruptively.

NOTE: Significantly exceeding the recommended dosage can cause nausea.

E. COLI.   Many of the most pathogenic forms of E. coli capable of causing diarrhea are immunologically B-like.[2] This makes you defenseless against the infection. Your best recourse is prevention.

- Never serve hamburger and other foods containing ground beef that is rare or raw. When properly cooked, the inside of ground beef should be brown rather than pink, with an internal temperature of 160 F, and the juices should run clear.
- Do not eat raw sprouts.
- Hands, utensils, and food-contact surfaces must be washed with warm, soapy water between contact with raw meat and foods that have already been cooked, or foods that will be served raw.
- Good hygiene is essential to prevent the spread of disease from infected persons. Hands should always be washed with warm water and soap after using the toilet or changing diapers. Persons with diarrhea should not prepare or serve food to others. Keep personal health items in your bathroom covered and in the medicine closet.

If you do succumb to an infection from *E.coli*, counter the dehydrating effects of diarrhea with plenty of fluids. Evidence suggests that it is the presence of both salt and sugars in the liquid replenishment of dehydration victims that allows the support of life. Make sure that liquids include fresh vegetable juices (such as carrot or celery) and fruit juices (such as blueberry). Bullion, broth, and gentle teas (such as chamomile) are also a good idea. Probiotic supplements and cultured foods are antagonistic to *E. coli* and most other GI pathogenic bacteria.

STREPTOCOCCAL DISEASE.   Streptococcal disease occurs more often in Type Bs than other blood types, resulting in strep throat, or more serious illnesses such as toxic shock syndrome, bacteremia, and pneumonia. A severe form of streptococcal disease occurs primarily among newborns. The consequences of this infection can be sepsis, pneumonia, and meningitis. Neurologic complications can also occur, resulting in loss of sight or hearing, and mental retardation. Death occurs in 6 percent of infants and 16 percent of adults.[3]

There is a connection between Blood Type B and neonatal group B streptococci infection. This association is strong enough to show even based on the mother's blood type. That is, a Type B infant with a Type B mother has double the risk.

Viral/Nervous System Disorders
I know of many cases of fibromyalgia that have dramatically improved through following the Blood Type Diet. Of the foods known to induce joint inflammation, grains certainly top the list. One researcher says of lectins: "Avoidance of these is frequently the only dietary maneuver required, especially in the early cases."[4] As seen, our most common grains contain lectins, and many of these lectins are specifically attracted to sugars, particularly N-acetyl glucosamine (NAG), that are found abundantly in connective tissue. Wheat germ lectin in particular has an affinity for NAG. My suspicion is that a substantial amount of the improvement in fibromyalgia is simply the result of wheat avoidance, particularly for Type B.

PREVENTIVE MEASURES:

- Follow the Type B Diet.
- Take elderberry. In experiments, elderberry has been shown to inhibit replication of all strains of human influenza viruses tested. In one placebo-controlled, double-blind study, an extract of

---

• FROM THE BLOOD TYPE OUTCOME REGISTRY •

John W.
Type B
Middle-aged male
Outcome: Chronic fatigue syndrome

"For several years I have suffered from many of the symptoms of CFS. I felt like I was improving at times, but the symptoms kept returning. I started the *ER4YT* diet in early March 1999, and noticed improvement almost immediately (within three days). Over the past two months I've been able to return to jogging, and more importantly, my cognitive abilities have returned to normal. I am convinced Dr. D. is on to something. I can only hope that his ideas will become more accepted by the medical profession and the public."

---

elderberry fruit was shown to be effective in treating influenza B. People using the elderberry extract got better much quicker—more than 70 percent were better after two days and over 90 percent completely resolved the infection within three days. In contrast, those given a placebo often needed as many as six days to feel well. Researchers found that those taking the elderberry were able to produce a higher level of recognition of the flu bug, seeing it as an enemy. In my clinic, patients who take an elderberry, blueberry, cherry, and apple concentrate mixture seem to pass easily through the flu season. However, be advised that when it comes to daily use of elderberry, more is not always better. Large doses will lead to nausea. If you are trying to avoid a flu, a small amount daily might help. I recommend elderberry especially for Type Bs and Type ABs because of their general susceptibility to the virus. For treatment, we use 2 tablespoons, 3–4 times daily for adults and proportionately less for children depending on their body weight.

- Eat exotic mushrooms. Shitake, maitake, and reishi mushrooms are very effective in supporting long-term antiviral resistance.
- Take B vitamins—particularly riboflavin and thiamine to encourage nerve health.
- Arginine (250 mg) can help boost nitric oxide levels and increase efficiency of anti-viral activity.
- Take Astragalus *(A. membranaceus)* root extract (0.8-1 percent isoflavones). This is an outstanding immune-balancing herb with

a demonstrated ability to increase NK cell activity, balance immune performance, and promote antistress and antiviral activity.
- Licorice root promotes antiviral immune sytem function.
- Probiotic supplements promote a range of improved antiviral specific immune activity.
- Pectin, usually from apples, is rich in polysaccharides, which can inhibit viral and bacterial adhesion.

Autoimmune Diseases

Many of the autoimmune diseases are rare, but as a whole, afflict millions of Americans. The brunt of the autoimmune diseases strike women more often than men. In particular, they affect women of working age and during their childbearing years. This seems to clearly point to the possibility that hormonal triggers are involved. Some autoimmune diseases occur more frequently in certain population groups than in others. Lupus is far more common among African-American and Hispanic women than it is in the population of Caucasian women of European descent. Rheumatoid arthritis and scleroderma affect many more members of certain Native American communities than it does the overall population of the United States.[5]

Type Bs are especially susceptible to autoimmune diseases such as rheumatoid arthritis, lupus, and scleroderma. In general, non-secretors are far more likely to suffer

To learn more about staying healthy and well balanced, log on to the blood type Web site: www.dadamo.com.

from an autoimmune disease than secretors, especially when it is provoked by an infection. Non-secretors also have genetically induced difficulties in removing immune complexes from their tissues, which increases their risk of attacking tissue that contains them. If you are a Type B non-secretor, you have an especially high risk.

In addition to the Type B Diet, the following supplementation will help strengthen the Type B immune system:

- Magnesium (300–500 mg daily).
- Licorice root extract—known to function as an antiviral agent, and helps prevent and treat chronic fatigue syndrome.
- Lecithin—Helps keep cell membranes fluid.
- Larch arabinogalactan—a safe, gentle immune modulator.

Chronic Fatigue Syndrome (CFS)
There are a number of nutritional strategies for CFS, and they are becoming more widely used, even in conventional medicine. Magnesium deficiency and oxidative stress have both been identified in more than 50 percent of cases. A detailed review of the literature suggests a number of marginal nutritional deficiencies may have some relevance to CFS. These include deficiencies in various B vitamins, vitamin C, magnesium, sodium, zinc, L-tryptophan, L-carnitine, coenzyme Q10, and essential fatty acids. Any of these nutrients might be marginally deficient in CFS patients, a finding that appears to be primarily due to the progression of the illness rather than an inadequate diet.[6] Here is a simple and effective treatment plan for Type Bs:

- Methylcobalamin, 500 mcg twice daily: Note that this is not the standard vitamin B12, but rather the "active B12" form.
- Magnesium, 500 mg twice daily: Note this can act as a laxative. If the stools become loose at this dose, lower the dose and gradually work back up as you get used to it.
- A good multivitamin.
- Essential Fatty Acids: These are probably more than adequately provided by the Membrane Fluidizer Drink. If you miss your daily cocktail, a few capsules of black currant seed oil can fill in.
- Licorice: Licorice can produce some side effects in a few individuals, such as water retention. It should be used under the guidance of a skilled herbalist or physician trained in herbology. The commonly available forms (called DGL licorice) will probably not work.

Live Right 4 Type AB

Type AB Profile

BELIEVED TO HAVE existed for only a thousand years or so and constituting only between 2 and 5 percent of the population, Type AB may be considered transitional—a work in progress. Since it is the only blood type whose existence is the result of intermingling rather than environment, Type AB has its own unique "spin" on immunity.

Type AB has a chameleonlike quality. Depending on the circumstances, this blood type can appropriate the characteristics of each of the other blood types. Type AB's stress hormone profile most resembles that of Type O—yet it shares some of Type B's chemical response to nitric oxide. The Type AB digestive profile is A-like, yet there is a shared Type B preference for meat. So, although Type AB needs a bit more

continued on page 290

Type AB Health Risk Profile

CHARACTERISTICS	MANIFESTATIONS
MIND/BODY Tendency to build-up higher levels of catecholamines (noradrenaline and adrenaline) during stress, due to low levels of the enzyme MAO	• Tendency to feel angry and alienated from others • Imbalance of the neurochemical, dopamine • Extreme introversion
Tend to clear nitric oxide rapidly, through the B gene allele's influence on enzymatic production of NO	*When out of balance:* • Overly emotional reaction to stressful situations
DIGESTION Low stomach acid production	• Makes it difficult to digest protein • Blocks action of digestive enzymes • Promotes excess bacterial growth in stomach and upper intestine • can impair vitamin and mineral absorption
Lack of enzyme, intestinal alkaline phosphatase	• Produces high serum cholesterol, especially LDL. • Makes it difficult to break down fat
METABOLISM High levels of blood clotting factors	• Blood clots more easily
IMMUNITY Low antibody IgA levels	• Creates vulnerability to ear and respiratory infections • Creates susceptibility to GI infections
Low antibody IgE levels	• Promotes asthma and allergies
Lacks anti-A and anti-B capabilities	• Impairs immune system's ability to discriminate between friend and foe • Need to maintain higher NK cell activity

INCREASED RISKS	VARIATIONS
• Bipolar (manic-depressive) disease • Depression • Heart disease (if "*Type A* personality") • Parkinson's disease • Schizophrenia • Substance abuse	
• Hypertension	
• Stomach cancer • Gallstones • Jaundice • Intestinal toxicity	NON-SECRETOR Slightly higher levels of stomach acid make animal protein more digestible
• Coronary artery disease • Osteoporosis • Colon cancer • Hypercholesterolemia	NON-SECRETOR Extremely low levels of intestinal alkaline phosphatase
• Coronary artery disease • Cerebral thrombosis • Problematic in cancer	ELDERLY • Increases risk of strokes from embolisms • Increases risk of occlusive heart diseases
• Celiac disease • Rheumatic heart disease • Kidney disease • "Leaky gut"	NON-SECRETOR Higher risk, especially children
• Poor defense against parasites	
• Most cancers • Chronic viral infections • Risk of low grade infections	SECRETORS • Higher risk of low grade infections • Lower NK cell levels ELDERLY • NK cell activity declines with age

animal protein than Type A, it lacks enough stomach acid to digest it efficiently. Similarly, Type AB has difficulty metabolizing protein, because of low levels of intestinal alkaline phosphatase. The Type AB immune system is also A-like, and it shares Type A's high risk of developing cancer.

Type AB blunts cortisol more effectively than Type A and may have a higher level of endurance for exercise. This added measure of strength may be caused by the unusual genetic inheritance Type AB contains. What precise measure is provided by the admixture of genetic materials will be revealed as more research is completed, but genetic and personality studies indicate that, at its best, Type AB is intuitive and spiritual, with an ability to look beyond the rigid confines of society. The conflicting desire to be independent and social can create conflicts, but Type AB possesses many of the characteristics that are most valued in our modern, less parochial, environment.

Type AB Prescription

The Type AB prescription is a combination of dietary, behavioral, and environmental therapies to help you live right for your type:

- LIFESTYLE STRATEGIES to structure your life for health and longevity
- ADAPTED LIFESTYLE STRATEGIES for children, the elderly, and non-secretors
- EMOTIONAL EQUALIZERS and stress relievers
- SPECIALIZED DIET PLAN: Tier One for maximum health
- TARGETED DIET PLAN: Tier Two to overcome disease
- INDIVIDUALIZED THERAPIES for chronic conditions
- THERAPEUTIC SUPPLEMENT PROGRAM for extra support

Lifestyle Strategies

Keys

🔑 Cultivate your social nature in welcoming environments. Avoid situations that are highly competitive.

🔑 Avoid ritualistic thinking and fixating on issues, especially those you can't control or influence.

🔑 Develop a clear plan for goals and tasks—annual, monthly, weekly, daily.

🗝 Make lifestyle changes gradually, rather than trying to tackle everything at once.

🗝 Engage in forty-five to sixty minutes of aerobic exercise at least twice a week, balanced by daily stretching, meditation, or yoga.

🗝 Engage in a community, neighborhood, or other group activity that gives you a meaningful connection to a group.

🗝 Practice visualization exercises daily.

🗝 Also carve out time alone. Have at least one sport, hobby, or activity that you perform independently of others.

1. Eat Right for Wellness

Type ABs should abide by this simple rule of thumb: Most foods that should be avoided by Type A and Type B should also be avoided by Type AB. This makes for a mixed dietary picture. Here are the keys:

- Avoid caffeine and alcohol, especially when you're in stressful situations. Caffeine can be particularly harmful, because of its tendency to raise adrenaline and noradrenaline—already high for Type ABs.
- Derive your protein primarily from sources other than red meat. Fish and seafood are your best choices.
- Don't undereat or skip meals. Use appropriate blood type snacks between meals if you get hungry. Avoid low calorie diets. Remember, food deprivation is a huge stress. It raises stress hormone levels, lowers metabolism, encourages fat storage, and depletes healthy muscle mass.
- Eat a balanced breakfast, with more protein-containing food. For Type ABs breakfast should be thought of as the "King of Meals," particularly if you're trying to lose weight. It is the most important meal of the day for balancing your metabolic needs and your stress response.
- Smaller, more frequent meals will counteract digestive problems caused by inadequate stomach acid and peptic enzymes. Your stomach initiates the digestive process with a combination of digestive secretions, and the muscular contractions that mix food with them. When you have low levels of digestive secretions, food tends to stay in the stomach longer. In addition, be attentive to food combining. You'll digest and metabolize foods more efficiently if you avoid eating starches and proteins at the same meal. The use of digestive bitters thirty minutes prior to a meal can also help rev up your digestion.

2. Combine Intense Physical Exercise
with Calming Exercises

Type ABs require both calming activities and more intense physical exercise. Vary your routine to include a mix of the following—two days calming, three days aerobic:

CALMING.   *Hatha Yoga:* Hatha yoga has become increasingly popular in Western countries as a method for coping with stress, and in my experience is an excellent form of exercise for Type ABs.

Healthy Type ABs should try to balance their exercise regimen in the following way:

CARDIOVASCULAR ACTIVITY	WEIGHTS	FLEXIBILITY/STRETCHING
25 minutes	20 minutes	30 minutes
2–3 times weekly	3–4 times weekly	2–3 times weekly

ADAPTED LIFESTYLE STRATEGIES	TYPE AB CHILDREN

Structure your Type AB child's life to include these essential strategies for healthy growth, wellness, and diminished risk for disease.

Young Children

- Create a non-restrictive environment. For example, allow your child to select his or her own clothes, even if the colors clash or you don't like the styles.
- Be flexible about rules, where possible—for example, bedtimes and meal times.
- Make sure your child spends plenty of time outdoors. Fresh air and sunshine help keep NK levels high.
- As early as age two or three, a child can join you in a daily deep breathing, stretching, and meditation.
- Emphasize social interaction in an environment that is noncompetitive. Type AB children tend to be highly social, but they are easily alienated in high-pressure settings.
- There is a tendency for Type ABs to internalize emotions. Be extrasensitive to signs that your child is upset or troubled.

Older Children

- Educate your child about the dangers of alcohol, tobacco, and drugs, while modeling positive behavior yourself. Like Type Os, Type ABs are especially vulnerable to developing addictive behaviors. These activities are harmful to NK cell activity.
- Encourage your child to choose sports activities that are not highly competitive, but allow for artistic expression, such as dance.
- Enable your Type AB child's need for independence and self-reliance with part-time jobs outside the home or an independent study program.

| ADAPTED LIFESTYLE STRATEGIES | TYPE AB SENIORS |

- Stomach acid production, already low in Type ABs, decreases even more in about 20 percent of elderly people. It is particularly important to follow the Type AB Diet to keep your stomach acid at a level that enables proper digestion. Take a supplement of L-histidine twice daily, drink a weak tea of bitter herbs before a meal, and avoid carbonated beverages.
- After age sixty, your sense of smell begins to decline, sometimes dramatically. Your sense of smell also plays a role in taste, both of which serve to activate your digestive juices and announce, "It's time to eat." Often people with a declining sense of taste and smell tend to undereat. Inability to smell strong odors can also be dangerous, as you are less likely to detect food that has spoiled. Undereating is a special problem for Type AB seniors. Your immune system also makes you more sensitive to bacterial infections. If your sense of smell seems to be diminishing, consider taking a trace mineral supplement.

Emotional Equalizers

Keys

- Plan your days and weeks to minimize surprises and avoid rushing.
- Break up your workday with physical activity, especially if your job is sedentary. You'll feel more energized.
- Set up small "rewards" you can give yourself when you accomplish tasks.

🖋 Stop smoking and avoid stimulants.

🖋 Spend some time "giving back." Type ABs are natural philan-
thropists and have a gift for empathy. Donate money or other resources to help others.

1. Identify Your Tendencies

Type ABs often receive mixed messages about emotional health. While
you tend to be drawn to other people and are friendly and trusting,
there is a side of you that feels alienated from the larger community. At
your best, you're intuitive and spiritual, with an ability to look beyond
the rigid confines of society. You are passionate in your beliefs, but you
also want to be liked by others, and this can create conflicts.

When it comes to stress hormones, you most resemble Type O in
your tendency to overproduce catecholamines like adrenaline. Yet
you have the additional complexity of Type B's rapid clearing of nitrous
oxide, so you suffer the physical consequences of high emotions. Your
greatest danger is the tendency to internalize your emotions—especially anger and hostility, which is much more damaging to your health
than the externalizing anger and aggressiveness of Type O. Evaluate
whether or not you fit any of these personality characteristics. It is not
my intention to label you. Your personality is quite individual, and genetic predispositions only form a small part of the picture. You might

---

▪ FROM THE BLOOD TYPE OUTCOME REGISTRY ▪

Gwen S.
Type AB
Middle-aged female
Improved: Smoking cessation

"I think that the most signifigant change was that I lost interest in
cigarettes only one week into trying the AB diet. To me this seemed
like a miracle because I'm a professional artist who enjoyed the nar-
cotic effects of nicotine while doing creative work. The calming effects of the tryptophan rich dark meat turkey and the calcium rich
foods in the diet are just the ticket for me. I've been off of cigarettes
now for four months and I rarely think of them. Pretty good after
eighteen years of such a bad habit! I just hope that it's not too late
for me with my sensitive AB immune system. I love the diet and
find it easy to follow for the most part. My heart feels stronger and
healthier from not smoking and probably from the diet."

consider, though, what this data means to you. In my experience, these prototypical behaviors tend to emerge most strikingly when resistance is low and stress is high.

2. Use Adaptogens to Improve Your Stress Response

The term "adaptogen" has been used to categorize plants that improve the nonspecific response to stress. Many of these plants have a bidirectional or normalizing influence on your physiology—if something is too low, they bring it up; too high, they bring it down. The following adaptogens are well-suited for Type AB.

RHODIOLA ROSEA AND RHODIOLA SP.   In addition to its anti-stress activity, *Rhodiola* has a significant ability to prevent stress-induced catecholamine activity in the heart and promote stable heart contractility. Rhodiola can also prevent abnormalities in cardiopulmonary function, when you're at high altitudes.

B VITAMINS.   Type ABs generally need an ample supply of B vitamins to promote a balanced stress response. Of particular importance are B_1, pantethine, and B_6. When you're dealing with stress, take them at levels several times the RDA.

LIPOIC ACID.   Lipoic acid is important in catecholamine metabolism, making it beneficial for the Type AB stress response.

3. Use These Supplements for Neurochemical Balance

L-TYROSINE.   Boosting your levels of the amino acid L-tyrosine can increase dopamine concentrations in the brain. In one study, military cadets using a tyrosine-rich drink during a demanding military combat training course performed better on memory and tracking tasks than a comparable group supplied with a carbohydrate-rich drink. These findings suggest tyrosine may, in circumstances characterized by psychosocial and physical stress, reduce the effects of stress and fatigue on cognitive tasks.

CITRULLINE.   This amino acid is involved in the energy cycle and nitric oxide synthesis. A good source is watermelon.

DANSHEN ROOT.   50 mg. This traditional Chinese herb helps regulate nitric oxide, as do two other Chinese herbs—CORDYCEPS SINENSIS (100 mg) and GYNOSTEMMA PENTAPHYLLUM (50 mg).

SANGRE DE GRADO.   50 mg. This herb from the Amazon helps regulate nitric oxide.

LIVE RIGHT 4 YOUR TYPE

GLUTAMINE. Glutamine is an amino acid that is transformed into the GABA class of neurotransmitters. It can be particularly helpful for Type ABs with a sweet tooth. Mix one gram in a glass of water when you feel the need for a carbohydrate.

FOLIC ACID. Most people will not respond well to pharmaceutical antidepressent drugs (Prozac, Zoloft) if they are deficient in this vitamin. Type ABs who suffer from mood swings should always supplement with extra folic acid, along with other B-complex vitamins. Folic acid also lowers homocystine levels, which can influence Type AB susceptibility to cardiovascular disease.

Type AB Two-Tier Diet

The Two-Tier Diet is designed to offer a more individualized program. It has been my experience that some people do very well on the basic Tier One Diet—that is, a moderate degree of adherence to the primary beneficial and avoid foods, with heavy reliance on neutral foods for general nutritional supplementation. Others need a more rigid plan, especially if they suffer from chronic conditions. Adding the Tier Two Diet will help increase the compliance to overcome disease and restore a state of well-being.

Your secretor status can influence your ability to fully digest and metabolize certain foods. For this reason, each food list contains a separate column of rankings for secretors and non-secretors. Although the majority of people are secretors and can safely follow the recommendations in the secretor column, the variations can make a big difference if you are among the approximately 20 percent who are non-secretors.

> SECRETOR or NONSECRETOR?
> Before you start the diet, take the easy home saliva test to determine your secretor status. See page 358.

In rare cases, your A_1, A_2, Rh, and MN status will influence a food ranking. Those distinctions are listed below the appropriate chart.

The Blood Type Diet Tier System

Tier One: Maximize Health
Make these choices as soon as possible to maximize your health. Using Tier One choices in combination with neutral foods for general nutritional supplementation will suffice for most healthy individuals.

Tier Two: Overcome Disease

Add these choices if you are suffering from a chronic disease or wish to follow the diet at a higher compliance level. If you are adhering to the Tier Two Diet, use caution when you incorporate neutral foods for general nutritional supplementation.

> BENEFICIAL: These foods possess components that enhance the metabolic, immune, or structural health of your blood type.
>
> NEUTRAL: These foods usually have no direct benefit or harmful effect, based on your blood type, but many of them supply nutrients needed for a well-balanced diet.
>
> AVOID: These foods contain components that are harmful for your blood type.

Individualized Dietary Guidelines

If you are a healthy Type AB, the Tier One Diet will provide the combination of foods you need for good health. To make the most of it, pay special attention to these guidelines.

Keys

- Limit red meat and avoid chicken. Low levels of hydrochloric acid and intestinal alkaline phosphatase make it difficult for Type AB to digest and can create a range of metabolic problems.
- Derive your primary protein from soy products and fresh seafood.
- Include modest amounts of cultured dairy foods in your diet, but avoid fresh milk products, which cause excess mucous production. Cultured dairy products have a probiotic effect; they promote healthy intestinal flora and a stronger immune environment.
- Include regular portions of richly oiled cold-water fish. Fish oils can boost your metabolism.
- Consume vitamin A-rich foods such as carrots, spinach, and broccoli, to boost intestinal alkaline phosphatase levels.

Type AB Dietary Strategies

These strategies are designed to help the healthy Type AB avoid the problems that can arise from your specific neurological, digestive, metabolic, and immune makeup.

Increase Your Stomach Acid Levels

These strategies will help counter low stomach acid.

TAKE 500 MILLIGRAMS OF L-HISTIDINE, an amino acid supplement, twice a day. It improves gastric acid production, especially if you have allergic symptoms.

USE BITTER HERBS.   Herbs such as Gentian *(Gentiana* spp.*)* have long been used by naturopaths to stimulate gastric secretions. They can be taken as a weak tea thirty minutes before a meal.

AVOID CARBONATED BEVERAGES, such as mineral water, seltzer, and soda. The carbonation decreases gastrin production, already marginal in Type ABs, which decreases stomach acidity.

TAKE BETAINE.   In the form of betaine hydrochloride, it can increase the acidity of the stomach, and it has some extra benefits. Betaine is also recommended to reduce blood levels of a substance called homocystine (associated with heart disease). It is used by the body to generate S-adenosylmethionine (SAM-e), a substance that has been receiving media attention as a natural antidepressant and as a healing agent for the liver. In traditional Chinese medicine, anxiety and depression are associated with imbalances of liver energy, or *chi*. Kola nuts contain substantial amounts of betaine, as well as a few other liver protectants, such as d-catechin, l-epicatechin, kolatin, and kolanin. They also contain caffeine, so use them sparingly, and not at all if you have digestive problems.

TAKE DENDROBIUM.   This increases acid output and gastrin concentration.

Prevent Lectin Damage

AVOID LECTINS THAT ARE TYPE AB RED FLAGS.   The worst are:

chicken
certain types of whitefish
corn
buckwheat
lima beans
kidney beans

Type ABs can help block the actions of dietary lectins by using polysaccharide sacrificial molecules, such as those found in:

- NAG (N-Acetylglucosamine)
- Fucus vesiculosis—kelp
- Laminaria
- Larch arabinogalactan

Meat and Poultry

ALTHOUGH A BIT more adapted to animal-based proteins than Type As (mainly because of their B gene's effects on fat absorption), Type ABs still have to beware of elevated cholesterol—a problem somewhat mollified if you are a Type AB non-secretor. Emphasize free-range, chemical- and pesticide-free meats.

BLOOD TYPE AB: MEATS AND POULTRY			
Portion: 4–6 oz. (men); 2–5 oz. (women and children)			
	African	**Caucasian**	**Asian**
Secretor	2–5	1–5	1–5
Non-Secretor	3–5	2–5	2–5
A₂B	Increase by 1 serving weekly		
MM	Decrease by 2 servings weekly		
	Times per week		

Variants: A₂B—partridge, quail, squab, and venison are Neutral. MM—lamb, liver, and mutton are Avoid.

Tier One

FOOD	TYPE AB SECRETOR	TYPE AB NON-SECRETOR
Bacon/ham/pork	Avoid	Avoid
Chicken	Avoid	Avoid
Cornish hens	Avoid	Avoid
Duck	Avoid	Avoid
Grouse	Avoid	Avoid
Guinea hen	Avoid	Avoid
Horse	Avoid	Avoid
Partridge	Avoid	Avoid
Quail	Avoid	Neutral
Squab	Avoid	Avoid
Squirrel	Avoid	Avoid
Turkey	Beneficial	Beneficial
Turtle	Avoid	Avoid

Tier Two

FOOD	TYPE AB SECRETOR	TYPE AB NON-SECRETOR
Beef	Avoid	Avoid
Buffalo	Avoid	Avoid
Goose	Avoid	Avoid
Heart/sweetbreads	Avoid	Avoid
Lamb	Neutral	Beneficial
Mutton	Neutral	Beneficial
Rabbit	Neutral	Beneficial
Veal	Avoid	Avoid
Venison	Avoid	Neutral

Neutral: General Nutritional Supplementation

FOOD	TYPE AB SECRETOR	TYPE AB NON-SECRETOR
Liver (calf)	Neutral	Neutral
Ostrich	Neutral	Neutral
Pheasant	Neutral	Neutral

Fish and Seafood

FISH AND SEAFOOD represent a primary source of protein for most Type ABs, increasing active tissue mass, while also providing the protein source needed to keep Natural Killer (NK) cells optimized. In general, many of the seafood avoids for Type ABs concern lectins with either A or B specificity, or polyamines commonly found in these foods. Avoid using frozen fish, as the content of polyamines in it is much higher than fresh. Because of a higher risk of cancer, Type ABs should consume regular servings of *Helix pomatia* (escargot).

BLOOD TYPE AB: FISH AND SEAFOOD			
Portion: 4–6 oz. (men); 2–5 oz. (women and children)			
	African	Caucasian	Asian
Secretor	4–6	3–5	3–5
Non-Secretor	4–7	4–6	4–6
A_2B	Increase by 2 servings weekly		
	Times per week		

Variants: A$_2$B—flounder, halibut, and whiting are Neutral. Carp, croaker, orange roughy, perch, scrod, weakfish, and whitefish are Beneficial.

Tier One

FOOD	TYPE AB SECRETOR	TYPE AB NON-SECRETOR
Anchovy	Avoid	Avoid
Barracuda	Avoid	Avoid
Bass (all types)	Avoid	Avoid
Beluga	Avoid	Avoid
Clam	Avoid	Avoid
Conch	Avoid	Avoid
Crab	Avoid	Avoid
Eel	Avoid	Avoid
Flounder	Avoid	Avoid
Frog	Avoid	Avoid
Haddock	Avoid	Avoid
Hake	Avoid	Avoid
Halibut	Avoid	Avoid
Mackerel	Beneficial	Beneficial
Mahimahi	Beneficial	Beneficial
Octopus	Avoid	Avoid
Oyster	Avoid	Avoid
Red snapper	Beneficial	Beneficial
Salmon	Beneficial	Beneficial
Sardine	Beneficial	Beneficial
Shad	Beneficial	Beneficial
Snail (*Helix pomatia*/ escargot)	Beneficial	Beneficial
Sole	Avoid	Avoid
Trout (brook)	Avoid	Neutral
Trout (rainbow)	Avoid	Neutral
Trout (sea)	Avoid	Neutral
Tuna	Beneficial	Beneficial
Whiting	Avoid	Avoid
Yellowtail	Avoid	Avoid

Tier Two

FOOD	TYPE AB SECRETOR	TYPE AB NON-SECRETOR
Cod	Beneficial	Beneficial
Grouper	Beneficial	Beneficial
Lobster	Avoid	Avoid
Monkfish	Beneficial	Beneficial
Pickerel	Beneficial	Beneficial
Pike	Beneficial	Beneficial
Porgy	Beneficial	Beneficial
Sailfish	Beneficial	Beneficial
Shrimp	Avoid	Avoid
Sturgeon	Beneficial	Beneficial

Neutral: General Nutritional Supplementation

FOOD	TYPE AB SECRETOR	TYPE AB NON-SECRETOR
Abalone	Neutral	Neutral
Bluefish	Neutral	Neutral
Bullhead	Neutral	Neutral
Butterfish	Neutral	Neutral
Carp	Neutral	Neutral
Catfish	Neutral	Neutral
Caviar	Neutral	Neutral
Chub	Neutral	Neutral
Croaker	Neutral	Neutral
Cusk	Neutral	Neutral
Drum	Neutral	Neutral
Halfmoon fish	Neutral	Neutral
Harvest fish	Neutral	Neutral
Herring	Neutral	Beneficial
Mullet	Neutral	Neutral
Muskellunge	Neutral	Neutral
Mussels	Neutral	Neutral
Opaleye fish	Neutral	Neutral
Orange roughy	Neutral	Neutral
Parrot fish	Neutral	Neutral
Perch (all types)	Neutral	Neutral
Pollack	Neutral	Neutral

Pompano	Neutral	Neutral
Rosefish	Neutral	Neutral
Scallop	Neutral	Neutral
Scrod	Neutral	Neutral
Scup	Neutral	Neutral
Shark	Neutral	Neutral
Smelt	Neutral	Neutral
Squid	Neutral	Neutral
Sucker	Neutral	Neutral
Sunfish	Neutral	Neutral
Swordfish	Neutral	Neutral
Tilapia	Neutral	Neutral
Tilefish	Neutral	Neutral
Weakfish	Neutral	Neutral
Whitefish	Neutral	Neutral

Dairy and Eggs

DAIRY PRODUCTS can be used with discretion by many Type ABs, especially if they are secretors. Eggs, a good source of DHA (as is fish), can complement the protein profile in this blood type, helping to build active tissue mass. Type ABs of African ancestry may need to minimize noncultured forms of dairy, such as milk.

BLOOD TYPE AB: EGGS

Portion: 1 egg

	African	Caucasian	Asian
Secretor	2–5	3–4	3–4
Non-Secretor	3–6	3–6	3–6
	Times per week		

BLOOD TYPE AB: MILK AND YOGURT

Portion: 4–6 oz. (men); 2–5 oz. (women and children)

	African	Caucasian	Asian
Secretor	2–6	3–6	1–6
Non-Secretor	0–3	0–4	0–3
	Times per week		

BLOOD TYPE AB: CHEESE			
Portion: 3 oz. (men); 2 oz. (women and children)			
	African	**Caucasian**	**Asian**
Secretor	2–3	3–4	3–4
Non-Secretor	0	0–1	0
A_2B	Increase eggs by 2 weekly. Decrease milk, cheese, and yogurt by 2 servings weekly		
MM	Decrease milk and yogurt by 2 servings weekly		
	Times per week		

Variants: A_2B—duck eggs are Neutral. Cheddar, Swiss, Jarlsberg, and Gruyère cheeses are Avoid.

Tier One

FOOD	TYPE AB SECRETOR	TYPE AB NON-SECRETOR
Brie	Avoid	Avoid
Duck egg	Avoid	Avoid
Egg white (chicken)	Beneficial	Beneficial
Goat cheese	Beneficial	Neutral
Kefir	Beneficial	Beneficial
Mozzarella cheese	Beneficial	Beneficial
Ricotta cheese	Beneficial	Beneficial
Salmon roe	Avoid	Avoid
Yogurt	Beneficial	Neutral

Tier Two

FOOD	TYPE AB SECRETOR	TYPE AB NON-SECRETOR
American cheese	Avoid	Avoid
Blue cheese	Avoid	Avoid
Butter	Avoid	Avoid
Buttermilk	Avoid	Avoid
Camembert	Avoid	Avoid
Cottage cheese	Beneficial	Beneficial
Farmer cheese	Beneficial	Beneficial
Feta cheese	Beneficial	Beneficial
Half & half	Avoid	Avoid
Ice cream	Avoid	Avoid
Milk (cow-whole)	Avoid	Avoid

Milk (goat)	Beneficial	Beneficial
Parmesan cheese	Avoid	Avoid
Provolone cheese	Avoid	Avoid
Sour cream (low/ non-fat)	Beneficial	Beneficial

Neutral: General Nutritional Supplementation

FOOD	TYPE AB SECRETOR	TYPE AB NON-SECRETOR
Casein	Neutral	Neutral
Cheddar cheese	Neutral	Neutral
Colby cheese	Neutral	Neutral
Cream cheese	Neutral	Neutral
Edam cheese	Neutral	Neutral
Egg yolk (chicken)	Neutral	Beneficial
Emmenthal cheese	Neutral	Avoid
Ghee (clarified butter)	Neutral	Beneficial
Goose egg	Neutral	Neutral
Gouda	Neutral	Neutral
Gruyère	Neutral	Neutral
Jarlsberg cheese	Neutral	Neutral
Milk (cow-skim or 2%)	Neutral	Neutral
Monterey Jack cheese	Neutral	Neutral
Muenster cheese	Neutral	Neutral
Neufchatel cheese	Neutral	Neutral
Paneer	Neutral	Neutral
Quail egg	Neutral	Neutral
Quark cheese	Neutral	Neutral
String cheese	Neutral	Neutral
Swiss cheese	Neutral	Avoid
Whey	Neutral	Neutral

Beans and Legumes

TYPE ABs CAN DO WELL on proteins found in many beans and legumes, although this food category does contain more than a few beans with problematic A- or B-specific lectins. In general, this category is only marginally sufficient to build active tissue mass in Type ABs, particularly non-secretors.

BLOOD TYPE AB: BEANS AND LEGUMES			
Portion: 1 cup dry			
	African	**Caucasian**	**Asian**
Secretor	3–6	3–6	4–6
Non-Secretor	2–5	2–5	3–6
MM	Increase by 3 servings weekly		
	Times per week		

Variants: MM—broad beans, tamarind, tofu, and all soy products are Beneficial.

Tier One

FOOD	TYPE AB SECRETOR	TYPE AB NON-SECRETOR
Adzuki beans	Avoid	Avoid
Black bean	Avoid	Avoid
Black-eyed pea	Avoid	Avoid
Fava bean	Avoid	Neutral
Garbanzo bean	Avoid	Avoid
Kidney bean	Avoid	Avoid
Lentil (green)	Beneficial	Beneficial
Lima bean	Avoid	Avoid
Mung bean (sprouts)	Avoid	Avoid
Pinto bean	Beneficial	Beneficial
Soy, miso	Beneficial	Neutral
Soy, tempeh	Beneficial	Neutral

Tier Two

FOOD	TYPE AB SECRETOR	TYPE AB NON-SECRETOR
Navy bean	Beneficial	Neutral
Soy bean	Beneficial	Neutral
Soy, tofu	Beneficial	Neutral

Neutral: General Nutritional Supplementation

FOOD	TYPE AB SECRETOR	TYPE AB NON-SECRETOR
Broad bean	Neutral	Neutral
Cannellini bean	Neutral	Neutral
Copper bean	Neutral	Neutral
Green bean	Neutral	Neutral
Jicama	Neutral	Avoid
Lentil (domestic)	Neutral	Neutral
Lentil (red)	Neutral	Neutral
Northern bean	Neutral	Neutral
Snap bean	Neutral	Neutral
Soy cheese	Neutral	Avoid
Soy flakes	Neutral	Neutral
Soy granules	Neutral	Neutral
Soy milk	Neutral	Avoid
Tamarind bean	Neutral	Neutral
White bean	Neutral	Neutral

Nuts and Seeds

NUTS AND SEEDS are a good secondary protein source for Type AB. Several nuts, such as walnuts, can help lower polyamine concentrations by inhibiting the enzyme ornithine decarboxylase. Flaxseeds are particularly rich in lignins, which can help lower the number of receptors for Epidermal Growth Factor, a necessary component of many common cancers, which can be stimulated by the A antigen.

BLOOD TYPE AB: NUTS AND SEEDS			
Portion: Seeds (handful) Nut Butters (1–2 tbsp)			
	African	**Caucasian**	**Asian**
Secretor	5–10	5–10	5–9
Non-Secretor	4–8	4–9	5–9
MM	Increase by 2 servings weekly		
	Times per week		

Variants: MM—almonds are Beneficial.

Tier One

FOOD	TYPE AB SECRETOR	TYPE AB NON-SECRETOR
Filbert (hazelnut)	Avoid	Avoid
Peanut	Beneficial	Neutral
Peanut butter	Beneficial	Neutral
Poppy seed	Avoid	Avoid
Pumpkin seed	Avoid	Avoid
Sesame butter/tahini	Avoid	Avoid
Sesame seed	Avoid	Avoid
Sunflower butter	Avoid	Avoid
Sunflower seed	Avoid	Avoid
Walnut (black)	Beneficial	Beneficial
Walnut (English)	Beneficial	Beneficial

Tier Two

FOOD	TYPE AB SECRETOR	TYPE AB NON-SECRETOR
Chestnut	Beneficial	Beneficial

Neutral: General Nutritional Supplementation

FOOD	TYPE AB SECRETOR	TYPE AB NON-SECRETOR
Almond	Neutral	Neutral
Almond butter	Neutral	Neutral
Almond cheese	Neutral	Neutral
Almond milk	Neutral	Neutral
Beechnut	Neutral	Neutral
Brazil nut	Neutral	Avoid
Butternut	Neutral	Neutral
Cashew/cashew butter	Neutral	Avoid
Flaxseed	Neutral	Neutral
Hickory	Neutral	Neutral
Litchi	Neutral	Neutral
Macadamia	Neutral	Neutral
Pecan/pecan butter	Neutral	Neutral
Pine nut (pignola)	Neutral	Neutral

Pistachio	Neutral	Avoid
Safflower seed	Neutral	Neutral

Grains and Starches

IN CONTRAST TO animal proteins, where Type AB non-secretors have a bit of an edge because of their insulin sensitivities, Type AB non-secretors should be careful of their consumption of complex carbohydrates, a concern not generally applicable to Type AB secretors. This leaves Type AB secretors many possible choices of grains. In particular, Type AB non-secretors should watch their consumption of wheat and corn products, as these foods contain lectins capable of exerting an insulinlike effect on their bodies, lowering active tissue mass and increasing total body fat. Amaranth, an ancient grain, should be included in the basic Type AB diet; it contains a lectin that may be beneficial in preventing colon cancer.

BLOOD TYPE AB: GRAINS AND STARCHES			
Portion: 1/2 cup dry (grains or pastas); 1 muffin, 2 slices of bread			
	African	**Caucasian**	**Asian**
Secretor	6–8	6–9	6–10
Non-Secretor	5–7	4–6	6–8
A_2B	Decrease by 1 serving weekly		
	Times per week		

Variants: A_2B—wheat products are Avoid. MM—quinoa is Beneficial.

Tier One

FOOD	TYPE AB SECRETOR	TYPE AB NON-SECRETOR
Amaranth	Beneficial	Beneficial
Artichoke pasta (pure)	Avoid	Avoid
Buckwheat/kasha	Avoid	Avoid
Corn (white/yellow/ blue)	Avoid	Avoid
Cornmeal	Avoid	Avoid
Essene bread (manna bread)	Beneficial	Beneficial
Ezekiel bread (commercial)	Beneficial	Neutral

Millet	Beneficial	Beneficial
Oat flour	Beneficial	Beneficial
Oat/oat bran/ oatmeal	Beneficial	Beneficial
Popcorn	Avoid	Avoid
Rice (puffed)/rice bran	Beneficial	Beneficial
Rice (white/brown/ basmati)/bread	Beneficial	Beneficial
Rice (wild)	Beneficial	Beneficial
Rice cake/flour	Beneficial	Beneficial
Rice milk	Beneficial	Beneficial
Soba noodles (100% buckwheat)	Avoid	Avoid
Sorghum	Avoid	Avoid
Tapioca	Avoid	Avoid
Teff	Avoid	Avoid

Tier Two

FOOD	TYPE AB SECRETOR	TYPE AB NON-SECRETOR
Kamut	Avoid	Avoid
Rye flour	Beneficial	Beneficial
Rye/100% rye bread	Beneficial	Beneficial
Soy flour bread	Beneficial	Avoid
Spelt	Beneficial	Neutral
Wheat (refined unbleached)	Avoid	Avoid
Wheat bread (sprouted commercial— not Ezekiel)	Beneficial	Beneficial

Neutral: General Nutritional Supplementation

FOOD	TYPE AB SECRETOR	TYPE AB NON-SECRETOR
Barley	Neutral	Neutral
Couscous (cracked wheat)	Neutral	Neutral
Gluten flour	Neutral	Neutral

Gluten-free bread	Neutral	Neutral
Quinoa	Neutral	Neutral
Rice (cream of)	Neutral	Neutral
Spelt flour/products	Neutral	Neutral
Wheat (bran)	Neutral	Neutral
Wheat (germ)	Neutral	Avoid
Wheat (gluten flour products)	Neutral	Avoid
Wheat (semolina flour products)	Neutral	Avoid
Wheat (white flour products)	Neutral	Avoid
Wheat (whole wheat products)	Neutral	Avoid

Vegetables

VEGETABLES PROVIDE a rich source of antioxidants and fiber, in addition to helping to lower the production of polyamines in the digestive tract. Onions are also a powerful friend to Type ABs: They contain significant amounts of the antioxidant quercetin, a very powerful antimutagen. If you have been typed as an AB secretor with the MM subtype, make the regular consumption of tier one beneficials part of your anticancer prevention program. Although not technically a vegetable, the common domestic mushroom contains cancer-fighting lectins. Artichoke is quite beneficial to the liver and gallbladder, weak spots for Type ABs. Parsnips contain polysaccharides, which are a great stimulant to the immune system.

BLOOD TYPE AB: VEGETABLES			
Portion: 1 cup cooked or raw			
	African	**Caucasian**	**Asian**
Secretor	Unlimited	Unlimited	Unlimited
Non-Secretor	Unlimited	Unlimited	Unlimited
MM	Try to use mostly Tier One Beneficials		
	Times per week		

Variants: A_2B—red pepper is Neutral. MM—onions, bok choy, chickory, and tomatoes are Beneficial.

Tier One

FOOD	TYPE AB SECRETOR	TYPE AB NON-SECRETOR
Acacia (Arabic gum)	Avoid	Avoid
Aloe/aloe tea/aloe juice	Avoid	Avoid
Artichoke (domestic/globe/ Jerusalem)	Avoid	Avoid
Beet	Beneficial	Neutral
Beet greens	Beneficial	Beneficial
Broccoli	Beneficial	Beneficial
Cauliflower	Beneficial	Beneficial
Collard greens	Beneficial	Beneficial
Cucumber	Beneficial	Beneficial
Dandelion	Beneficial	Beneficial
Garlic	Beneficial	Beneficial
Kale	Beneficial	Beneficial
Mushroom (maitake)	Beneficial	Beneficial
Olive (black)	Avoid	Avoid
Pepper (green/ yellow/ jalapeno)	Avoid	Avoid
Potato (sweet)	Beneficial	Beneficial
Radish	Avoid	Avoid
Radish sprouts	Avoid	Avoid
Rhubarb	Avoid	Avoid

Tier Two

FOOD	TYPE AB SECRETOR	TYPE AB NON-SECRETOR
Alfalfa sprouts	Beneficial	Beneficial
Cabbage juice	Beneficial	Beneficial
Caper	Avoid	Avoid
Carrot juice	Beneficial	Beneficial
Celery/celery juice	Beneficial	Beneficial
Chili pepper	Avoid	Avoid
Eggplant	Beneficial	Beneficial
Mushroom (abalone)	Avoid	Avoid

Mushroom (shiitake)	Avoid	Avoid
Mustard greens	Beneficial	Beneficial
Parsnip	Beneficial	Beneficial
Pepper (red/cayenne)	Avoid	Avoid
Pickle (in brine)	Avoid	Avoid
Pickle (in vinegar)	Avoid	Avoid
Yam	Beneficial	Beneficial

Neutral: General Nutritional Supplementation

FOOD	TYPE AB SECRETOR	TYPE AB NON-SECRETOR
Agar	Neutral	Avoid
Arugula	Neutral	Neutral
Asparagus	Neutral	Neutral
Bamboo shoot	Neutral	Neutral
Bok choy	Neutral	Neutral
Brussel sprout	Neutral	Neutral
Cabbage (Chinese/ red/white)	Neutral	Neutral
Carrot	Neutral	Neutral
Celeriac	Neutral	Neutral
Chervil	Neutral	Neutral
Chicory	Neutral	Neutral
Cilantro	Neutral	Neutral
Cucumber juice	Neutral	Neutral
Daikon radish	Neutral	Neutral
Endive	Neutral	Neutral
Escarole	Neutral	Neutral
Fennel	Neutral	Neutral
Fiddlehead fern	Neutral	Neutral
Ginger	Neutral	Beneficial
Horseradish	Neutral	Neutral
Juniper	Neutral	Avoid
Kelp	Neutral	Neutral
Kohlrabi	Neutral	Neutral
Leek	Neutral	Neutral
Lettuce (bibb/ Boston/iceberg/ mesclun)	Neutral	Neutral

Lettuce (romaine)	Neutral	Neutral
Mushroom (silver-dollar)	Neutral	Neutral
Mushroom (enoki)	Neutral	Neutral
Mushroom (straw)	Neutral	Neutral
Okra	Neutral	Neutral
Olive (Greek/Spanish)	Neutral	Neutral
Olive (green)	Neutral	Neutral
Onion (all kinds)	Neutral	Neutral
Pea (green/pod/ snow)	Neutral	Neutral
Pimento	Neutral	Neutral
Poi	Neutral	Avoid
Potato (white/red/ blue/yellow)	Neutral	Neutral
Pumpkin	Neutral	Neutral
Radicchio	Neutral	Neutral
Rappini	Neutral	Neutral
Rutabaga	Neutral	Neutral
Sauerkraut	Neutral	Neutral
Scallion	Neutral	Neutral
Seaweed	Neutral	Neutral
Senna	Neutral	Neutral
Shallots	Neutral	Neutral
Spinach/spinach juice	Neutral	Neutral
Squash (summer/ winter)	Neutral	Neutral
String bean	Neutral	Neutral
Swiss chard	Neutral	Neutral
Taro	Neutral	Avoid
Tomato/tomato juice	Neutral	Beneficial
Turnip	Neutral	Neutral
Water chestnut	Neutral	Neutral
Watercress	Neutral	Neutral
Yucca	Neutral	Neutral
Zucchini	Neutral	Neutral

Fruits and Fruit Juices

FRUITS ARE RICH in antioxidants, and many, such as blueberries, elderberries, cherries, and blackberries contain pigments that block the liver enzyme ornithine decarboxylase. This has the effect of lowering the production of polyamines, chemicals that act with insulin to encourage weight gain and act to enhance the potential for cells to mutate. If you are a Type AB secretor, make the regular consumption of Tier One beneficials part of your anticancer prevention program.

A diet rich in proper fruits and vegetables can help weight loss by tempering the effects of insulin while also helping to shift the balance of water in the body from high extracellular concentrations (bad) to high intracellular concentrations (good). Many fruits, such as pineapple, are rich in enzymes that can help reduce inflammation and encourage proper water balance. If you are a non-secretor, you'll need to watch your intake of high glucose-containing fruits, especially if you are sensitive to sugar.

BLOOD TYPE AB: FRUITS			
Portion: 1 cup or 1 piece			
	African	**Caucasian**	**Asian**
Secretor	3–4	3–6	3–5
Non-Secretor	1–3	2–3	3–4
A₂B	Decrease by 1 serving daily		
MM	Try to use mostly Tier One Beneficials		
			Times per week

Variants: A₂B—honeydew melon and tangerines are Avoid. Coconut is Neutral. MM—currants, blueberries, and elderberries are Beneficial.

Tier One

FOOD	TYPE AB SECRETOR	TYPE AB NON-SECRETOR
Avocado	Avoid	Avoid
Banana	Avoid	Avoid
Bitter melon	Avoid	Avoid
Cherry (all)	Beneficial	Beneficial
Cherry juice (black)	Beneficial	Beneficial

Dewberry	Avoid	Avoid
Fig (fresh/dried)	Beneficial	Beneficial
Grape (all types)	Beneficial	Beneficial
Grapefruit	Beneficial	Beneficial
Guava/guava juice	Avoid	Avoid
Kiwi	Beneficial	Beneficial
Loganberry	Beneficial	Beneficial
Persimmon	Avoid	Avoid
Pineapple	Beneficial	Beneficial
Plum (dark/green/ red)	Beneficial	Beneficial
Pomegranate	Avoid	Avoid
Prickly pear	Avoid	Avoid
Quince	Avoid	Avoid
Sago palm	Avoid	Avoid
Watermelon	Beneficial	Beneficial

Tier Two

FOOD	TYPE AB SECRETOR	TYPE AB NON-SECRETOR
Coconut	Avoid	Avoid
Cranberry/cranberry juice	Beneficial	Beneficial
Gooseberry	Beneficial	Beneficial
Lemon/lemon juice	Beneficial	Beneficial
Mango/mango juice	Avoid	Avoid
Orange/orange juice	Avoid	Avoid
Starfruit (carambola)	Avoid	Avoid

Neutral: General Nutritional Supplementation

FOOD	TYPE AB SECRETOR	TYPE AB NON-SECRETOR
Apple	Neutral	Neutral
Apple cider/apple juice	Neutral	Neutral
Apricot/apricot juice	Neutral	Neutral

Asian pear	Neutral	Neutral
Blackberry/black- berry juice	Beneficial	Neutral
Blueberry	Neutral	Beneficial
Boysenberry	Neutral	Neutral
Breadfruit	Neutral	Neutral
Canang melon	Neutral	Neutral
Cantaloupe	Neutral	Avoid
Casaba melon	Neutral	Neutral
Christmas melon	Neutral	Neutral
Crenshaw melon	Neutral	Neutral
Currants (black/red)	Neutral	Neutral
Date (all types)	Neutral	Neutral
Elderberry (dark blue/purple)	Neutral	Beneficial
Grapefruit juice	Neutral	Neutral
Honeydew	Neutral	Avoid
Kumquat	Neutral	Neutral
Lime/lime juice	Neutral	Beneficial
Mulberry	Neutral	Neutral
Musk melon	Neutral	Neutral
Nectarine/nectarine juice	Neutral	Neutral
Papaya	Neutral	Neutral
Peach	Neutral	Neutral
Pear/pear juice	Neutral	Neutral
Pineapple juice	Neutral	Neutral
Plantain	Neutral	Neutral
Prune/prune juice	Neutral	Avoid
Raisin	Neutral	Neutral
Raspberry	Neutral	Neutral
Spanish melon	Neutral	Neutral
Strawberry	Neutral	Neutral
Tangerine/tangerine juice	Neutral	Avoid
Water & lemon	Neutral	Neutral
Youngberry	Neutral	Neutral

Oils

TYPE ABs WILL WANT to ensure that their oils are fresh and free of rancidity. In general, Type ABs do best on monounsaturated oils (such as olive oil) and oils rich in omega series fatty acids (such as flax oil). Type AB secretors have a bit of an edge in breaking down oils over non-secretors, and probably benefit more from their consumption, as they enhance the absorption of calcium via the small intestine.

BLOOD TYPE AB: OILS			
Portion: 1 tbsp			
	African	**Caucasian**	**Asian**
Secretor	4–7	5–8	5–7
Non-Secretor	3–6	3–6	3–4
A_2B	Increase by 2 servings weekly		
	Times per week		

Variants: Rh– —borage oil is Avoid. A_2B—coconut oil is Neutral.

Tier One

FOOD	TYPE AB SECRETOR	TYPE AB NON-SECRETOR
Corn oil	Avoid	Avoid
Cottonseed oil	Avoid	Avoid
Olive oil	Beneficial	Beneficial
Sesame oil	Avoid	Avoid
Sunflower oil	Avoid	Avoid
Walnut oil	Beneficial	Beneficial

Tier Two

FOOD	TYPE AB SECRETOR	TYPE AB NON-SECRETOR
Coconut oil	Avoid	Avoid
Safflower oil	Avoid	Avoid

Neutral: General Nutritional Supplementation

FOOD	TYPE AB SECRETOR	TYPE AB NON-SECRETOR
Almond oil	Neutral	Neutral
Black currant seed oil	Neutral	Neutral
Borage seed oil	Neutral	Neutral
Canola oil	Neutral	Neutral
Castor oil	Neutral	Neutral
Cod liver oil	Neutral	Neutral
Evening primrose oil	Neutral	Neutral
Flaxseed (linseed) oil	Neutral	Neutral
Peanut oil	Neutral	Neutral
Soy oil	Neutral	Neutral
Wheat germ oil	Neutral	Neutral

Herbs, Spices, and Condiments

MANY SPICES HAVE mild to moderate medicinal properties, often by influencing the levels of bacteria in the lower colon. Many common gums, such as Guar gum, should be avoided as they can enhance the effects of lectins found in other foods. Molasses is a beneficial sweetener for Type ABs: it can provide some additional dietary iron. Turmeric (a spice in curry powder) contains a powerful phytochemical called curcumin, which helps lower levels of intestinal toxins. Brewer's yeast is a beneficial food for Type AB non-secretors; it enhances glucose metabolism and helps insure a healthy flora balance in the intestinal tract.

Variants: A_2B— stevia and brewer's yeast are Avoid. Red pepper is Neutral. MM— turmeric is Beneficial.

Tier One

FOOD	TYPE AB SECRETOR	TYPE AB NON-SECRETOR
Almond extract	Avoid	Avoid
Anise	Avoid	Avoid
Aspartame	Avoid	Avoid

Barley malt	Avoid	Avoid
Carrageenan	Avoid	Avoid
Corn syrup	Avoid	Avoid
Cornstarch	Avoid	Avoid
Curry	Beneficial	Beneficial
Dextrose	Avoid	Avoid
Fructose	Avoid	Avoid
Gelatin plain	Avoid	Avoid
Guar gum	Avoid	Avoid
Guarana	Avoid	Avoid
Ketchup	Avoid	Avoid
Maltodextrin	Avoid	Avoid
Parsley	Beneficial	Beneficial
Pepper (black/white)	Avoid	Avoid
Pepper (peppercorn/ red flakes)	Avoid	Avoid
Pickle relish	Avoid	Avoid
Sucanat	Avoid	Avoid
Vinegar (balsamic/ cider/red wine/ white/rice)	Avoid	Avoid
Worcestershire sauce	Avoid	Avoid

Tier Two

FOOD	TYPE AB SECRETOR	TYPE AB NON-SECRETOR
Allspice	Avoid	Avoid
MSG	Avoid	Avoid

Neutral: General Nutritional Supplementation

FOOD	TYPE AB SECRETOR	TYPE AB NON-SECRETOR
Apple pectin	Neutral	Neutral
Arrowroot	Neutral	Neutral
Basil	Neutral	Neutral
Bay leaf	Neutral	Beneficial
Bergamot	Neutral	Neutral
Caraway	Neutral	Neutral

Cardamom	Neutral	Neutral
Carob	Neutral	Neutral
Chili powder	Neutral	Neutral
Chives	Neutral	Neutral
Chocolate	Neutral	Neutral
Cinnamon	Neutral	Neutral
Clove	Neutral	Neutral
Coriander	Neutral	Neutral
Cream of tartar	Neutral	Neutral
Cumin	Neutral	Neutral
Dill	Neutral	Neutral
Dulse	Neutral	Neutral
Honey	Neutral	Avoid
Licorice root	Neutral	Neutral
Mace	Neutral	Neutral
Maple syrup	Neutral	Avoid
Marjoram	Neutral	Neutral
Mayonnaise	Neutral	Neutral
Molasses	Neutral	Neutral
Mustard (prepared, vinegar free)	Neutral	Neutral
Mustard (dry)	Neutral	Neutral
Nutmeg	Neutral	Neutral
Paprika	Neutral	Neutral
Peppermint	Neutral	Neutral
Rice syrup	Neutral	Avoid
Rosemary	Neutral	Neutral
Saffron	Neutral	Neutral
Sage	Neutral	Neutral
Savory	Neutral	Neutral
Sea salt	Neutral	Neutral
Soy sauce	Neutral	Neutral
Spearmint	Neutral	Neutral
Stevia	Neutral	Neutral
Sugar (brown/white)	Neutral	Avoid
Tamari, wheat free	Neutral	Neutral
Tamarind	Neutral	Neutral
Tarragon	Neutral	Neutral
Thyme	Neutral	Neutral
Turmeric	Neutral	Beneficial

Vanilla	Neutral	Neutral
Wintergreen	Neutral	Neutral
Yeast (brewer's)	Neutral	Neutral

Beverages

TYPE AB NON-SECRETORS may wish to have a glass of wine occasionally with their meals; they derive substantial benefit to their cardiovascular system from moderate use. Green tea should be part of every Type AB's health plan; it contains polyphenols that block the production of harmful polyamines.

Tier One

FOOD	TYPE AB SECRETOR	TYPE AB NON-SECRETOR
Tea (green)	Beneficial	Beneficial

Tier Two

FOOD	TYPE AB SECRETOR	TYPE AB NON-SECRETOR
Coffee (regular/ decaf)	Avoid	Avoid
Liquor (distilled)	Avoid	Neutral
Soda (misc./diet/ cola)	Avoid	Avoid
Tea (black regular/ decaf)	Avoid	Avoid

Neutral: General Nutritional Supplementation

FOOD	TYPE AB SECRETOR	TYPE AB NON-SECRETOR
Beer	Neutral	Avoid
Seltzer water	Neutral	Neutral
Soda (club)	Neutral	Neutral
Wine (red)	Neutral	Beneficial
Wine (white)	Neutral	Neutral

Individualized Therapies
for Chronic Conditions

As you can see by referring to your Risk Profile, Type AB is more susceptible to certain chronic conditions and diseases than the other blood types. However, the picture is more complex for Type AB, since you contain both the A and B antigens—comparable to natural enemies sharing the gatekeeper function. This heightens your vulnerability to immune conditions, making it especially important for you to adhere to the Type AB Diet.

See Type AB Health Risk Profile, page 288.

In my experience, Type AB is more A-like than B-like when it comes to most chronic conditions. That is most likely because the A antigen is so vulnerable to attacks on all fronts—be they digestive, cardiovascular, or immune. Type AB appears to have little of Type B's propensity for slow-growing bacterial or viral infections. On the other hand, the Type AB cancer risk is sometimes more severe than that of Type A.

To learn more about staying healthy and well balanced, log on to the blood type Web site: www.dadamo.com.

Overall, Type ABs can do well by following the diet and prescriptions in this chapter—and by observing the therapeutic guidelines outlined for Type A. (See page 119 for Individualized Therapies for Chronic Conditions.)

However, there is one area that Type ABs need to pay special attention to, in the area of immunity. It has been shown that Type AB is particularly susceptible to diminished Natural Killer (NK) cell activity. The following guidelines deliver a special protection for Type ABs.

Many dietary factors have been linked to NK cell activity. Failure to eat breakfast, irregular eating habits, low vegetable intake, inadequate protein, excessive wheat intake, high fat diets (especially those with excessive amounts of polyunsaturated fatty acids) have all been associated with poor NK cell activity.

- As a general rule, exposure to toxic chemicals and heavy metals will decrease NK cell activity. After weeks or months, it will rebound to normal in some individuals, but others suppress the effects for much longer. It's important to minimize your exposure.
- Deficiencies in a range of nutrients can result in decreased NK

cell activity. In particular, selenium, zinc, vitamin C, CoQ10, beta-carotene, vitamin A, vitamin E, and vitamin D deficiencies should be addressed.

- Tamoxifen appears to have an indirect but positive influence on NK cell activity. In studies of women with postmenopausal stage I breast cancer who took tamoxifen for one month, there was a statistically significant increase in NK activity.
- The periodic use of L-arginine for three days to a week (from 3 up to 30 grams per day) can be helpful. Use of this type of high-dose L-arginine supplementation is particularly recommended for women about to undergo a dose of chemotherapy. Several studies have shown this to be a reasonably effective strategy for maintaining white blood cell count through chemotherapy.
- To boost NK cell activity, I routinely use larch arabinogalactan; however, many polysaccharides have some NK cell–modifying activity. Many of the common immune-boosting herbs can also be supportive—including ginseng, astragalus, licorice, and echinacea. Most of the water-soluble extracts of medicinal mushrooms, such as cordyceps, reishi, maitake, and coriolis have been shown to positively influence NK cell function.

A final word on herbs. They work best to boost your NK cell function before it has bottomed out. Once you are chronically ill, a small dose is unlikely to produce a dramatic result. Use herbs proactively to help you tolerate stress and keep your immune system in good health.

For Best Effects in Using Herbs and Medicinal Mushrooms

- The longer you take them the better.
- They are dose-dependent, so higher doses equal greater results. The Chinese always use several grams (at least 3 and often as much as 15 grams twice per day), and most experts believe a minimum of 1½ to 3 grams of the polysaccharide components are needed to get a high enough rate of absorption to have any benefit.
- The water-soluble compounds (not alcohol extracts) have the NK–stimulating activity. I can't tell you how many people I have met who are taking alcohol extracts of herbs such as astragalus and ginseng, when this type of extract was not used in Chinese traditional medicine and probably has little to no immune-boosting usefulness.

JEFFREY BLAND, PH.D

FOUNDER, INSTITUTE FOR FUNCTIONAL MEDICINE

AUTHOR, *Genetic Nutritioneering*

EFORE THE PUBLICATION OF DR. PETER D'ADAMO'S book, *Eat Right 4 Your Type* in 1996, very few people had heard the concept that our blood type or secretor status could influence how our bodies respond to certain foods and environmental exposures. However, to those in the field of genetic metabolism disorders, it was not entirely new. In fact the medical literature goes back more than sixty years indicating how our ABO blood groups are under the control of our genes; they can influence our risks for many diseases including heart disease, certain forms of cancer, and allergic disorders.

In *Live Right 4 Your Type*, the research is taken to the next level of understanding and application. Since 1996 much has been learned by Dr. D'Adamo and other clinicians and researchers, including breakthrough information from the Human Genome Project. An important aspect of these investigations relates to the way that our genetic inheritance—in particular our ABO blood group—relates to factors that can influence our personality and mood, as well as our overall health. It is truly fascinating that medicine is moving from a period of the past one hundred years when disease was considered to be "hard wired" into our genes, to a time when we realize that we can play a role in strengthening our genetic inheritance through our daily living.

One might ask why the blood type science, as outlined in Dr. D'Adamo's work, is not generally agreed upon by all medical professionals. The answer is related in part to the types of training and insight that are involved in recognizing the associations among blood type, secretor status, diet, lifestyle, and health. Dr. D'Adamo is a second generation naturopathic physician whose mind was prepared for the chance of observation through his upbringing and education. He is also a scholar who has always asked difficult questions and has not been satisfied until he found evidence in the medical literature to support his premises. And lastly, he is a clinician who in working with chronically ill patients has seen what works and what doesn't. This represents a collection of experiences that most doctors do not have.

Dr. D'Adamo has done a masterful job in this book in describing how our genetic inheritance related to our ABO blood group relates to particular factors that can influence our personality and mood as well as our overall health.

Live Right 4 Your Type is a very practical application guide that demonstrates how we can modify the way our genes express their messages. By selecting the right diet and lifestyle for our genotype—related in part to our blood type—we can turn off the expression of certain genetic messages that trigger ill-health and turn on the expression of messages that foster good health. This is a powerful message that can enable us to both add life to our years and years to our life.

Appendices

Notes

There is abundant documentation supporting the central role that blood type plays in every bodily system. The primary scientific background was footnoted in the text and is referenced in the following pages. In addition, I have included some general references that you may find helpful. Researchers interested in accessing the full reference list of over 1,500 studies can log on to my Web site at *www.dadamo.com*.

CHAPTER ONE: THE UNMISTAKABLE YOU: THE BLOOD TYPE GENE

1. The Human Genome Project. Research archives; Washington DC: http://www.ornl.gov
2. Skolnick, M. H., E. A. Thompson, D. T. Bishop, and L. A. Cannon. "Possible linkage of a breast cancer–susceptibility locus to the ABO locus: sensitivity of LOD scores to a single new recombinant observation." *Genet Epidemiol,* 1984; 1(4): pp. 363–73.
3. Craig, S. P., V. J. Buckle, A. Lamouroux, et al. "Localization of the human dopamine beta hydroxylase (DBH) gene to chromosome 9q34." *Cytogenet Cell Genet,* 1988; 48(1): pp. 48–50.

Goldin, L. R., E. S. Gershon, C. R. Lake, et al. "Segregation and linkage studies of plasma dopamine beta hydroxylase (DBH), erythrocyte catechol-O-methyltransferase (COMT), and platelet monoamine oxidase (MAO): possible linkage between the ABO locus and a gene controlling DBH activity." *Am J Hum Genet,* March 1982; 34(2): pp. 250–62.

Sherrington, R., D. Curtis, J. Brynjolfsson, et al. "A linkage study of affective disorder with DNA markers for the ABO-AK1-ORM linkage group near the dopamine beta hydroxylase gene." *Biol Psychiatry,* October 1, 1994; 36(7): pp. 434–42.

Wilson, A. F., R. C. Elston, R. M. Siervogel, and L. D. Tran. "Linkage of a gene regulating dopamine beta hydroxylase activity and the ABO blood group locus." *Am J Hum Genet,* January 1988; 42(1): pp. 160–66.

4. Mohn, J. F., N. A. Owens, and R. W. Plunkett. "The inhibitory properties of group A and B non-secretor saliva." *Immunol Commun,* 1981;10(2): pp. 101–26.

Kapadia, A., T. Feizi, D. Jewell, et al. "Immunocytochemical studies of blood group A, H, I, and i antigens in gastric mucosae of infants with normal gastric histology and of patients with gastric carcinoma and chronic benign peptic ulceration." *J Clin Pathol,* March 1981; 34(3): pp. 320–37.

5. Cruz-Coke, R. "Genetics and alcoholism." *Neurobehav Toxicol Teratol,* March–April 1983; 5(2): pp. 179–80.

Kojic, T., A. Dojcinova, D. Dojcinova, et al. "Possible genetic predisposition for alcohol addiction." *Adv Exp Med Biol,* 1977; 85A: pp. 7–24.

6. Wahlberg T. B., M. Blomback, and D. Magnusson. "Influence of sex, blood group, secretor character, smoking habits, acetylsalicylic acid, oral contraceptives, fasting and general health state on blood coagulation variables in randomly selected young adults." *Haemostasis,* 1984; 14(4): pp. 312–19 and vWf.

Orstavik, K. H. "Genetics of plasma concentration of von Willebrand factor." *Folia Haematol Int Mag Klin Morphol Blutforsch,* 1990; 117 (4): pp. 527–31.

Orstavik, K. H., L. Kornstad, H. Reisner, and K. Berg. "Possible effect of secretor locus on plasma concentration of factor VIII and von Willebrand factor." *Blood,* March 1989; 73 (4): pp. 990–3.

Green, D., O. Jarrett, K. J. Ruth, A. R. Folsom, and K. Lui. "Relationship among Lewis phenotype, clotting factors, and other cardiovascular risk factors in young adults." *J Lab Clin Med*, March 1995; 125 (3): pp. 334–339.

CHAPTER TWO: IN SEARCH OF IDENTITY: IS THERE A BLOOD TYPE PERSONALITY?

1. Neumann, J. K. et al. "Effects of stress and blood type on cortisol and VLDL toxicity preventing activity." *Psychosom Med*, September–October 1992; 54(5): pp. 612–19.
2. Sato, T. Blood-typing: As a lay personality theory. *Japanese Journal of Social Psychology*, 1993; 8; pp. 197–208 (In Japanese).

   Sato, T. and Y. Watanabe. "Psychological Studies on Blood-typing in Japan." *Japanese Psychological Review*, 1993; 35; pp. 234–268 (In Japanese).
3. Sato, T. and Y. Watanabe. "The Furukawa theory of blood-type and temperament: The origins of a temperament theory during the 1920s." *The Japanese Journal of Personality*, 1995; 3; pp. 51–65 (In Japanese).

   Takuma, T. and Y. Matsui. "Ketsueki gata sureroetaipu ni tsuite [About blood type stereotype]," *Jinbungakuho* (Tokyo Metropolitan University), 1985; 44: pp. 15–30.
4. Nomi, T. and A. Besher. *You Are Your Blood Type*. New York: St. Martin's Press, 1983.
5. Constantine, P. *What's Your Type?* New York: Plume Books, 1997.
6. Cattell, R. B. "The relation of blood types to primary and secondary personality traits." *The Mankind Quarterly* 1980; 21: pp. 35–51.

   Cattell, R. B., H. B. Young, and J. D. Houndelby. "Blood groups and personality traits." *American Journal of Human Genetics*, 1964; 16–4: pp. 397–402.
7. Eysenk, H. J. "National differences in personality as related to ABO blood group polymorphism." *Psychological Reports*, 1977; 41: pp 1257–58.
8. Eysenk, H. J., "The biological basis of cross-cultural differences in personality: Blood group antigens." *Psychological Reports*, 1982. 51: pp. 531–40.
9. Jung, C. G. *Psychological Types*. Princeton, NJ: Princeton University Press, 1971.

10. Myers, I., and P. Myers. *Gifts Differing: Understanding Personality Type*. Consulting Psychologists Press, 1995.

11. Keirsey, D. *Please Understand Me II*. Del Mar CA: Prometheus Nemesis Book Company.

CHAPTER 3: STRESS AND EMOTIONAL STABILITY: BLOOD TYPE AS A MENTAL HEALTH MARKER

1. Rubello, D., N. Sonino, D. Casara, et al. "Acute and chronic effects of high glucocorticoid levels on hypothalamic-pituitary-thyroid axis in man." *J Endocrinol Invest*, June 15, 1992; 15(6): pp. 437–41.

    Pike J. L., T. L. Smith, R. L. Hauger, et al. "Chronic life stress alters sympathetic, neuroendocrine, and immune responsivity to an acute psychological stressor in humans." *Psychosom Med*, Jul–August 1997; 59(4): 447–57.

2. Masugi, F., T. Ogihara, K. Sakaguchi, et al. "High plasma levels of cortisol in patients with senile dementia of the Alzheimer's type." *Find Exp Clin Pharmacol*, November 1989; 11(11): pp. 707–10.

    Leproult R, O. Van Reeth, M. M. Byrne, et al. "Sleepiness, performance, and neuroendocrine function during sleep deprivation: effects of exposure to bright light or exercise." *J Biol Rhythms*, 1997 Jun; 12(3): 245–58

    Opstad, K. "Circadian rhythm of hormones is extinguished during prolonged physical stress, sleep and energy deficiency in young men." *Eur J Endocrinol*, 1994 Jul; 131(1): 56–66.

3. Neumann, J. K., B. W. Arbogast, D. S. Chi, and L. Y. Arbogast. "Effects of stress and blood type on cortisol and VLDL toxicity preventing activity." *Psychosom Med*, September 1992; 54(5): 612–19.

4. Locong, A. H. and A. G. Roberge. "Cortisol and catecholamines response to venisection by humans with different blood groups." *Clin Biochem*, February 1985; 18(1): 67–69.

5. Mao, X. et al. "Study on relationship between human ABO blood groups and type A behavior pattern." *Hua Hsi I Ko Ta Hsueh Hsueh Pao*, March 1991; 22(1): pp. 93–96. [article in Chinese].

    Neumann, J. K. et al. "Relationship between blood groups and behavior patterns in men who have had myocardial infarction." *South Med J.*, February 1991; 84(2): pp. 214–18.

6. Pu, S. et al. "Evidence showing that beta-endorphin regulates cyclic guanosine 3',5'-monophosphate (cGMP) efflux: anatomical and functional support for an interaction between opiates and nitric oxide." *Brain Res*, January 30, 1999; 817(1–2): pp. 220–25.

7. Locong, A. H., A. G. Roberge. "Cortisol and catecholamines response to venisection by humans with different blood groups." *Clin
Biochem*, February 1985; 18(1): pp. 67–69.

8. Bosco, C., J. Tihanyl, L. Rivalta, et al. "Hormonal responses in strenuous jumping effort." *Jpn J Physiol*, February 1996; 46(1): pp. 93–98.

Frey, H. "The endocrine response to physical activity." *Scand J Soc
Med Suppl*, 1982; 29: pp. 71–75.

Gallois, P., G. Forzy, J. L. Dhont. "Hormonal changes during relaxation." *Encephale*, 1984; 10(2): 79–82 [Article in French].

Jin, P. "Efficacy of Tai Chi, brisk walking, meditation, and reading
in reducing mental and emotional stress." *J Psychosom Res*, May
1992; 36(4): pp. 361–70.

Jin, P. "Changes in heart rate, noradrenaline, cortisol and mood during Tai Chi." *J Psychosom Res*, 1989; 33(2): pp. 197–206.

Keller, S. and P. Seraganian. "Physical fitness level and autonomic
reactivity to psychosocial stress." *J Psychosom Res*, 1984; 28: pp. 279–
87.

Lehmann, M., U. Gastmann, K. G. Petersen, et al. "Training-
overtraining: performance, and hormone levels, after a defined increase in training volume versus intensity in experienced middle-
and long-distance runners." *Br J Sports Med*, December 1992; 26(4):
pp. 233–42.

Platania-Solazzo, A., T. M. Field, J. Blank, et al. "Relaxation therapy reduces anxiety in child and adolescent psychiatric patients."
Acta Paedopsychiatr, 1992; 55(2): pp. 115–20.

Schell, F. J., B. Allolio, O. W. Schonecke. "Physiological and psychological effects of hatha-yoga exercise in healthy women." *Int J
Psychosom*, 1994; 41(1–4): pp. 46–52.

Schmidt, T., A. Wijga, A. Von Zur Muhlen, et al. "Changes in cardiovascular risk factors and hormones during a comprehensive resi-
dential three month kriya yoga training and vegetarian nutrition."
Acta Physiol Scand Suppl, 1997; 640: pp. 158–62.

Schurmeyer, T., K. Jung, and E. Nieschlag. "The effect of an 1,100
km run on testicular, adrenal and thyroid hormones." *Int J Androl*,
August 1984; 7(4): pp. 276–82.

Semple, C. G., J. A. Thomson, and G. H. Beastall. "Endocrine responses to marathon running." *Br J Sports Med*, September 1985;
19(3): pp. 148–51.

9. MEDLINE: The online database at Medscape (http://www.medscape.com).

10. Sherrington, R., D. Curtis, J. Brynjolfsson, E. Moloney, L. Rifkin, H. Petursson, and H. Gurling. "A linkage study of affective disorder with DNA markers for the ABO-AK1-ORM linkage group near the dopamine beta hydroxylase gene." *Biol Psychiatry*, October 1994 1; 36(7): pp. 434–42.

Goldin, L. R., et al. "Segregation and linkage studies of plasma dopamine beta hydroxylase (DBH), erythrocyte catechol-O-methyltransferase (COMT), and platelet monoamine oxidase (MAO): Possible linkage between the ABO locus and a gene controlling DBH activity." *Am J Hum Genet*, March 1982; 34(2): pp. 250–62.

Kleber, E., T. Obry, S. Hippeli, W. Schneider, E. F. Elstner. "Biochemical activities of extracts from *Hypericum perforatum* L. 1st Communication: inhibition of dopamine beta hydroxylase." *Arzneimittelforschung*, February 1999; 49(2): pp. 106–9.

Retezeanu, A., et al. "The ABO blood groups in affective and in schizophrenic psychosis." *Neurol Psychiatr (Bucur)*, October–December 1978; 16(4): pp. 271–75.

Rihmer, Z., and M. Arato. "ABO blood groups in manic-depressive patients." *J Affect Disord*, March 1981; 3(1): pp. 1–7.

Rinieris, P. M., C. N. Stefanis, E. P. Lykouras, and E. K. Varsou. "Affective disorders and ABO blood types." *Acta Psychiatr Scand*, September 1979; 60(3): pp. 272–78.

11. Arato, M., G. Bagdy, Z. Rihmer, Z. Kulcsar. "Reduced platelet MAO activity in healthy male students with blood group O." *Acta Psychiatr Scand*, February 1983; 67(2): pp. 130–34.

12. Sozmen, E. S. et al. "Platelet-rich plasma monoamine oxidase activities: A novel marker of criminality for young Turkish Delinquents?" *J. Medical Sciences*. 1996; 26(5): pp. 475–77.

13. Blanco, C., L. Orensanz-Munoz, C. Blanco-Jerez, and J. Saiz-Ruiz. "Pathological gambling and platelet MAO activity: A psychobiological study." *Am J Psychiatry*, January 1996; 153(1): pp. 119–21.

Sofuoglu, S., P. Dogan, K. Kose, E. Esel, M. Basturk, H. Oguz, and A. S. Gonul. "Changes in platelet monoamine oxidase and plasma dopamine beta hydroxylase activities in lithium-treated bipolar patients." *Psychiatry Res*, November 29, 1995; 59(1–2): pp. 165–70.

14. Susman, E. J., K. H. Schmeelk, B. K. Worrall, D. A. Granger, A.

Ponirakis, and G. P. Chrousos. "Corticotropin-releasing hormone and cortisol: Longitudinal associations with depression and antisocial behavior in pregnant adolescents." *J Am Acad Child Adolesc Psychiatry*, April 1999; 38(4): pp. 460–67.

Blood, G. W., I. M. Blood, S. B. Frederick, H. A. Wertz, and K. C. Simpson. "Cortisol responses in adults who stutter: Coping preferences and apprehension about communication." *Percept Mot Skills*, June 1997; 84(3 Pt 1): pp. 883–89.

Prüßner, J. et al. *Increasing Correlations between Personality Traits and Cortisol Stress Responses Obtained by Data Aggregation.* Seattle: Hogrefe & Huber Publishers. 1998.

Ritter, M. "[The Associated Press] Study links hormone, memory loss." *The Seattle Times Company.* Wednesday, April 15, 1998.

Scerbo, A. S. and D. J. Kolko. "Salivary testosterone and cortisol in disruptive children: Relationship to aggressive, hyperactive, and internalizing behaviors." *J Am Acad Child Adolesc Psychiatry*, October 1994; 33(8): pp. 1174–84.

15. Sapse, A. T. "Stress, cortisol, interferon and stress diseases. I. Cortisol as the cause of stress diseases." *Med Hypotheses,* January 1984; 13(1): pp. 31–44.

16. Glaser, R., J. K. Kiecolt-Glaser, W. B. Malarkey, and J. F. Sheridan. "The influence of psychological stress on the immune response to vaccines." *Ann NY Acad Sci*, May 1, 1998; 840: pp. 649–55.

17. Benkelfat, C., I. N. Mefford, C. F. Masters, T. E. Nordahl, A. C. King, R. M. Cohen, and D. L. Murphy. "Plasma catecholamines and their metabolites in obsessive-compulsive disorder." *Psychiatry Res*, June 1991; 37(3): pp. 321–31.

Gehris, T. L., R. G. Kathol, D. W. Black, and R. Noyes Jr. "Urinary free cortisol levels in obsessive-compulsive disorder." *Psychiatry Res*, May 1990; 32(2): pp. 151–58.

Monteleone, P., F. Catapano, A. Tortorella, and M. Maj. "Cortisol response to d-fenfluramine in patients with obsessive compulsive disorder and in healthy subjects: evidence for a gender-related effect." *Neuropsychobiology*, 1997; 36(1): pp. 8–12.

18. Catapano, F., P. Monteleone, A. Fuschino, M. Maj, and D. Kemali. "Melatonin and cortisol secretion in patients with primary obsessive-compulsive disorder." *Psychiatry Res*, December 1992; 44(3): pp. 217–25.

19. Rinieris, P. M., C. N. Stefanis, A. D. Rabavilas, and N. M. Vaidakis. "Obsessive-compulsive neurosis, anancastic symptomatology and ABO blood types." *Acta Psychiatr Scand*, May 1978; 57(5): pp. 377–81.

20. Rinieris, P., C. Stefanis, and A. Rabavilas. "Obsessional personality traits and ABO blood types." *Neuropsychobiology*, 1980; 6(3): pp. 128–31.

21. Boyer, W. F. "Influence of ABO blood type on symptomatology among outpatients: Study and replication." *Neuropsychobiology*, 1986; 16(1): pp. 43–46.

22. Pu, S., et al. "Evidence showing that beta-endorphin regulates cyclic guanosine 3',5'-monophosphate (cGMP) efflux: anatomical and functional support for an interaction between opiates and nitric oxide." *Brain Res*, 1999 Jan 30; 817(1–2): 220–5.

23. Expression of a blood group B antigen-related glycoepitope in human dorsal root ganglion cells. Yamada M, N. Yuki, T. Kamata, Y. Itoh, T. Miyatake, Department of Neurology, Faculty of Medicine, Tokyo Medical and Dental University, Japan. "Carbohydrate epitopes of glycoconjugates are expressed on sensory neurons of dorsal root ganglion (DRG). A possible role of antibodies directed at carbohydrate determinants of the glycoconjugates has been suggested in some patients with sensory neuropathy. We investigated expression of blood group antigen-related epitopes in human DRG immunohistochemically using monoclonal antibodies to A, B, and H antigens. A blood group B determinant [Gal alpha 1-3(Fuc alpha 1–2)Gal beta-]-related glycoepitope was demonstrated in the neurons and surrounding satellite cells of DRG obtained from subjects with any ABO blood group phenotype. The treatment with trypsin or chloroform/methanol prior to the immunostaining suggested that the glycoconjugate exhibiting the blood group B determinant-related epitope consisted mainly of glycoprotein and included glycolipid. The glycoconjugates with the blood group B determinant-related epitope may play a role in the physiological function and pathophysiology of human DRG neurons."

CHAPTER 4: DIGESTIVE INTEGRITY:
BLOOD TYPE'S SYSTEMIC INFLUENCE

1. Toft, A.D., C. C. Blackwell, A. T. Saadi, et al. "Secretor status and infection in patients with Graves' disease." *Autoimmunity*, 1990; 7(4): pp. 279–89.

2. Arneberg, P., L. Kornstad, H. Nordbo, and P. Gjermo. "Less dental caries among secretors than among non-secretors of blood group substance." *Scand J Dent Res*, November 1976; 84(6): pp. 362–66.

Holbrook, W. P., and C. C. Blackwell. "Secretor status and dental caries in Iceland." *FEMS Microbiol Immunol,* June 1989; 1(6–7): pp. 397–99.

Kaslick, R. S., T. L. West, and A. I. Chasens. "Association between ABO blood groups, HL-A antigens and periodontal diseases in young adults: A follow-up study." *J Periodontol,* June 1980; 51(6): pp. 339–42.

Nikawa, H., H. Kotani, S. Sadamori, and T. Hamada. "Denture stomatitis and ABO blood types." *J Prosthet Dent,* September 1991; 66(3): pp. 391–94.

3. Macartney, J. C. "Lectin histochemistry of galactose and N-acetyl-galactosamine glycoconjugates in normal gastric mucosa and gastric cancer and the relationship with ABO and secretor status." *J Pathol,* October 1986; 150(2): pp. 135–44.

4. Pals, G., J. Defize, J. C. Pronk, et al. "Relations between serum pepsinogen levels, pepsinogen phenotypes, ABO blood groups, age and sex in blood donors." *Ann Hum Biol,* September 1985; 12(5): pp. 403–11.

5. Melissinos, K., G. Alegakis, A. J. Archimandritis, and G. Theodoropoulos. "Serum gastrin concentrations in healthy people of the various ABO blood groups." *Acta Hepatogastroenterol* (Stuttg), December 1978; 25(6): pp. 482–86.

6. Springer, G. F. "Importance of blood-group substances in interactions between man and microbes." *Ann NY Acad Sci.,* February 1970 13;169(1): pp. 134–52.

7. Acarin, L., J. M. Vela, B. Gonzalez, and B. Castellano. "Demonstration of poly-N-acetyl lactosamine residues in ameboid and ramified microglial cells in rat brain by tomato lectin binding." *J Histochem Cytochem,* August 1994; 42(8): pp. 1033–41.

Gibbons, R. J. and I. Dankers. "Immunosorbent assay of interactions between human parotid immunoglobulin A and dietary lectins." *Arch Oral Biol,* 1986; 31(7): pp. 477–81.

Irache, J. M., C. Durrer, D. Duchene, Ponchel. "Bioadhesion of lectin-latex conjugates to rat intestinal mucosa." *Pharm Res,* November 1996; 13(11): pp. 1716–19.

8. Boyd, W. C. *Genetics and the Races of Man: An Introduction to Modern Physical Anthropology.* Boston: Little Brown, 1950.

9. Freed, D. J. *Dietary Lectins in Food Allergy and Intolerance.* Brostoff and Callacombe Editors; London: Bailliere Tindall Publishers.

10. Pusztai, A. "Dietary lectins are metabolic signals for the gut and modulate immune and hormone functions." *Eur J Clin Nutr,* October 1993; 47(10): pp. 691–99.

11. Falth-Magnusson, K., et al. "Elevated levels of serum antibodies to the lectin wheat germ agglutinin in celiac children lend support to the gluten-lectin theory of celiac disease." *Pediatr Allergy Immunol,* May 1995; 6(2): pp. 98–102.

12. Freed, D. L. J. Rheumatic Patches. http://www.elfstrom.com/arthritis/articles/r-patch.html.

13. Brady, P. G., A. M. Vannier, and J. G. Banwell. "Identification of the dietary lectin, wheat germ agglutinin, in human intestinal contents." *Gastroenterology,* August 1978; 75(2): pp. 236–39.

14. Hollander, D., C. M. Vadheim, E. Brettholz, G. M. Petersen, T. Delahunty, and J. I. Rotter. "Increased intestinal permeability in patients with Crohn's disease and their relatives. A possible etiologic factor." *Ann Intern Med,* December 1986; 105(6): pp. 883–85.

15. Jordinson, M., R. J. Playford Calam. "Effects of a panel of dietary lectins on cholecystokinin release in rats." *Am J Physiol,* October 1997; 273(4 Pt 1): pp. G946–50.

16. Jordinson, M., et al. "Soybean lectin stimulates pancreatic exocrine secretion via CCK-A receptors in rats." *Am J Physiol,* April 1996; 270(4 Pt 1): pp. G653–59.

17. Weinman, M. D., C. H. Allan, J. S. Trier, and S. J. Hagen. "Repair of microvilli in the rat small intestine after damage with lectins contained in the red kidney bean." *Gastroenterology,* 1989 Nov; 97(5): 1193–204.

18. Erickson, R. H., J. Kim J., M. H. Sleisenger, and Y. S. Kim. "Effect of lectins on the activity of brush border membrane-bound enzymes of rat small intestine." *J Pediatr Gastroenterol Nutr,* December 1985; 4(6): pp. 984–91.

19. Ponzio, G., A. Debant, J. O. Contreres, and B. Rossi. "Wheat-germ agglutinin mimics metabolic effects of insulin without increasing receptor autophosphorylation." *Cell Signal,* 1990; 2(4): pp. 377–86.

20. Hussain, N., P. U. Jani, and A. T. Florence. "Enhanced oral uptake of tomato lectin-conjugated nanoparticles in the rat." *Pharm Res,* May 1997; 14(5): pp. 613–18.

21. J. S. Chuang, J. M. Callaghan, P. A. Gleeson, and B. H. Toh. "Diagnostic ELISA for parietal cell autoantibody using tomato lectin-purified gastric H+/K(+)-ATPase (proton pump)." *Autoimmunity,* 1992; 12(1): pp. 1–7.

22. A. W. Burks, et al. "Identification of peanut agglutinin and soybean trypsin inhibitor as minor legume allergens." *Int Arch Allergy Immunol*, October 1994; 105(2): pp. 143–49.

S. M. Tariq, M. Stevens, S. Matthews, S. Ridout, R. Twiselton, and D. W. Hide. "Cohort study of peanut and tree nut sensitisation by age of 4 years." *BMJ*, August 31, 1996; 313(7056): pp. 514–17. http://www.foodallergy.org/research.html

23. Gan, R. L. "[Peanut lectin-binding sites in gastric carcinoma and the adjacent mucosa]." *Chung-hua Ping Li Hsueh Tsa Chih*, June 1990; 19(2): pp. 109–11.

Lin, M. et al. "Peanut lectin–binding sites and mucins in benign and malignant colorectal tissues associated with schistomatosis." *Histol Histopathol*, October 1998; 13(4): pp. 961–66.

Melato, M. et al. "The lectin-binding sites for peanut agglutinin in invasive breast ductal carcinomas and their metastasis." *Pathol Res Pract*, 1998; 194(9): pp. 603–8.

24. Agbedana, E. O. and M. H. Yeldu. "Serum total, heat and urea stable alkaline phosphatase activities in relation to ABO blood groups and secretor phenotypes." *Afr J Med Med Sci*, December 1996; 25(4): pp. 327–29.

Domar, U., K. Hirano, and T. Stigbrand. "Serum levels of human alkaline phosphatase isozymes in relation to blood groups." *Clin Chim Acta*, December 16, 1991; 203(2–3): pp. 305–13.

Mehta, N. .J, D. V. Rege, and M. B. Kulkarni. "Total serum alkaline phosphatase (SAP) and serum cholesterol in relation to secretor status and blood groups in myocardial infarction patients. *Indian Heart*, March 1989; 41(2): pp. 82–85.

CHAPTER 5: METABOLIC SYNCHRONY:
BLOOD TYPE'S BIOCHEMICAL INFLUENCE

1. Ponzio, G., A. Debant, J. O. Contreres, and B. Rossi. "Wheat-germ agglutinin mimics metabolic effects of insulin without increasing receptor autophosphorylation." *Cell Signal*, 1990; 2(4): pp. 377–86.

Shechter, Y. "Bound lectins that mimic insulin produce persistent insulinlike activities." *Endocrinology*, December 1983; 113(6): pp. 1921–26.

2. Clausen, J. O., H. O. Hein, P. Suadicani, et al. "Lewis phenotypes and the insulin resistance syndrome in young healthy white

men and women." *Am J Hypertens*, November 8, 1995; (11): pp. 1060–66.

Melis, C., P. Mercier, P. Vague, and B. Vialettes. "Lewis antigen and diabetes." *Rev Fr Transfus Immunohematol*, September 1978; 21(4): pp. 965–71 [Article in French].

Patrick, A. W. and A. Collier. "An infectious aetiology of insulin-dependent diabetes mellitus? Role of the secretor status." *FEMS Microbiol Immunol*, June 1989; 1(6–7): pp. 411–416.

Peters, W. H. and W. Gohler. "ABH-secretion and Lewis red cell groups in diabetic and normal subjects from Ethiopia." *Exp Clin Endocrinol*, November 1986; 88(1): pp. 64–70.

3. Rosskamp, R. "Hormonal findings in obese children: A review." *Klin Padiatr* 1987 Jul–Aug; 199(4):253–9 [Article in German]

4. Blfiore, F, and S. Iannello. "Insulin resistance in obesity: Metabolic mechanisms and measurement methods." *Mol Genet Metab*, 1998; 65: 121–8.

5. Grundy, S. M. "Hypertriglyceridemia, insulin resistance, and the metabolic syndrome." *Am J Cardiol*, May 13, 1999; 83(9B): pp. 25F–29F.

    Kotake, H. and S. Oikawa. "Syndrome X." *Nippon Rinsho*, March 1999; 57(3): pp. 622–26 [Article in Japanese].

6. Wong, F. L., K. Kodama, H. Sasaki, M. Yamada, and H. B. Hamilton. "Longitudinal study of the association between ABO phenotype and total serum cholesterol level in a Japanese cohort." *Genet Epidemiol*, 1992; 9(6): pp. 405–18.

7. George, V. T., R. C. Elston, C. I. Amos, L. J. Ward, and G. S. Berenson. "Association between polymorphic blood markers and risk factors for cardiovascular disease in a large pedigree." *Genet Epidemiol* ,1987; 4(4): pp. 267–275.

8. Tarjan, Z., M. Tonelli, J. Duba, and A. Zorandi. "Correlation between ABO and Rh blood groups, serum cholesterol and ischemic heart disease in patients undergoing coronarography." *Orv Hetil*, 1995 Apr 9; 136(15): 767–9.

9. Lamarche, B. et al. "Atherosclerosis prevention for the next decade: Risk assessment beyond low density lipoprotein cholesterol." *Can J Cardiol*, 1998 Jun; 14(6): 841–51.

10. Terrier, E., M. Baillet, and B. Jaulmes. "Detection of lipid abnormalities in blood donors." *Rev Fr Transfus Immunohematol*, 1979 Mar; 22(2):147–58.

11. Bayer, P. M., H. Hotschek, and E. Knoth. "Intestinal alkaline phosphatase and the ABO blood group system—a new aspect." *Clin Chim Acta*, November 20, 1980; 108(1): pp. 81–87.

CHAPTER 6: THE IMMUNE BATTLEGROUND:
BLOOD TYPE AS A WEAPON FOR SURVIVAL

1. [Breanndon Moore, The Mayo Clinic, Rochester, MN.]
2. Oriol, R., J. Le Pendu, and R. Mollicone. "Genetics of ABO, H, Lewis, X and related antigens." *Vox Sang*, 1986; 51(3): pp. 161–71.

   Sarafian, V., P. Dimova, I. Georgiev, and H. Taskov. "ABH blood group antigen significance as markers of endothelial differentiation of mesenchymal cells." *Folia Med*, (Plovdiv) 1997; 39(2): pp. 5–9.

   Szulman, A. E. "Evolution of ABH blood group antigens during embryogenesis." *Ann Inst Pasteur Immunol*, November–December 1987; 138(6): pp. 845–47.

3. Pamm, A. O. "Effects of antibiotics on intestinal microflora and production of metabolics." *Journal of Antibiotics*, 1989 June; 34: 409–414.

4. Nayak, S. K. "ABO blood groups in different diseases." *J. Ind Med*, 1971; 87: 449–52.

   Rybalka, A. N., P. V. Andreeva, L. F. Tikhonenko, and N. A. Koval'chuk. "ABO system blood groups and the rhesus factor in tumors and tumorlike processes of the ovaries." *Vopr Onkol*, 1979; 25(3): 28–30 [Article in Russian].

5. Ichikawa, D., K. Handa, and S. Hakomori. "Histo-blood group A/B antigen deletion/reduction vs. continuous expression in human tumor cells as correlated with their malignancy." *Int J Cancer*, April 1998 13; 76(2): pp. 284–89.

   Sarafian, V., A. Popov, and H. Taskov. "Expression of A, B and H blood-group antigens and carcinoembryonic antigen in human tumours." *Zentralbl Pathol*, November 1993; 139(4–5): pp. 351–54.

6. Kurtenkov, O., K. Klaamas, and L. Miljukhina. "The lower level of natural anti-Thomsen-Friedenreich antigen (TFA) agglutinins in sera of patients with gastric cancer related to ABO(H) blood-group phenotype." *Int J Cancer*, March 16, 1995; 60(6): 781–85.

   Yoshida, A., et al. "Different expression of Tn and sialyl-Tn antigens between normal and diseased human gastric epithelial cells." *Acta Med Okayama*, August 1998; 52(4): pp. 197–204.

7. Orstavik, K. H., L. Kornstad, H. Reisner, and K. Berg. "Possible effect of secretor locus on plasma concentration of factor VIII and von Willebrand factor." *Blood*, 1989 Mar; 73(4): 990–3.

   Koster, T., A. D. Blann, E. Briet, J. P. Vandenbroucke, and F. R. Rosendaal. "Role of clotting factor VIII in effect of von Willebrand factor on occurrence of deep-vein thrombosis." *Lancet*, 1995 Jan 21; 345(8943): 152–5.

8. Oleksowicz, L., N. Bhagwati, and M. DeLeon-Fernandez. "Deficient activity of von Willebrand's factor-cleaving protease in patients with disseminated malignancies." *Cancer Res*, 1999 May 1; 59(9): 2244–50.

9. Ciardiello, F. and G. Tortora. "Interactions between the epidermal growth factor receptor and type I protein kinase A: Biological significance and therapeutic implications." *Clin Cancer Res*, April 1998; 4(4): pp. 821–28.

10. Anderson, D. E., and C. Haas. "Blood type A and familial breast cancer." *Cancer*, November 1, 1984; 54(9): pp. 1845–49.

    Costantini, M., T. Fassio, L. Canobbio et al. "Role of blood groups as prognostic factors in primary breast cancer." *Oncology*, 1990; 47(4): pp. 308–12.

    Skolnick, M. II., E. A. Thompson, D. T. Bishop, and L. A. Cannon. "Possible linkage of a breast cancer–susceptibility locus to the ABO locus: Sensitivity of LOD scores to a single new recombinant observation." *Genet Epidemiol*, 1984; 1(4): pp. 363–73.

    Tryggvadottir, L., H. Tulinius, and J. M. Robertson. "Familial and sporadic breast cancer cases in Iceland: a comparison related to ABO blood groups and risk of bilateral breast cancer." *Int J Cancer*, October 15, 1988; 42(4): pp. 499–501.

11. Kaur, I., I. P. Singh, and M. K. Bhasin. "Blood groups in relation to carcinoma of cervix uteri." *Hum Hered*, 1992; 42(5): pp. 324–26.

    Llopis, B., J. L. Ruiz, G. Server et al. "ABO blood groups and bladder carcinoma." *Eur Urol*, 1990; 17(4): pp. 289–92.

    Marinaccio, M., A. Traversa, E. Carioggia et al. "Blood groups of the ABO system and survival rate in gynecologic tumors." *Minerva Ginecol*, March 1995; 47(3): pp. 69–76.

    Metoki, R., K. Kakudo, Y. Tsuji, et al. "Deletion of histo-blood group A and B antigens and expression of incompatible A antigen in ovarian cancer." *J Natl Cancer Inst*, 1989 Aug 2; 81(15): 1151–7.

Nayak, S. K. "ABO blood groups in different diseases." *J. Ind Med,* 1997; 1; 87: pp. 449–52.

Rybalka, A. N., P. V. Andreeva, L. F. Tikhonenko, N. A. Koval'chuk. "ABO system blood groups and the rhesus factor in tumors and tumorlike processes of the ovaries." *Vopr Onkol,* 1979; 25(3): pp. 28–30 [Article in Russian].

Tsukazaki, K., M. Sakayori, H. Arai, et al. "Abnormal expression of blood group-related antigens in uterine endometrial cancers." *Jpn J Cancer Res,* 1991 Aug; 82(8): 934–41.

12. Orlow, I., L. Lacombe, I. Pellicer et al. "Genotypic and phenotypic characterization of the histoblood group ABO(H) in primary bladder tumors." *Int J Cancer,* March 16, 1998; 75(6): pp. 819–24.

Orihuela, E. and R. S. Shahon. "Influence of blood group type on the natural history of superficial bladder cancer." *J Urol,* October 1987; 138(4): pp. 758–59.

Raitanen, M. P. and T. L. Tammela. "Relationship between blood groups and tumour grade, number, size, stage, recurrence and survival in patients with transitional cell carcinoma of the bladder." *Scand J Urol Nephrol,* 1993; 27(3): pp. 343–47.

Srinivas, V., S. A. Khan, S. Hoisington, A. Varma, and M. J. Gonder. "Relationship of blood groups and bladder cancer." *J Urol,* January 1986; 135(1): pp. 50–52.

13. Annese, V., M. Minervini, A. Gabbrielli, G. Gambassi, and R. Manna. "ABO blood groups and cancer of the pancreas." *Int J Pancreatol,* March 1990; 6(2): pp. 81–88.

Uchida, E., M. A. Tempero, D. A. Burnett, Z. Steplewski, and P. M. Pour. "Correlative studies on antigenicity of pancreatic cancer and blood group types." *Cancer Detect Prev Suppl,* 1987; 1: pp. 145–48.

14. Slater, G. et al. "Clinicopathologic correlations of ABO and Rhesus blood type in colorectal cancer." *Dis Colon Rectum,* January 1993; 36(1): pp. 5–7.

15. Itzkowitz, S. H. "Blood group–related carbohydrate antigen expression in malignant and premalignant colonic neoplasms." *J Cell Biochem Suppl,* 1992; 16G: pp. 97–101.

Jordinson, M. et al. "Vicia faba agglutinin, the lectin present in broad beans, stimulates differentiation of undifferentiated colon cancer cells." *Gut,* May 1999; 44(5): pp. 709–14.

16. David, L., D. Leitao, M. Sobrinho-Simoes, E. P. Bennett, T. White, U. Mandel, E. Dabelsteen, and H. Clausen. "Biosynthetic basis of incompatible histo-blood group A antigen expression: Anti-A transferase antibodies reactive with gastric cancer tissue of type O individuals." *Cancer Res*, 1993 Nov 15; 53(22): 5494–500.

 Torrado, J., B. Ruiz, J. Garay et al. "Blood group phenotypes, sulfomucins, and *Helicobacter pylori* in Barrett's esophagus." *Am J Surg Pathol*, September 1997; 21(9): pp. 1023–29.

17. Pyd, M., I. Rzewnicki, and U. Suwayach. "ABO blood groups in patients with laryngeal and hypopharyngeal cancer." *Otolaryngol Pol*, 1995; 49 Suppl 20: pp. 396–98.

 Xie, X., M. Boysen, O. P. Clausen, and M. A. Bryne. "Prognostic value of Le(y) and H antigens in oral tongue carcinomas." *Laryngoscope*, 1999.

18. Gnedkova, I. A., N. I., Lisianyi, Ala Glavatskii. "Efficacy of chemotherapy and immunochemotherapy in neuro-oncologic patients of various blood groups." *Zh Vopr Neirokhir*, January–February 1989; (1): pp. 17–20 [Article in Russian].

19. Gonzalez-Campora, R., J. A. Garcia-Sanatana et al. "Blood group antigens in differentiated thyroid neoplasms." *Arch Pathol Lab Med*, November 1998; 122(11): pp. 957–65.

 Klechova, L. and T. S. Gosheva-Antonova. "ABO and Rh blood group factors in thyroid gland diseases." *Vutr Boles*, 1980; 19: pp. 75–79.

 Larena, A., M. Vierbuchen, S. Schroder, A. Larena-Avellaneda, I. Hadshiew, and R. Fischer. "Blood group antigen expression in papillary carcinoma of the thyroid gland. An immunohistochemical and clinical study of expression of Lewis, ABO and related antigens." *Langenbecks Arch Chir*, 1996; 381(2): pp. 102–13.

20. Dintenfass, L. "Some aspects of haemorrheology of metastasis in malignant melanoma." *Haematologia* (Budap), 1977; 11(3–4): pp. 301–7.

21. Manthorpe, R., L. Staub Nielsen et al. "Lewis blood type frequency in patients with primary Sjogren's syndrome: A prospective study including analyses for A1A2BO, Secretor, MNSs, P, Duffy, Kell, Lutheran and rhesus blood groups." *Scand J Rheumatol*, 1985; 14(2): pp. 159–62. Among individuals with multiple sclerosis, a similar trend for over representation of the Lewis negative (Le (a-b)) phenotype also occurs.

22. Hafner, V., M. Coatmelec, and R. Niculescu. "Temporary changes and permanent changes in the erythrocyte blood group antigens in malignant hemopathies." *Rom J Intern Med,* July–December 1996; 34(3–4): pp. 183–88.

Uchikawa, M. "Alterations of ABH antigens in leukemic patients." *Nippon Rinsho,* September 1997; 55(9): pp. 2369–73.

CHAPTER 7: RESTORING BALANCE:
BIOLOGICAL HARMONY AND DETOXIFICATION

1. Anderson, R. L., J. K. Maurer, W. R. Francis, and S. L. Buring. "Trypsin inhibitor ingestion-induced urinary indican excretion and pancreatic acinar cell hypertrophy." *Nutr Cancer,* 1986; 8(2): pp. 133–39.

Mayer, P. J. and W. L. Beeken. "The role of urinary indican as a predictor of bacterial colonization in the human jejunum." *Am J Dig Dis,* November 1975; 20(11): pp. 1003–9.

2. Pusztai, A. and S. Bardocz. "Biological effects of plant lectins on the gastrointestinal tract: Metabolic consequences and applications." *Trends In Glycoscience and Glycotechnology,* Volume 8, Number 41 May 1996.

3. Mikkat, U., I. Damm, G. Schroder, K. Schmidt, C. Wirth, H. Weber, and L. Jonas. "Effect of the lectins wheat germ agglutinin (WGA) and Ulex europaeus agglutinin (UEA-I) on the alpha-amylase secretion of rat pancreas *in vitro* and *in vivo.*" *Pancreas,* May 1998; 16(4): pp. 529–38.

4. Wu, G., W. G. Pond, S. P. Flynn, T. L. Ott, and F. W. Bazer. "Maternal dietary protein deficiency decreases nitric oxide synthase and ornithine decarboxylase activities in placenta and endometrium of pigs during early gestation." *J Nutr,* December 1998; 128(12): pp. 2395–402.

Wu, G., and S. M. Morris Jr. "Arginine metabolism: nitric oxide and beyond." *Biochem J,* November 15, 1998; 336 (Pt 1): pp. 1–17.

5. Naidu, A. S., W. R. Bidlack, and R. A. Clemens. "Probiotic spectra of lactic acid bacteria (LAB)." *Crit Rev Food Sci Nutr,* January 1999; 39(1): pp. 13–126.

Schaafsma, G., W. J. Meuling, W. van Dokkum, and C. Bouley. "Effects of a milk product, fermented by Lactobacillus acidophilus and with fructo-oligosaccharides added, on blood lipids in male volunteers." *Eur J Clin Nutr,* June 1998; 52(6): pp. 436–40.

CHAPTER 9: LIVE RIGHT 4 TYPE O

1 Smith, D. F. "Type A personalities tend to have low platelet monoamine oxidase activity." *Acta Psychiatr Scand,* February 1994; 89(2): pp. 88–91.

2. Ota, H. et al. "Intestinal metaplasia with adherent *Helicobacter pylori:* A hybrid epithelium with both gastric and intestinal features." *Hum Pathol,* August 1998; 29(8): pp. 846–50.

3. Hein, H. O. et al. "[Genetic markers for stomach ulcer. A study of 3,387 men aged 54–74 years from The Copenhagen Male Study]." *Ugeskr Laeger,* August 24, 1998; 160(35):5045–49.

Heneghan, M. A. et al. "Effect of host Lewis and ABO blood group antigen expression on *Helicobacter pylori* colonisation density and the consequent inflammatory response." *FEMS Immunol Med Microbiol,* April 1998; 20(4): pp. 257–66.

McNamara, D. et al. "*Helicobacter pylori* and gastric cancer." *Ital J Gastroenterol Hepatol,* October 30, 1998; 30 Suppl 3: pp. S294–98.

4. Springer, G. F. "Relation of blood group active plant substances to human blood groups." *Acta Haem,* 1958; 20: pp. 147–55.

5. "Observations on abnormal thyroid-stimulating hormone levels and on a possible association of blood group O with hyperthyroidism." *Arch Intern Med,* August 1982; 142(8):pp. 1465–69.

6. Robbins, J. "Factors altering thyroid hormone metabolism." *Environ Health Perspect,* April 1981; 38: pp. 65–70.

CHAPTER 10: LIVE RIGHT 4 TYPE A

1. Beale, N. and S. Nethercott. "Job-loss and family morbidity: a study of a factory closure." *J R Coll Gen Pract,* 1985 Nov; 35(280):510–4.

Cohen, B.G., M. J. Colligan, W. Wester, 2d, M. J. Smith. "An investigation of job satisfaction factors in an incident of mass psychogenic illness at the workplace." *Occup Health Nurs,* 1978 Jan; 26(1): 10–6

Eysenck, H. J. "Personality, stress and cancer: prediction and prophylaxis." *Br J Med Psychol,* 1988 Mar; 61 (Pt 1):57–75.

Kiecolt-Glaser, J.K., R. Glaser, et al. "Marital stress: Immunologic, neuroendocrine, and autonomic correlates." *Ann NY Acad Sci,* 1998 May 1; 840: 656–63.

Martin, R. A. and J. P. Dobbin. "Sense of humor, hassles, and immunoglobulin A: Evidence for a stress-moderating effect of humor." *Int J Psychiatry Med,* 1988; 18(2): 93–105.

Rein, G., M. Atkinson, and R. McCraty. "The physiological and psychological effects of compassion and anger." *J Advanc Med,* 1995; 8:87–105.

2. Mockel, M., T. Stork, J. Vollert et al. "Stress reduction through listening to music: Effects on stress hormones, hemodynamics and mental state in patients with arterial hypertension and in healthy persons." *Dtsch Med Wochenschr,* 1995 May 26; 120(21): 745–52 [Article in German].

   VanderArk, S. D. and D. Ely. "Cortisol, biochemical, and galvanic skin responses to music stimuli of different preference values by college students in biology and music." *Percept Mot Skills,* 1993 Aug; 77(1): 227–34.

3. Wan X. S., Lu L. J., Anderson K. E., Kennedy A. R. "Urinary excretion of Bowman-Birk inhibitor in humans after soy consumption as determined by a monoclonal antibody-based immunoassay." *Cancer Epidemiol Biomarkers Prev.,* Jul 2000; 9(7): 741–7.

   Clawson, G. A. "Protease inhibitors and carcinogenesis: A review." *Cancer Invest,* 1996; 14(6): 597–608.

4. Steuer M. K., Hofstadter F., Probster L. et al. "Are ABH antigenic determinants on human outer ear canal epithelium responsible for Pseudomonas aeruginosa infections?" *ORL J Otorhinolaryngol Relat Spec,* 1995;57: 148–152.

   Mortensen E. H. Lildholdt T., Gammelgard N. P., Christensen P. H. "Distribution of ABO blood groups in secretary otitis media and cholesteatoma." *Clin Otolaryngol,* 1983;8:263–265.

   Gannon, M. M. Jagger C., Haggard M. P. "Material blood group in otitis media with effusion." *Clin Otolaryngol,* 1994;19:327–331.

5. Billington, B. P. "A note on the distribution of ABO blood groups in bronchiectasis and portal cirrhosis." *Aust Annal Med,* 1956; 5: pp. 20–22.

6. Samuels, M. H. and P. A. McDaniel. "Thyrotropin levels during hydrocortisone infusions that mimic fasting-induced cortisol elevations: A clinical research center study." *J Clin Endocrinol Metab,* November 1997; 82(11): pp. 3700–4.

7. Bertolini, S., C. Donati, N. Elicio, et al. "Lipoprotein changes induced by pantethine in hyperlipoproteinemic patients: adults and children." *Int J Clin Pharmacol Ther Toxicol,* 1986; 24: pp. 630–37.

8. Melato, M. et al. "The lectin-binding sites for peanut agglutinin in

invasive breast ductal carcinomas and their metastasis." *Pathol Res Pract*, 1998; 194(9): pp. 603–8.

9. Schumacher, U., D. Higgs, M. Loizidou, R. Pickering, A. Leathem, and I. Taylor. "Helix pomatia agglutinin binding is a useful prognostic indicator in colorectal carcinoma." *Cancer*, 1994 Dec 15; 74(12): 3104–3107.

10. Andersen, B.L., W. B. Farrar, D. Golden-Kreutz, et al. "Stress and immune responses after surgical treatment for regional breast cancer." *J Natl Cancer Inst*, January 7 1998 ;90(1): pp. 30–36.

Irwin, M., T. Patterson, T. L. Smith, et al. "Reduction of immune function in life stress and depression." *Biol Psychiatry*, January 1, 1990; 27(1): pp. 22–30.

Sieber, W. J., J. Rodin, L. Larson, et al. "Modulation of human natural killer cell activity by exposure to uncontrollable stress." *Brain Behav Immun*, June 1992; 6(2): pp. 141–56.

11. Defize, L. II., D. J. Arndt-Jovin, T. M. Jovin, J. Boonstra, J. Meisenhelder, T. Hunter, H. T. de Hey, and S. W. de Laat. "A431 cell variants lacking the blood group A antigen display increased high affinity epidermal growth factor–receptor number, protein-tyrosine kinase activity, and receptor turnover." *J Cell Biol*, September 1988; 107(3): pp. 939–49.

CHAPTER 11: LIVE RIGHT 4 TYPE B

1. Kinane, D. F., C. C. Blackwell, R. P. Brettle, et al. "ABO blood group, secretor state, and susceptibility to recurrent urinary tract infection in women." *Br Med J* (Clin Res Ed), July 3, 1982; 285(6334): pp. 7–9.

2. Blackwell, C. C. "The role of ABO blood groups and secretor status in host defences. *FEMS Microbiol Immunol*, June 1989; 1(6–7): pp. 341–49.

Gabr, N. S. and A. M. Mandour. "Relation of parasitic infection to blood group in El Minia Governorate, Egypt." *J Egypt Soc Parasitol*, December 1991; 21(3): pp. 679–83.

3. Haverkorn, M. J. and W. R. Goslings. "Streptococci, ABO blood groups, and secretor status." *Am J Hum Genet*, July 1969; 21(4): pp. 360–75.

4. Freed, D. J. Rheumatic Patches. http://www.elfstrom.com/arthritis/articles/r-patch.html

5. Tang, W., A. Matsumoto, K. Shikata, F. Takeuchi, T. Konishi, M.

Nakata, T. Mizuochi. "Detection of disease-specific augmentation of abnormal immunoglobulin G in sera of patients with rheumatoid arthritis."

6. Manuel Y., Keenoy, B., Moorkens, G., Vertommen, J. Noe, M., Neve, J. J. De Leeuw, I. "Magnesium status and parameters of the oxidant-antioxidant balance in patients with chronic fatigue: effects of supplementation with magnesium." *J Am Coll Nutr,* Jun 2000; 19(3):374–82.

Werbach, M. R. "Nutritional strategies for treating chronic fatigue syndrome." *Altern Med Rev,* Apr 2000; 5(2):93–108. Review.

GENERAL REFERENCE WORKS ON BLOOD TYPE

Brues, A. M. "Tests of Blood Group Selection." *Amer. J. Forensic Medicine* (1929), 287 9.

Childe, V. G. *Man Makes Himself.* London: Watts and Co. 1936.

Coon, C. S. *The Races of Europe.* New York: MacMillan Co 1939.

D'Adamo, J. *The D'Adamo Diet.* Montreal: McGraw Hill Ryerson (Canada). 1989.

———. *One Man's Food,* New York: Richard Marek, 1980. (out of print)

D'Adamo, Peter. *Cook Right 4 Your Type: The Practical Kitchen Companion to Eat Right 4 Your Type.* New York: G.P. Putnam's Sons, 1998.

———. *Eat Right 4 Your Type: The Individualized Diet Solution to Staying Healthy, Living Longer and Achieving Your Ideal Weight.* New York: G.P. Putnam's Sons 1996.

———. "Gut ecosystems III: The ABO and other polymorphic systems." *Townsend Ltr. for Doctors,* August 1990.

Gates, R. R. *Human Ancestry.* Cambridge, MA: Harvard Univ Press, 1948.

Livingstone, F. R. *Natural selection disease and ongoing human evolution as illustrated by the ABO groups.* Source unknown. Copy in author's possession.

Marcus, D. M. "The ABO and Lewis Blood-Group System." *New England J. Med.* 280: 994–1005 1969.

Mourant, A. E. *Blood Relations; Blood Groups and Anthropology.* Oxford Science Publications, Oxford University Press, 1983.

Mourant, A. E., A. C. Kopec, and K. Domaniewska-Sobczak, *Blood Groups and Disease.* New York: Oxford Press, 4th edition, 1984.

Muschel, L. "Blood groups, disease and selection." *Bacteriological Rev.* 30(2) 1966; 427–41.

Nomi, T. and A. Besher, *You are Your Blood Type.* Pocket Books USA, 1983.

Race, R. R., and R. Sanger. *Blood Groups in Man.* Oxford: Blackwell Scientific Publications, 1975.

Sheppard, P. M. "Blood groups and natural selection." *Brit. Med. Bull,* 15; 132–9: 1959.

Snyder, L. H. *Blood Grouping in Relation to Clinical and Legal Medicine.* Williams and Wikin Publishers, 1929.

Wyman, L. C. and W. C. Boyd, "Blood group determinations of prehistoric American Indians." *Amer. Anthropol,* 39; 583–592: 1937.

Wyman, L. C. and W. C. Boyd, "Human blood groups and anthropology." *Amer. Anthropol,* 37; 181: 1935.

Your Genetic
Typography

Your blood type serves as the primary architect of your cellular structure. It does this through its antigens, which are chemical markers on our cells that help distinguish friend from foe. Blood type antigens are extremely powerful; in conditions of optimum health, they can effectively block foreign substances, such as dangerous bacteria, from entering your system. In addition, strong evidence exists showing that blood type antigens serve as "differentiation markers," paving the way for the development of nerves and blood vessels in the growing fetus—much in the way that a surveyor works ahead of a highway construction crew, determining the best site for a new road to be laid.

Each blood type possesses a different antigen with its own special chemical structure. Your blood type is named for the blood type antigen you possess on your red blood cells. There is nothing special about the use of letters to name the blood types, other than the fact that the O antigen was given the letter O to indicate the number zero.

Your immune system creates antibodies to reject foreign antigens, including blood type antigens foreign to you. Your own blood type antigen prevents you from making antibodies to your own blood type anti-gen. People with Type A blood have an antibody to Type B in their blood plasma. This anti-B antibody helps the body destroy any Type B blood cells that might enter the system. Likewise, people with Type B blood have an antibody to Type A in their blood plasma, which helps destroy any Type A blood cells that might enter the system. Blood Type O has both anti-A and anti-B antibodies, and Blood Type AB carries *no* opposing blood group antibodies.

If you were studying blood types in medical school, this would be the end of your education. Medical training is usually limited to the rel-evance of blood types to transfusions. So once you know that Type A and Type B cannot exchange blood; Type AB can receive blood from any type, but donate blood to none of them; and Type O can give blood to anyone, but receive it only from Type Os; you're as knowledgeable as most physicians. Mother Nature must be shaking her head in disbelief that we have made such limited use of this fantastic genetic tool. Blood type provides us with an agent that is present on every red blood cell. Using blood type, we can monitor immune function, metabolic activity, digestion, and neurological signals. That's an extremely powerful pre-dictor of function, and yet blood type is still primarily relegated to the transfusion lab. Fortunately, as this book documents, medical science is slowly but surely coming around to the idea that blood type might have a pervasive role in the human system.

Your Blood Type Lineage

WHAT DETERMINES your blood type? Blood type genetics is really quite simple. You're the physical result of your genes; this is called your phenotype. You get these genes from your parents, and the combination of each of your parent's genes is called your genotype. One of the two genes will usually be dominant, which is the key to your differences. For example, the gene for Type A is dominant to the gene for Type O, so if you've received an A from your mother and an O from your father, your genotype will be *Ao*, but your phenotype will be Type A. However, you carry a latent O, which in turn can be passed on to your offspring. The distinction between phenotype and genotype is what confuses so many people about blood type genetics. It explains why a Type A mother and a Type O father can have a Type O child, even though you can only become Type O if you receive an O gene from each parent.

		MOM	
		O	o
D A D	A	Ao = Type A	Ao = Type A
	o	Oo = Type O	Oo = Type O

		DAD	
		A	B
MOM	o	Ao = Type A	Bo = Type B
	o	Ao = Type A	Bo = Type B

Here's a simple illustration. The box above, called a Punnett square, is used by geneticists to determine possible combinations of phenotype from genotype. Mom (the top) is phenotype O (Blood Type O) and genotype *Oo*. Dad (along the right side) is phenotype A (Blood Type A) and genotype *Ao*. As we can see, each offspring has a 50 percent chance of being either Blood Type A *(Ao)* or Blood Type O *(Oo)*. Since neither parent carries a B allele, it is impossible for the offspring of these two parents to be either Blood Type B or Blood Type AB. This is why blood type can be useful in determining paternity. It cannot confirm that a person *is* the father of a child; however, in certain circumstances it can confirm that a person is *not* the father. Here's an interesting combination: Mom is Blood Type O and Dad is Blood Type AB. In this circumstance, the offspring will be either Blood Type A or Blood Type B, as both A and B alleles are dominant to O. No offspring will possess the blood type of their mother. However, both will possess a recessive O al-

		DAD	
		B	O
M O M	A	AB = Type AB	Ao = Type A
	o	Bo = Type B	Oo = Type O

lele that can be passed on to their own offspring, potentially producing Type O children. Grandma's revenge! This answers another question—why Type O doesn't disappear over time, since Type A and Type B are dominant. There are enough O alleles in the human gene pool to allow Blood Type O to continue into the foreseeable future.

In a third scenario, we can see how a Type B father and a Type A mother are capable of producing offspring of every type. Thus, although it is a long shot, it is possible for each member of a family to have a different blood type.

From this we can see that two individuals who are the same blood type phenotype can have different genotypes. For example, both of my parents are Type A. I presume that I received an A allele from each parent (making me genotype *Aa*) because my two daughters are both Type A. My wife Martha is Type O and can only have two O alleles, so it is certain that our daughters are genotypically *Ao*.

Your blood type genotype and phenotype comprise only two layers of your genetic uniqueness. To give added dimension and meaning, we must examine the subtypography of your blood type heritage.

Secondary Systems

YOUR BLOOD TYPE profile includes as many as 300 subtypes, which are like genealogical microrefinements. However, for our purposes, only three of them have any real impact. Your phenotype accounts for more than 90 percent of all factors, with your secretor status accounting for about 5 percent. Two others can be useful in special situations. These are the Rh Factor and the MN Blood Group System.

The Rh Factor

When your blood is typed, you also learn whether you are "negative" or "positive." Many people don't realize that this is an additional blood type called the Rhesus or Rh system, and it really has nothing to do with your ABO blood type. The Rh system is named for the rhesus monkey, a commonly used laboratory animal in whose blood it was first discovered. For many years it remained a mystery to doctors why some women who had normal first pregnancies developed complications in their second and subsequent pregnancies, which often resulted in miscarriage and even the death of the mother. In 1940, it was discovered by Dr. Karl Landsteiner (who previously had discovered the entire system of ABO antigens and antibodies) that these women were carrying different blood types from their babies, who took their blood types from their fathers. The babies were Rh+, which meant that they carried the Rh antigen on their blood cells. Their mothers were Rh-, which meant that this antigen was missing from their blood.

Unlike the ABO system, where the antibodies to other blood types develop from birth, Rh- people do not make an antibody to the Rh antigen unless they are first, "sensitized." This sensitization usually occurs when blood is exchanged between the mother and infant during birth, so the mother's immune system does not have enough time to react to the first baby. However, should a subsequent conception result in another Rh+ baby, the mother, now sensitized, will produce antibodies to the baby's blood type. Reactions to the Rh factor can only occur in Rh- women who conceive the children of Rh+ fathers. Rh+ women, who comprise 85 percent of the population, have nothing to worry about. Even though the Rh system doesn't figure prominently when it comes to diets or diseases, it's certainly a factor for childbearing women and their partners.

The MN Blood Group System

The MN blood group system is virtually unknown, since it has no role in transfusions or transplants. However, there is evidence that your MN status may play a role in certain aspects of cardiovascular disease and cancer. In this system, you can type out as MM, NN or MN, depending upon whether your cells have only the "M" antigen (which would make you MM), the "N" antigen (NN), or both (MN). Around 28 percent of the population type out as MM, 22 percent as NN, and 50 percent as

MN. Most health problems are associated with the two "purebred" types (NN and MM), not with the mixed type (MN), a phenomenon known in genetics as hybrid vigor.

It appears that the MN system may play a role in breast cancer. Up until his recent death, Dr. George Springer, a research scientist with the Bligh Cancer Center at the University of Chicago School of Medicine, had been working on a vaccine whose basis is a molecule called the T antigen. The T antigen, which is a common tumor marker found in many cancers, especially those of breast cancer, is the immediate precursor to the antigens that produce the M antigen of the MN blood type. Although the T antigen is manufactured from the blood group M antigen, by the time of its completion, the T antigen looks more like the Blood Type A antigen than it does the M antigen. In healthy tissue, these antigens are normally occluded by the finishing touches, which are added to the T antigen to produce the MN blood type antigen. Healthy, cancer-free people usually carry antibodies against the T antigen, so it is almost never seen in them. In general, if I subtype a patient with a family history of cancer as TypeA / MM, I tend to advise that he or she adopt an aggressive cancer-prevention lifestyle.

There is also a potential role for the MN System in cardiovascular disease. A 1983 study in the journal *Clinical Genetics* showed that people who typed NN had significantly higher cholesterol and triglyceride levels in their blood immediately after being given a standard test meal. The researchers concluded that people who have at least one M gene (blood types MM and MN) seem to be better protected against rapid rises in their triglycerides and cholesterol.

The subtypography is a wide and diverse landscape, much of it unexplored. Although you will not need to travel there often, if ever, it is best to be prepared. Your best preparation is knowledge and understanding.

A_1 or A_2?

There is a further variation for Type A and Type AB that has certain implications for your health and dietary strategies. The distinction between whether one is A_1 or A_2 (and consequently A_1B or A_2B) is done by testing the blood with a solution containing a lectin from the plant *Dolichos biflorus*. Dolichos biflorus lectin reacts more strongly with A_1 red blood cells than with A_2 cells. This is available as a reagent from several chemical supply companies, and A_1-A_2 determination can usually be performed by many diagnostic labs.

The distinction between A_1 and A_2 is becoming increasingly important with regard to certain microbial lectins, some of which seem to possess a preference for one type of A or the other. There are several other minor variations of A_1 but virtually no work has been done on their connection to lectins, disease, or diet.

Your Blood Type Pedigree Includes

GENOTYPE: Blood Type gene inherited from your father + your mother

PHENOTYPE: Your blood type—O, A, B, AB

SECRETOR STATUS: Lewis a-b+ (secretor) Lewis a+b- (non-secretor)

Lewis a-b- (secretor or non-secretor)

RHESUS FACTOR: Rh+ or Rh-

MN BLOOD TYPE: MM, NN, MN

Learn Your
Secretor Status

I HOPE YOU'RE CONVINCED THAT ONE OF THE MOST IMPORTANT things you can do to achieve the highest possible benefits from the blood type prescription is to find out your secretor status. In particular, if you are among the 15 to 20 percent of the population who are non-secretors, you will want to make the appropriate adjustments in your diet and health regimen to counteract the additional risk factors.

We now have available a simple home saliva-based test that can determine your secretor status. The cost for the submission kit and instructions is $32.95 plus $5.25 shipping and handling. Results take approximately two weeks.

To order the Secretor/Non-secretor Test Kit, log onto our website at *www.dadamo.com* or contact:

North American Pharmacal, Inc.
5 Brook Street
Norwalk, CT 06851
Tel: 203-866-7664
Fax: 203-838-4066
Toll free: 877-ABO TYPE (877-226-8973)

Blood Type
and Infectious
Disease

*I*T'S A JUNGLE IN THERE.

Within every being, the age-old battle rages. Virulent diseases—the Black Plague, smallpox, cholera, influenza, tuberculosis—have cut a swath through the evolutionary cycles of time, encouraging "survival of the fittest." Susceptibility has always chosen its victims from among the easiest of pickings—the elderly and the newborns. Add the genetic variables, overall health of the immune system, and the underlying lack of hygiene and sanitation. These further enhance resistance to or decrease the likelihood of disease susceptibility.

Infectious diseases still kill about 13 million people a year worldwide. Even in the United States, 180,000 people died of infectious diseases in 1998. Six infectious diseases killed about 90 percent of all persons who died before the age of forty-four—AIDS, tuberculosis, malaria, measles, diarrhea, and pneumonia. Blood type associations exist for tuberculosis, malaria, measles, and diarrheal diseases.

Most anthropologists view infectious diseases as a form of natural selection. If that's true, the factor doing most of the selecting has always been our blood type. Blood type is an integral part of the body's hard wiring, a program that determines many of the outcomes between its systems and its exterior environment.

Infection has two factors—susceptibility and survivability. You may be susceptible to a particular infectious disease, but have a high level of survivability against it. You may have a natural resistance to a certain type of infectious disease, but if you contract it, your system breaks down and your survivability becomes questionable.

Your blood type dictates the severity of an infection. It also has the ability to adapt to an onslaught, build defenses against it, and repel it the next time it attempts to attack. Blood type allows the body to fend off some infectious diseases and impairs and limits its response against other infectious diseases.

The story of the human struggle with infectious disease is the story of survival. It is the key to understanding blood type—the first line of defense against killer diseases. Many of the most problematic infectious diseases of both our past and present actually do create more problems for some blood types, while other blood types are relatively protected. Many experts have made strong arguments that the pressure applied by infectious diseases along blood type lines has been one, if not the primary, factor, influencing natural selection and blood type distributions. In this section, we will explore some of the evidence connecting blood type and infectious diseases.

Why Didn't Type O Die Out?

IN GENETICS, we have often observed that early forms of life evolve and are eventually replaced by later forms. Yet today, Type O remains the most common blood type. There are several probable explanations for the survival of Type O. An obvious one is the sheer amount of the O gene in the gene pool, and the fact that, to a certain degree, it is self-replicating.

A recent article may explain from a more practical perspective why the gene for Type O blood persists. It appears that individuals with a rare disorder called Leukocyte Adhesion Deficiency type II (characterized by recurrent infections, persistent high white blood count, and severe mental and growth retardation) are unable to mobilize their white blood cells to the sites of inflammation. LAD II patients exhibit a deficiency in the expression of cell surface structures the include the Blood Type O (actually H) antigen. Thus it may be that the manufacture of H antigen (the only antigen Type O manufactures, but also made to varying degrees by all of the blood types) helps the cells of our immune system travel to sites where repair is needed. If so, the maintenance of genes necessary to manufacture H antigen is vitally important to our continued existence and may explain why human breast milk is so rich in fucose (the H antigen). It helps an infant's developing immune system fight off infection efficiently until it matures sufficiently to do so by itself.

The Clash of the Titans

WHEN I SPEAK in front of groups, the question inevitably comes up, in one form or another: "Which blood type is best?" I've heard people joke about "blood type envy" and complain that they received the short end of the stick. This is especially true for Type As and ABs because of their general predisposition to poorer outcomes with heart disease and cancer. However, the anthropological truth is much more complex. No blood type is inherently better or worse than another; they all have particular advantages and disadvantages.

If Type As and ABs feel more vulnerable today, Type Os were certainly more vulnerable 100 or 200 years ago. If I could transport myself back in time and speak to audiences at different points in history and in different regions of the world, the Type Os in my audience would be wishing they could swap their disease challenges with those of another blood type. In fact, they would probably all willingly swap poorer outcomes with heart disease and cancer for their health challenges—which included the devastating scourge of tuberculosis. Even today, in different regions of the world, I would find many audiences more willing to be Type A than another blood type. Depending upon the place and the time in our history, different blood types offered significant advantages. And these advantages were a direct result of the relative degree of protection your blood type can offer against developing severe forms of infectious diseases, which over the course of human history has been among the single largest challenge to human health and survival.

The plague of the Middle Ages killed a third of the entire population of Europe. Those who fled spread the plague to Africa and Asia, where untold millions died. The Black Death was a specific infectious disease, *Yersinia*. It produced an O-like antigen, a pathogenic liar that Type Os viewed as friendly. Many of those who died in the sweeping plagues of medieval times were Type O. In another epidemic redress, survival of the fittest tipped the scales toward a higher relative population of Type As than there had previously been. Consider this: The single greatest challenge to human survival may also have been the greatest single motivator of diversity and change, leading to an increase in the numbers of survivors with other blood types.

A century ago, more Europeans died from cholera, an infection of the digestive tract causing extreme fluid loss often leading to death, than from any other illness. Again and again, studies have shown that this disease shows a great preference for Type O over the other types. Thus, as little as one hundred years ago, a common, lethal disease was blood type specific.

At one point in time, smallpox was among the most feared diseases in Europe. We rarely hear of smallpox today, because it has been virtually eradicated. Types O and B always had a greater resistance to and better outcomes with this disease. However, smallpox showed a marked selective effect against Types A and AB, meaning that these two blood types got much more severe forms of the infection. Some researchers have even suggested that because of this selective pressure to eliminate Types A and AB, certain regions of the world, such as Iceland, which were somewhat isolated and exposed to repeated smallpox epidemics, still have a low frequency of A and high frequency of O blood group genes. This is an example of blood type interacting with an infectious agent to promote natural selection.

These are not isolated examples, nor are they remote. Infectious diseases still act selectively, applying genetic pressure for adaptation along blood type lines. And, while recent articles suggest that Type Os now have the survival advantage, the wild card public health factor of infectious disease could at some point shift this advantage to another blood type.

Strong proof for the theory that blood type was a supercritical influence on the survival of early mankind is the fact that virtually every infectious disease known to influence population demographics (malaria, cholera, typhus, influenza, and tuberculosis) has a "preferred" blood type that is especially susceptible, and an opposing blood type that is resistant. Especially interesting in this age of spectacular medical advances is the fact that as recently as a hundred years ago, blood type was still influencing the survival of large numbers of people, and that certain blood type–related infections, such as tuberculosis, are increasingly becoming drug resistant.

The Blood Type Advantage

EVERY INFECTIOUS disease has blood type preferences that can tip the balance. Knowing your susceptibility is definitely a factor in protecting yourself. However, I can't stress enough that no one is free of risk for any infectious disease. A weakened immune system, combined with exposure, can put anyone in danger. The best defense for every blood type is living right for your type. That means eating the most beneficial foods, taking immune-boosting and probiotic supplements, reducing stress, and all the other recommendations that are part of your individual prescription.

Let's take a look at the infectious diseases that currently stalk our world and examine your genetic blood type–related risk factors.

Influenza: The Flu Bug

Influenza is a perennial killer, appearing every winter like clockwork. On several occasions in the twentieth century, influenza has reached epidemic proportions. The Spanish flu of 1918–1919 killed 500,000 people in the United States, and 20 million worldwide. The Asian flu of 1957–1958 caused 70,000 deaths in America alone. The Hong Kong flu of 1968–1969 took 34,000 lives. As we enter the twenty-first century, the flu remains deadly to thousands. As many as 20,000 Americans still die from it every year—the victims mostly among the elderly, the immuno-suppressed, and those with preexisting conditions, such as diabetes, asthma, or heart disease.

People often use the term "flu" to describe a wide range of symptoms that include anything from a cough to a fever. The influenza virus is a very specific bug, delivering the illness combination platter from hell. Influenza causes a fever; respiratory symptoms such as a cough, sore throat, and runny nose; headache; muscle ache; and deep fatigue. Influenza is usually designated as a type $\underline{A}$ or a type $\underline{B}$. This delineation has no relation to blood type; rather, it describes particular strains. To differentiate influenza strain A or B from blood type A or B, the influenza strain $\underline{A}$ or $\underline{B}$ is underlined.

Blood Type and the Flu
A number of different researchers have investigated connections between blood types and influenza. These are the results of examining the different immune responses:

BLOOD TYPE O.   Has a relatively good ability to generate antibody response against the two common type $\underline{A}$ viruses—$\underline{A}$ (H1N1) and $\underline{A}$ (H3N2). Tends to get sick more easily from $\underline{A}$ (H1N1) than $\underline{A}$ (H3N2). Less dramatic antibody response is generated against the influenza $\underline{B}$ virus. Type O tends to be highly susceptible to the most virulent strains.

In those years when the influenza virus is especially powerful and is making people *very* sick, Type O will be among the hardest hit.

BLOOD TYPE A.   Demonstrates an ability to generate a quick and substantial antibody response against influenza type $\underline{A}$ (H1N1), and even more so against type $\underline{A}$ (H3N2). The response against the influenza $\underline{B}$ virus is less strong. Overall, Blood Type A tends to get only the less virulent forms of the virus. If they get sick, they get sick less severely than do others.

BLOOD TYPE B.   Has the weakest defense against $\underline{A}$ (H3N2), and a slightly better defense against $\underline{A}$ (H1N1). The type $\underline{A}$ (H3N2) antigen can still be found in healthy Blood Type Bs as long as five months after their recovery from the flu. There may be no symptoms, but the virus has nevertheless been given a safe harbor. Blood Type B, however, has an extremely strong advantage against influenza $\underline{B}$ strains, more than any of the other blood types. The immune response happens much more quickly and persists far longer than that of the other blood types.

BLOOD TYPE AB.   Has a relatively poor ability to generate antibodies against any of the influenza viruses. The flu is problematic every year for Type ABs, as they're pretty much defenseless against all of the influenza types.

Many of my patients ask me every year if they should get flu shots, the assumption being that they'll be fully protected from the virus if they do. Under normal circumstances, this is true. Each year's flu shot is produced from the most common flu viruses in circulation from the year before. When the influenza virus from the year before hasn't changed a lot over the current year, the flu shot will offer reasonable protection.

That's a big caveat, however. The reason the influenza virus remains so deadly is its chameleonlike nature. It can change just enough to make the flu shot ineffective. In the case of certain type $\underline{A}$ strains, we've seen entirely new mutations emerge that no one's immune system is prepared for. In those years, the flu became a pandemic, a worldwide epidemic that killed millions and millions of people.

Recently, there has been some excitement generated by a new class of drugs under development at biotechnology and pharmaceutical companies. Selective viral neuroaminidase inhibitors (Zanamivir), designed to halt the cellular path of the virus, show early promise in reducing the symptoms if you're already infected, and potentially preventing infection altogether. However, the drug will no doubt be very expensive, and since it doesn't work well orally, will probably require an inhaler.

In my practice, I've found that elderberry, used by herbalists for centuries, works very well, and research has backed up my experience. In studies, elderberry has been shown to inhibit replication of all strains of influenza viruses. In a double-blind study, using influenza type B, people taking the elderberry extract shook off the flu much more quickly than the placebo group. Seventy percent were better after forty-eight hours; 90 percent were better after seventy-two hours.

We offer our patients a concentrate mixing blueberry, cherry, apple, and elderberry, which seems to help many of them glide through the flu season—even Type ABs, who have so few defenses against influenza.

Diarrheal Diseases

Diarrheal diseases are the number-one killers worldwide by infectious organisms. And, while we seldom hear about it in the United States, cholera is still an epidemic disease in many poorer regions of the world. Other common causes of diarrhea include *E. coli* infection, dysentery, giardiasis, and shigellosis. All of us have suffered from a bout of diarrhea at one time or another. And most of us have our own ideas of exactly what diarrhea is. For those of us in the Western world, the usual amount of water in our stool each day is generally no more than about a cupful. When it is consistently more than that, it is considered to be diarrhea.

Diarrhea in a previously healthy person is usually the result of disease. In fact, more than one hundred different diseases may cause the condition. The following are the most common.

Cholera
Cholera still accounts for enormous numbers of deaths worldwide, and as little as one hundred years ago was common in the slums of many modern cities, such as London and New York. In ancient times cholera epidemics routinely decimated large cities. Several highly lethal plagues that were the scourge of the Roman world are now thought to have been in fact cholera.

Cholera offers a huge selective disadvantage to Blood Type O. Effectively speaking, Blood Type O is almost guaranteed to be the blood type that gets the most severe form of this once dreaded epidemic infection. It has been speculated that the low incidence of Type O over type A in Mediterranean cities with ancient roots may in fact have been the selective effect of Type O people dying more frequently from cholera. The constant selective pressure of cholera against Type Os may account in part for the extremely low prevalence of Type O genes and the high prevalence of Type B genes found among the people living in

---

▪ FROM THE BLOOD TYPE OUTCOME REGISTRY ▪

Janet R.
Type A
Middle-aged female
Improved: Intestinal infection

"After a trip to the Mediterranean, I spent two years with severe intestinal problems. I could not get through a meal without running to the bathroom. Every medical test possible was performed, with no tangible results. They could not find what was wrong, and I began to be viewed as someone with questionable symptoms. I lost muscle mass and was aging prematurely as my body was unable to absorb necessary nutrients. A new gym opened nearby, and they were promoting your book as their bible. Within two days of starting the diet plan for Type As, my digestion and elimination was back to normal. My husband immediately began the plan for Type B. He has beat the odds on a rare autoimmune disease he was diagnosed with five years ago, but he feels wonderful on his diet of his favorite foods. We have only been following this plan a couple weeks, but we are believers so far!"

---

the Ganges Delta in India. Type ABs appear to have the highest degree of protection from cholera infections.

Worse for Type Os, their outcome after infection is poor. In a household survey conducted in Trujillo, Peru, in 1991, at the onset of a Latin American cholera epidemic, Type O was strongly associated with severe cholera: Infected Type Os had more diarrhealike stools per day than persons of other blood groups, were more likely to report vomiting and muscle cramps, and were almost eight times more likely to require hospital treatment. In an independent study, similar findings were reported. Individuals with the most severe diarrhea compared with those with asymptomatic infection were more often Type O.

Poverty and lack of basic sanitation measures are among the main contributing factors to the current and past epidemics of cholera. Cholera is most commonly spread by contact with infected feces (generally by drinking water or eating food contaminated with the cholera bacterium). So, the disease spreads most rapidly in areas with inadequate treatment of sewage and drinking water. The cholera bacterium can also live in brackish rivers and coastal waters, so raw shellfish have been a source of cholera. In the United States, cases of cholera have developed after eating raw or undercooked shellfish from the Gulf of Mexico. If you are Type O and plan to visit areas where diarrheal diseases are common, make sure that you take appropriate preventive measures.

Typhoid

Typhoid infection skyrockets in times of war and deprivation, when sanitary habits tend to fall. In ancient times, typhoid was a killer of people on a massive scale. Not surprisingly, like most infections that influence demographics on a massive scale, typhoid shows some blood type specificity. In a study done in Uzbekistan, the data demonstrated the A blood group was especially prone to chronic typhoid carrier state, a trait especially linked to inhabitants of the Asian part of the country. In comparison with control, there were significantly fewer Type Os.

E. coli

The very mention of a bacteria such as *E. coli (Escherichia coli)*, is enough to send the population into a panic. Most people view *E. coli* as a deadly foreign invader—and it can be that. What they don't realize is that within a normal lower intestinal tract, huge numbers of *E. coli* adhere and live in a mutually profitable relationship with us: Our digestive tracts provide them with nutrition, and they in turn provide us with disease resistance.

So how can *E. coli* be both good and bad?

As you develop from an infant to a child to an adult, your intestine becomes colonized with "good" *E. coli*. The good normally serve to crowd out the "bad" by out-reproducing them, competing for food, and denying the bad access to places on the intestinal wall where they might attach.

There are many variant strains of *E. coli*, and the vast majority are tolerated by the immune system. The reason there are so many different strains of *E. coli* is because they're excellent at exchanging genetic information, and they can mutate at an astounding rate. Some strains of *E. coli* have surface antigens similar to the human blood type antigens. These are carbohydrates associated with membrane lipopolysaccharides. An extensive study has shown that *E. coli* strains Y1089 and Y1090 possess the Type O antigen, which can also be converted to the Type A antigen. This illustrates how, by converting one blood type antigen to another, gut bacteria can produce opposing blood type immunization and adapt to a different host by altering elements of their "blood type." The highly dangerous variant of *E. coli* bacteria, O157:H7 is the one that most of us are now familiar with. It was first recognized as a cause of human disease in 1982. Since then, large outbreaks of *E. coli* O157:H7 have been reported in the United States, including an outbreak in 1993 linked to undercooked ground beef hamburgers that resulted in more than 600 reported cases of severe illness, and four deaths. In 1996, more than six thousand schoolchildren in Japan became severely ill with an *E. coli* O157:H7 infection after eating contaminated radish sprouts.

Even though the vegetarian purists like to emphasize meat as a cause of *E. coli* infection, that obviously isn't always the case. Since 1995, thirteen outbreaks of foodborne disease due to *E. coli* or salmonella have been directly linked to commercially sold raw sprouts. Contamination of the sprouts, rather than improper handling, is believed to be the source of the problem.

In most cases, the infection is limited to diarrhea and cramps, although in advanced cases the diarrhea can be bloody and debilitating. In fewer than 2 to 7 percent of those infected, particularly in the very young and the very old, a disorder called hemolytic uremic syndrome (HUS) sometimes develops. A bacterial toxin damages small blood vessels in the kidney, reduces platelet counts, and destroys red blood cells. Kidney function can be impaired to the degree that dialysis may be necessary. Once infected with this particular organism, there are no treatments available that can prevent HUS.

Many of the deadlier strains of *E. coli* have developed a taste for different blood types. Even the invasion strategies they employ differ among blood types:

TYPE O: INTERACTION.   There is an association between Type O blood and the severity of the diarrhea that results from *E. coli* infection. During research on diarrhea caused by *E. coli* with 316 adult volunteers, ABO and Rh blood types were sampled to look for the degree of severity in the reactions of the different blood types. Type O volunteers had a significantly more intense bout of diarrhea than did those of the other blood types. The researchers speculated that there was a greater reaction between a substance in the Type O blood and the toxin produced by the strain of bacteria.

TYPE A: ATTACHMENT.   Many of the more pathogenic forms of *E. coli* will produce ropelike bundles of filaments, referred to as bundle-forming pili (BFP), which allow the *E. coli* to attach to the lining of the intestines. These particular *E. coli* have lectins on their pili shaped like tiny suction cups that attach themselves to the various sugars (glycoproteins or glycolipids) comprising the polysaccharides of the intestinal mucous lining. Many of these sugars are specific to ABO antigens. Certain *E. coli* strains that colonize the human digestive tract express lectins specific for various glycolipids. One of these, globo_A, is made only by individuals who are Blood Type A, with a positive secretor status.

Type B And Type AB: Mimicry.   Many forms of *E. coli* that cause diarrhea are Type B–like, immunologically. They possess an antigen on their surface that resembles the Type B antigen. Several studies indicate that a higher number of Type Bs and Type ABs are afflicted with *E. coli*–caused gastroenteritis than are those blood types that are hostile to B-like antigens.

Parasites

There is a story, famous in medical history, that involved a man who thought that the cholera ravaging the countryside around him was caused by the use of a certain well that he was convinced harbored the deadly bacteria. He tore off the well's pump handle, and the cholera epidemic was stopped in its tracks.

There is another, less well-known story. It also is true. There was a man who violently opposed the entire theory that germs caused cholera and so drank a water glass full of cholera organisms. The man didn't get cholera.

Both were on to something. *Candida, Giardia,* and other parasites can and do cause problems when they infect and attack our digestive systems.

But these bugs can only gain a foothold when our digestive systems are weak and the powerful curative powers of the immune system compromised. To keep your intestines free of pathogenic microorganisms, the best path to follow is clearly marked. Eat the diet that your system is best suited to absorb. That diet is easy on the system and free from irritants; it also conditions the gut to allow for the healthy growth of friendly flora.

There are some strong associations between the blood types and various parasitic infections. Many, however, are expressed through connections to other minor blood grouping systems such as the *Kell, Duffy,* and *P1 antigen.*

ABO is by far the most significant of the blood grouping systems, but it's also only one of about twenty-three systems by which we can be blood typed. Since we seek to limit discussion to the ABO and secretor systems, with the occasional tip of the hat to the Rh and MN systems, we'll limit our focus.

Not surprisingly, parasites have blood type preferences.

Hookworm: Type O

Hookworm was common in America as recently as seventy years ago, especially in the South. There seems to be a preference for Type O rather than the other blood types. Hookworm is still a common disease of pets, and because of this can be transmitted to humans. Transmission usually occurs through unwashed hands and a hookworm-infested yard—that is, your dog's stools, with hookworms in them, are left all over the yard. If you garden, be sure to wear gloves, and wash your hands thoroughly if you're digging around in the soil.

Giardia: Type A

A number of studies have shown that *Giardia* ("Montezuma's Revenge") has a surface antigen that mimics the A antigen. So it more frequently infects those who are Type A, and the Giardia infection in a Type A is more severe and threatening than in the other blood types. Giardia may be found in wild animals, contaminated streams, and well water. Giardia outbreaks can occur in communities where water supplies are contaminated with raw sewage. It can be contracted by drinking water from lakes or streams inhabited by water-dwelling animals, such as beavers and muskrats, or where domestic animals, such as sheep, have caused contamination. It's also spread by direct contact, which has caused outbreaks among the children and the workers in day-care centers. Its most common symptom is diarrhea, which by itself can be serious and debilitating.

Amoeba Infection: Type B

Though two studies showed that amoebae did not seem to adhere to the red blood cells of any particular blood type over another, a separate study showed that the percentage of amoebae scavenged by the immune system was higher if they were attached to Type A or Type AB red blood cells, as opposed to Type O or Type B. So, though no particular blood type seemed to contract amoeba more than any of the others, Type A and Type AB mounted a better immune response. This probably explains why amoebic infection was seen to be associated with Type B blood in one study.

Malaria

On a global scale, malaria is a very dangerous killer; as many as two and a half million people die from it every year. Malaria has clearly influenced blood type percentages in those areas of the world where this infectious disease has dominated over time, and to some extent still does today. Among the hot spots are sub-Saharan Africa, south and southeast Asia, Central and South America, Mexico, Haiti, the Dominican Republic, and some of the Pacific Islands—Papua New Guinea, the Solomon Islands, and Vanuatu.

As little as thirty years ago, the eradication of malaria seemed within reach. But spraying programs have proved ineffective in stopping the mosquito, and more and more drug resistant strains of malaria are being discovered all the time. Drug resistance outpaces drug development, as resistance to anti-malarial drugs continues to rise.

Transmitted by the *Anopheles* mosquito, the bite injects parasites—*Plasmodium falciparum*, *P. malariae*, *P. vivax*, and *P. ovale*—carried by the mosquito into our bloodstreams. The parasites then reproduce within our red blood cells.

Of the four, only *P. falciparum* is potentially life threatening. A severe attack can cause liver and kidney failure, convulsions, and coma. Usually because of delayed treatment, about 2 percent of those infected with *P. falciparum* will die.

Blood type plays a large role in susceptibility and how badly you'll react to malaria:

TYPE O.   Predisposition to infection with the *P. vivax* parasite, and a slightly higher degree of protection against *P. falciparum* than other blood types. Has a better outcome once infected than the other blood types. Type O has the most protection against rosette formation, an autoimmune reaction in the blood mounted against the parasite.

TYPE A.   Predisposition to infection with the *P. vivax* parasite, and a slightly higher degree of protection against *P. falciparum* than Type B or AB. Once infected, outcome poorer—including cerebral complications.

TYPE B.   Predisposition to infection with *P. falciparum* infection. Better outcomes once infected than A or AB.

TYPE AB.   Protected somewhat from several forms of the parasite. Once infected, a poor outcome similar to Type A.

Tuberculosis

At the turn of the last century, tuberculosis was the leading cause of death in the United States. This infection is caused by bacteria called *Mycobacterium tuberculosis,* which can attack any part of your body, but usually attack the lungs. In the 1940s, scientists discovered the first of several drugs now used to treat TB, which resulted in a slow and steady decline in TB infection within the United States. However, TB has been making a comeback. Since 1984, the number of TB cases reported in the United States has begun to increase, with more than 25,000 cases reported in 1993.

Almost in opposition to malaria, tuberculosis runs a much more aggressive and detrimental course in Type Os, while Type As are afforded the highest degree of protection. A further complicating factor appears to be racial background. Type Os of European descent have a greater susceptibility and a poorer outcome than other Type Os. Among Asians, Type Bs have higher rates of infection and severer forms. Your Rh status might have some impact on tuberculosis survival, as well. Research demonstrates that more Rh- persons died from tuberculosis, while a higher percent of Rh+ persons survived.

Just as we have found with several other diseases, blood type plays a significant role as a genetic adaptation favoring either survival or severity of infection. So, it is quite possible that over the course of human history and particularly during the nineteenth century, when tuberculosis was among the biggest killers, tuberculosis has been playing a chess match against blood type genetics.

TB is spread through the air from one person to another, generally by an infected person either coughing or sneezing. When you are initially infected with the TB bacteria, you will usually not feel sick, generally do not have any symptoms, and cannot spread TB. However, after infection you might develop TB at some point in the future. In most people who breathe in TB bacteria and become infected, the body keeps the bacteria, at least initially, in check. The bacteria become inactive, but they remain alive in the body and can become active later. Many people who have TB infection never develop TB disease. In these people, the TB bacteria remain inactive for a lifetime without causing disease. But in other people, especially people who have weak immune systems, the bacteria become active and cause TB disease.

Symptoms of TB include a bad cough that lasts longer than two weeks, pain in the chest, coughing up blood or sputum (phlegm from deep inside the lungs), weakness or fatigue, weight loss, no appetite, chills, fever, and sweating at night. A TB skin test is the only way to find out if you have the TB infection. You can get a skin test at the health department or at your doctor's office.

References: Blood Type and Infectious Disease

Alonso, P. et al. "Phagocytic activity of three Naegleria strains in the presence of erythrocytes of various types." *J Protozool,* 1985 Nov; 32(4):661–4.

Becker, D. J., J. B. Lowe, "Leukocyte adhesion deficiency type II. *Biochim Biophys Acta,* 1999 Oct 8;1455(2–3): 193–204.

Black, R. E., Levine, M. M., Clements, M. L., Hughes, T. and S. O'Donnell. "Association between O blood group and occurrence and severity of diarrhoea due to *Escherichia coli.*" *Trans R Soc Trop Med Hyg,* 1987;81(1):120–3.

Bouree, P., and G. Bonnot, "Study of relationship of ABO and Rh blood group, and HLA antigens with parasitic diseases." *J Egypt Soc Parasitol,* 1989 Jun;19(1):67–73.

Cameron, B. J., et al. "Blood group glycolipids as epithelial cell receptors for Candida albicans." *Infect Immun,* 1996 Mar;64(3):891–6.

de Manueles, Jimenez J. et al. "Histocompatibility antigens and *Giardia lamblia parasitosis.*" *An Esp Pediatr,* 1992 Jan;36(1):41–4. Review. Spanish.

Essery, S. D. et al. "Detection of microbial surface antigens that bind Lewis(a) antigen." *FEMS Immunol Med Microbiol,* 1994 Jun; 9(1):15–21.

Glass, R. I., J. Holmgren, C. E. Haley, M. R. Khan, A. M. Svennerholm, B. J. Stoll, Hossain Belayet, K. Kaneko, et al. "Prevalence of O agglutinins against the epizootic strains of Yersinia pseudo tuberculosis serovars IB and IVA in barn rats." *Nippon Juigaku Zasshi,* 1982 Apr;44(2):375–7.

K. M., R. E. Black, M. Yunus, and D. Barua. "Predisposition for cholera of individuals with O blood group. Possible evolutionary significance." *Am J Epidemiol,* 1985 Jun;121(6):791–6.

Lindstedt, R., G. Larson, P. Falk, U. Jodal, H. Leffler, and C. Svanborg. "The receptor repertoire defines the host range for attaching *Escherichia coli* strains that recognize globo-A." *Infect Immun*, 1991 Mar;59(3):1086–92.

Lopez-Revilla, R., et al. "Adhesion of *Entamoeba histolytica trophozoites* to human erythrocytes." *Infect Immun*, 1982 Jul;37(1):281–5.

Mourant, A. E. *Blood Types and Disease.* New York: Oxford University Press, 1979.

Roberts-Thomson, I. C. "Genetic studies of human and murine giardiasis." *Clin Infect Dis*, 1993 Mar;16 Suppl 2:S98–104. Review.

Sinha, A. K., S. K. Bhattacharya, D. Sen, P. Dutta, D. Dutta, M. K. Bhattacharya, and S. C. Pal. "Blood group and shigellosis." *J Assoc Physicians India*, 1991 Jun;39(6):452–3.

Springer, G. F. "Role of human cell surface structures in interactions between man and microbes." *Naturwissenschaften*, 1970 Apr;57(4): 162–71.

Swerdlow, D. L., E. D. Mintz, M. Rodriguez, E. Tejada, C. Ocampo, L. Espejo, T. J. Barrett, J. Petzelt, N. H. Bean, L. Seminario, et al. "Severe life-threatening cholera associated with blood group O in Peru: Implications for the Latin American epidemic." *J Infect Dis*, 1994 Aug;170(2):468–72.

Thom, S. M. et al "Non-secretion of blood group antigens and susceptibility to infection by Candida species." *FEMS Microbiol Immunol*, 1989 Jun;1(6–7):401–5.

Tosh, F .D., et al. "Characterization of a fucoside-binding adhesin of *Candida albicans*." *Infect Immun*, 1992 Nov;60(11):4734–9.

Villalobos, J. J., et al. "A 10-year prolective study on cancer of the digestive system." *Rev Gastroenterol Mex*, 1990 Jan–Mar;55(1):17–24. Spanish.

Wittels, E. G., Lichtman, H. C. "Blood group incidence and *Escherichia coli* bacterial sepsis." *Transfusion*, 1986 Nov–Dec;26(6):533–5.

Yamamoto, M., et al. "Structure and action of saikosaponins isolated from *Bupleurum falcatum* L. II. Metabolic actions of saikosaponins, especially a plasma cholesterol-lowering action." *Arzneimittelforschung*, 1975 Aug;25(8):1240–3.

Yang, N., and B. Boettcher, "Development of human ABO blood group A antigen on Escherichia coli Y1089 and Y1090." *Immunol Cell Biol*, 1992 Dec;70 (Pt 6):411–6.

Zhukov-Berezhnilov, N. N., et al. "Heterogenetic antigens of plague and cholera microbes, similar to antigens of human and animal tissues." *Biull Eksp Biol Med*, 1972 Apr;73(4):63–5. Russian.

Support and Resources

*D*R. PETER D'ADAMO AND HIS STAFF CONTINUE TO accept new patients on a limited basis. To find out more about scheduling an appointment, please contact:

> The D'Adamo Clinic
> 2009 Summer Street
> Stamford, CT 06905
> 203-348-4800

Note: Please do not submit questions regarding Dr. D'Adamo's work or send questions seeking personal advice on health matters to his clinic.

Dr. D'Adamo maintains an Internet Web site (http://www.dadamo. com) that has an interactive message board and archives of past posts and questions to the board. This is currently the only vehicle available for additional information regarding Dr. D'Adamo's ongoing research on blood type and individuality.

www.dadamo.com

The World Wide Web has proven to be a valuable venue for exploring and applying the tenets of the Blood Type Diet and Lifestyle.

Since January 1997, hundreds of thousands have visited the site to participate in the ABO chat groups, to peruse the scientific archives, to share experiences and recipes, and to learn more about the science of blood type.

One of the most important features on the Web page is the Blood Type Outcome Registry, which has facilitated the collection of data on the measurable effects of the Blood Type Diet on a wide range of medical conditions.

I invite you to share your outcome at the Web site. It is actually quite simple. When you visit www.dadamo.com, scroll down the main page until you locate "Share Your Outcome." Click on "Share Your Outcome," and you will be taken to the Blood Type Outcome Registry.

I appreciate your taking the time to provide feedback about experiences you have had with the program. Your feedback can be critical in showing indicators and trends, which can then be further studied. All information shared on the Web site Blood Type Outcome Registry will be held in complete confidence.

Self Testing

Home Blood Typing Kits

North American Pharmacal, Inc. is the official distributor of Home Blood Type Testing Kits. Each kit costs $7.95 and is a single-use disposable educational device capable of determining one individual's ABO and rhesus blood type. Results are obtained within about 4 to 5 minutes. If you have several friends or family members who need to learn their blood type, you will need to order a separate home blood-typing kit for each individual.

All U.S. orders are shipped via UPS ground (shipping and handling cost is $5.25 per order irrespective of the number of kits ordered). Expedited shipping methods (UPS second day or next day) are available but cost more. Please contact the customer service department to inquire about rates for expedited shipping to your area.

If you are ordering a kit to be shipped outside of the U.S., shipping rates can vary dramatically and can be quite expensive. Please contact our customer service department prior to placing your order for an estimate of shipping charges for non-U.S. orders.

To order a single Home Blood Typing Kit, please enclose $7.95 plus $5.25 for shipping and handling and send to:

North American Pharmacal, Inc.
5 Brook Street
Norwalk, CT 06851
Tel: 203-866-7664
Fax: 203-838-4066
Toll free: 877-ABO TYPE (877-226-8973)
www.4yourtype.com

Health Products and Supplements

North American Pharmacal, Inc., is the official distributor of Blood Type Specialty Products. The product line includes supplements, books, tapes, teas, meal replacement bars, cosmetics, and support material that makes "eating and living right 4 your type" easier.

Included in this product line are: New Chapter® D'Adamo 4 Your Type Products™. These whole-food vitamins, herbs, and other food supplements have been specifically crafted to address the unique requirements of each blood type.

Also included are Sip Right 4 Your Type™ teas, Deflect™ lectin-blocking formulas, and a range of additional blood type specific and blood-type friendly health products, which have been formulated in partnership with The Republic of Tea and New Chapter.

Product information and price lists are available from our website or by contacting North American Pharmacal.

DR. PETER D'ADAMO'S father, James D'Adamo, N.D., who pioneered the early clinical work on blood type, continues to practice. He may be reached at:

Dr. James D'Adamo, N.D.
44-46 Bridge Street
Portsmouth, NH 03801

Index